Nursing in Haematology Oncology

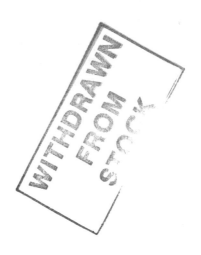

Especial thanks to Ros Bratt-Wyton, without whose help, support and expertise this book might never have seen the light of day

For Baillière Tindall:

Senior Commissioning Editor: Ninette Premdas
Project Manager: Gail Murray
Project Development Manager: Katrina Mather
Designer: George Ajayi

Nursing in Haematological Oncology

Edited by

Maggie Grundy

MSc RGN RM DipNursEd (Clinical Teaching) DipNurs (Lond) PGTC
Macmillan Lecturer in Cancer Nursing, The Robert Gordon University, Aberdeen, UK

Foreword by

Dame Gill Oliver

DBE FRCN
Director of Patient Services, Clatterbridge Centre for Oncology, Wirral, UK

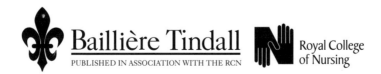

Baillière Tindall

PUBLISHED IN ASSOCIATION WITH THE RCN

Royal College
of Nursing

EDINBURGH ● LONDON ● NEW YORK ● PHILADELPHIA ● ST LOUIS ● SYDNEY ● TORONTO ● 2000

BAILLIÈRE TINDALL
An imprint of Harcourt Publishers Limited

© Harcourt Publishers Limited 2000

 is a registered trademark of Harcourt Publishers Limited

The right of Maggie Grundy to be identified as editor of this work has been asserted
by her in accordance with the Copyright, Designs and Patents Act 1988

First published 2000

Reprinted 2001, 2002

ISBN 0 7020 2323 X

British Library Cataloguing in Publication Data
A catalogue record for this book is available from the
British Library

Library of Congress Cataloging in Publication Data
A catalog record for this book is available from the Library
of Congress

Note
Medical knowledge is constantly changing. As new
information becomes available, changes in treatment,
procedures, equipment and the use of drugs become necessary.
The editor, contributors and the publishers have taken care to
ensure that the information given in this text is accurate and up
to date. However, readers are strongly advised to confirm that the
information, especially with regard to drug usage, complies
with the latest legislation and standards of practice.

Printed in China by RDC Group Limited
B/03

The
publisher's
policy is to use
**paper manufactured
from sustainable forests**

Contents

Colour plate section is between pages 144 and 145.

Contributors

Roslyne Bratt-Wyton BScN RGN DPSN
Clinical Nurse Specialist, Oncology Unit,
Russells Hall Hospital,
Dudley, UK

Gosia Brykczynska BA BSc MPhil RN RSCN RNT
CertEd ENB 237
Lecturer, Royal College of Nursing Institute,
London, UK

Tracey Burgoyne BSc(Hons)
Lecturer/Practitioner,
University of Central England,
Birmingham, UK

Evelyn Dannie BSc(Hons) MSc RGN ENB 998 A27
C&G 370 BMT NursCert
Senior Sister/Clinical Nurse Specialist,
Department of Haematology,
Hammersmith Hospitals NHS Trust,
London, UK

Shelley Dolan BA BSc(Hons) RGN ENB 100, 237, 998
Clinical Nurse Specialist,
The Royal Marsden Hospital,
Sutton, UK

Maura Dowling MSc BNS(Hons) RNT RGN SCM
OncCert
Nurse Tutor, School of Nursing,
University College Hospital, Galway,
Ireland

Julia Downing BN(Hons) MMedSci DipCN RGN
Lecturer in Cancer Care,
Centre for Cancer and Palliative Care Studies,
Institute of Cancer Research,
London, UK

Helen C. Hamilton RGN
Director TPN and Vascular Access Services,
Department of Parenteral Nutrition,
John Radcliffe Hospital,
Oxford, UK

Sarah Hart BSc(Hons) MSc RGN FETC
Clinical Nurse Specialist Infection
Control/Radiation Protection,
The Royal Marsden Hospital NHS Trust,
London and Sutton, UK

Jan Hawthorn BSc PhD
London, UK

Samantha Heath BSc(Hons) MA PGDE RGN RSCN
Lecturer/Nurse Consultant,
The University of Auckland and
Starship Children's Hospital, Auckland,
New Zealand

Damian Heron BA(Hons) RGN
Macmillan Lead Cancer Nurse for
North Wales and Cancer Lead, North Wales
Health Authority, Mold, UK

Timothy Jackson SRN RM RNMS OncCert ENB 237,
998, 931, 934
Divisional Nurse Director, Clinical Services,
The Royal Marsden Hospital, NHS Trust,
London and Sutton, UK

Alison Knight RGN ENB 237 ENB N14
Senior Sister, Bone Marrow Transplant Unit,
University Hospital, Birmingham, UK

Robert Lloyd-Richards MA DipTheol DipCouns
Managing Chaplain,
University Hospital of Wales;
Honorary Teacher, University of
Wales College of Medicine;
Associate Lecturer, Cardiff University;
Associate Lecturer, Open University,
Cardiff, UK

Alexander Molassiotis BSc MSc PhD BMT(Cert) CounsCert RN
Assistant Professor, Department of Nursing,
Chinese University of Hong Kong,
Hong Kong

Helen Outhwaite BSc(Hons) RGN OncCert PGDip Healthcare Ethics
Haematology Nurse Specialist,
Guy's and St Thomas's Hospital Trust,
London, UK

Helen Porter MSc RGN OncCert
Lead Cancer Nurse,
University Hospital Birmingham NHS Trust,
Birmingham, UK

Joanne Read BSc(Hons) RGN OncCert DNCert
District Nursing Sister,
Christie Hospital NHS Trust,
Manchester, UK

Diane Spreadborough RGN OncCert
Chemotherapy Sister,
Christie Hospital NHS Trust,
Manchester, UK

Evelyn Thomson MBA MSc RGN
Service Development Manager,
Macmillan Cancer Relief,
Glasgow, UK

Breege Traynor BNurs MSc RGN NDNCert OncCert
Senior Product Safety Manager,
AMGEN Ltd, Cambridge, UK

Paula Wilkins RGN OncCert Cert Management
Haematology Clinical Nurse Specialist,
Guy's and St Thomas's Hospital Trust,
London, UK

Foreword

It is with great pleasure that I write the foreword to this new addition to the cancer nursing literature. As we move into the 21st century there has never been a more exciting time for those working in cancer services. Nurses and nursing have crucial and integral roles to play in the development and expansion of existing services and the implementation of innovative practice for the benefit of all those affected by the disease.

The publication of the Policy Framework for Commissioning Cancer Services, which became widely known as 'Calman/Hine', was the catalyst for the production of a whole range of guidance at local, regional and national levels. In all of these, the pivotal role of nursing is made clear. While nurses are key players in the management of patients affected by haematological malignancies, they work alongside patients and their families and in close collaboration with members of all professions and disciplines. It is good to recognise this collaboration in the list of contributors to this new text.

If people affected by cancer are to receive the excellent treatment and care that is their right, then those who provide that care must be assured of the appropriate education and training. Texts such as this, written by nurses, and principally for nurses, will play a significant part in this process. The experience and skill of the contributors to this new book demonstrate the breadth of knowledge available within the profession of nursing. This text will enable and encourage the sharing of that knowledge, making it available to a wide audience. It will not be solely nurses who benefit but the publication will be of interest and use to a range of health care professionals beyond nursing. In fact, all of those people who may be called upon in their professional life to contribute to the care and support of anyone suffering from a haematological malignancy or the effects of its treatment will find information and help within the pages of this book.

Haematological malignancies comprise a small proportion of the overall cancer incidence. They form, however, a complex group of diseases which often require long-term treatment and management, affect lifestyle and socialisation, and demand specialist and expert skills from the professionals who provide treatment and care. It is now well recognised that a diagnosis of malignant disease is just one part of an individual's life and increasingly now emphasis is being re-aligned to consider issues of living with cancer. The holistic approach promoted by successive models of nursing care enables nurses to consider all aspects of a patient's circumstances, accurately assessing needs and referring onwards for additional specialist help as necessary. It is good to see that the largest section of this new text addresses nursing issues. While not underestimating the importance of an understanding of patterns of disease and the treatment modalities that can be used, the strength of this particular text lies in its broad approach to total patient care.

As the organisation and structure of cancer services nationally are reviewed, plans are being developed to ensure that the highest quality of treatment and care is available for patients wherever they may live and whatever their circumstances or background. Networks of hospitals, community units, and voluntary and charitable organisations will come together to ensure that these goals can be met. The agreement and establishment of multi-professional teams will ensure that the most up-to-date and best treatment and care decisions are made for each individual patient. Each team member will contribute the experience and expertise developed often over many years of practice and study. Different professions and disciplines are working increasingly closely together and the patient can only benefit as research-based decisions are made, using all the available evidence.

In a health service that is subject to constant change, the pressures on staff cannot be overlooked and it is a credit to the editor of this text that this particular issue is addressed. In highlighting education and training as essential elements of a supportive and developmental working environment, this addition to the literature is thus helping to meet the need it identifies.

Cancer services remain at the top of the agenda in political, professional and public circles; it is likely that this will remain the case for a considerable time. In all parts of the UK work is progressing on the production of clinical guidance and existing services are subject to comprehensive review and assessment against ever more detailed criteria. As national

standards and performance indicators are developed with specific input from professionals within the field, the benefits to people affected by cancer will be more readily amenable to audit. National attention has been focused on cancer services and the appointment of a National Cancer Director and Cancer Action Team has added strength to the work already under way.

This new text *Nursing in Haematological Oncology* has its part to play in the overall development of cancer services. Professional teamwork is an essential part of the delivery of excellent care to people with a haematological cancer. The education and training that those staff need in order to play their part to the full are provided in many and varied ways. This text is one of them. In recognising the key role of expert nursing in the management of these cancers, the authors have contributed to a publication which will be of use and interest not just to nurses but to all those who are concerned in improving the multi-professional care provided for anyone experiencing the effects of one of these complex types of cancer.

Dame Gill Oliver

Preface

Haematology is a rapidly advancing and exciting field of medicine. Haematological malignancies are, however, comparatively rare and specialist units tend to be geographically distant; it is therefore not unusual for patients to be treated in general medical wards. Nurses working in these wards may encounter haematological diseases relatively infrequently, yet they still need to be able to provide physical, psychosocial and spiritual care for patients and their families. In order to do this, they need to understand the disease process, treatment regimens, problems that patients are likely to encounter during their disease trajectory, and the associated nursing issues.

Most texts on this subject are written primarily for doctors and tend to focus on cell biology and laboratory methods, and the depth of content is frequently off-putting to nurses. Additionally, there are several North American nursing texts which address aspects of haemato-oncology in depth, for example blood and marrow transplantation. This book provides an overview of haematological oncology and is the first British textbook addressing the subject to have been written specifically for nurses. The idea for the book came from the Royal College of Nursing, Haematology and Bone Marrow Transplant Forum Steering Committee, which identified the need for a textbook for qualified nurses. The Forum Steering Committee also contributed to the outline and content of the book, which is primarily intended for qualified nurses working with or having an interest in haematological malignancies. However, it will also be useful to student nurses and those undertaking specialist courses.

This book is divided into three separate but complementary sections. The first section examines the diseases, the second treatment, and the third and largest section discusses nursing issues. The emphasis of the book is on the patient and nursing management, but to manage patients effectively, knowledge of both normal and abnormal haematopoiesis and medical management is necessary. The first chapter, therefore, concentrates on the normal physiology of the blood and is followed by five chapters which review the differing haematological malignancies and their related pathophysiology.

Many treatments such as chemotherapy and blood and marrow transplants are common to a number of haematological malignancies, as are many aspects of nursing care, so to avoid repetition separate chapters are devoted to individual treatment modalities and nursing issues are grouped in a section of their own. Although this book deals mainly with adults, it would not be complete without making some reference to the special problems of children with haematological malignancies and these are covered in Chapter 7.

Considerable expertise is required to support individuals with haematological malignancies and the nursing issues section provides essential information. Venous access is a particular problem for patients as veins tend to fibrose owing to the huge number of venepunctures and the enormous quantity of drugs which require to be given intravenously. Chapter 12 therefore deals with the particular issues associated with the differing vascular devices available and guidelines for their care. Further chapters discuss the potentially life-threatening issues of infection and haemorrhage and other important aspects of care including oral care, nutrition, fertility issues and the reduction of nausea and vomiting. The immunosuppression experienced by patients results in prolonged periods of isolation and this, combined with the life-threatening nature of the disease and aggressive chemotherapy regimens, means that psychological care is an important aspect of care, and issues such as reaction and adaptation to diagnosis, treatment and relapse are also included.

Advances in the treatment of haematological malignancies have resulted in an increased life expectancy for many patients, which in turn may lead to discrimination in employment and financial problems. Social issues, quality of life and survivorship are therefore addressed in Chapter 20. Despite these advances in treatment, many patients will die from their disease and Chapter 21 is devoted to death, bereavement and spiritual issues. Furthermore, many ethical dilemmas may arise when nursing patients with haematological malignancies and these issues are explored in Chapter 22.

Nurses working with individuals with a life-threatening illness can suffer from stress and burnout. This can be especially so in haematology as patients are frequently hospitalised for prolonged periods of time, on numerous occasions. Nurses get to know patients and their families extremely well, and may become emotionally attached to them, nursing them through one or more relapses and episodes of acute illness. When a patient dies, nurses can experience a grief-like reaction and eventually this can lead to stress and dissatisfaction with the job. Staff support strategies may help to reduce stress, improve staff retention and prevent burnout. Chapter 23, therefore, deals with the issues of staff support and retention. The final chapter explores future developments in this rapidly evolving specialty.

The division of this book into three separate sections should allow nurses to easily find a specific topic of interest. There are many areas of overlap between the different disorders and consequently much cross-referencing between chapters. This should enable readers to dip into the book at different points to find the information they require without having to read the book sequentially. Reflection points and case studies are included in every chapter except for the first and final chapters. These text features are included to help the reader focus on patient needs and nursing management. Discussion questions are also included at the end of each chapter to stimulate reflection on practice and encourage readers to discuss, with colleagues, issues within their own practice. The chapters are all relatively short and readers may want to explore issues in greater depth. To facilitate this, a list of suggested reading is included at the end of each chapter.

A number of different authors have contributed their knowledge and clinical expertise to this book. We hope that this knowledge and expertise will benefit others caring for individuals with haematological malignancies.

Aberdeen 2000   Maggie Grundy

Acknowledgements

Grateful thanks to the many colleagues and friends who have provided help, support, advice, expertise and encouragement and in doing so have contributed, in their own unique ways, to the publication of this book.

SECTION ONE
The Diseases

Haematopoiesis

BREEGE TRAYNOR

Key points
- Haematopoiesis, the process of blood cell production, is a diverse and productive process
- The bone marrow produces all cells required by the body for an intact immune system, coagulation and oxygenation
- All mature myeloid and lymphoid cells originate from pluripotent stem cells
- The features of self-renewal and differentiation make haematopoietic stem cells unique
- Different blood cells have varying specialised functions
- Haematopoietic growth factors play a complex role in controlling haematopoiesis
- The immune system is the body's natural defence mechanism and has the ability to distinguish between self and non-self
- The complement system plays an important part in the inflammatory response and microbial killing
- A number of genetic rearrangements are associated with bone marrow disease

INTRODUCTION

Blood...
hot, temperate, red humor whose office is to nourish the whole body to give it strength and color being dispersed by the veins through every part of it

Burton 1628

The bone marrow is a complex and sophisticated organ and haematopoiesis – blood cell production – is a diverse and productive process. The marrow gives rise to all the cells which an individual requires to have an intact immune system, coagulation and oxygenation. Many factors influence the marrow. A series of progenitor cells and a complex array of regulatory proteins maintain haematopoiesis and allow a measured production of cells under 'steady-state' conditions (Dexter 1990, Robinson 1993). Furthermore, increasing understanding of cytogenetics have helped to begin to piece together both normal and abnormal haematopoiesis which can maintain health or contribute to disease development. This chapter describes how myeloid and lymphoid cells are formed, how haematopoiesis is positively and negatively controlled and highlights known genetic aberrations which may contribute to myelo- or lympho-proliferative disorders.

Blood is a fluid tissue which constitutes approximately 7% of body weight. Total volume is around 5.5 litres in adult humans and some 2.5 litres of blood cells – erythrocytes, leucocytes, platelets – circulate in 3 litres of protein-rich plasma. One of the largest organs of the body, blood supports the activities of all other tissues and provides nutrients, oxygen, hormones, cleansing of waste and body defence (Babior & Stossel 1994, Pallister 1994).

Blood cells each have varying specialised functions and a finite life-span. The number of circulating cells is maintained within extremely narrow limits and cells are replaced at a rate equal to their loss. Erythrocytes are subjected to mechanical and oxidant stress, leucocytes are destroyed during the process of dealing with micro-organisms and platelets are consumed during coagulation (Babior & Stossel 1994). As a result, some 5×10^{11} myeloid cells need to be manufactured daily to account only for cells lost through the normal ageing process

(Molineux & Dexter 1994). In times of need, however, erythropoiesis can be increased 20–30-fold, granulopoiesis at least 20-fold and thrombopoiesis at least three-fold (Emerson 1992).

Fetal haematopoiesis

Fetal haematopoiesis, in particular erythropoiesis, begins extra-embryonically in the walls of the yolk sac in the second week of gestation. Leucopoiesis and thrombopoiesis commence at approximately 6 weeks' gestation. By 10 weeks' gestation the yolk sac ceases to produce blood cells and the liver becomes the major site of blood cell production, feeding fetal bone marrow stroma with stem cells. The human fetal spleen is a secondary haematopoietic organ and plays a role in blood production from 10 weeks' gestation into the second trimester (Pallister 1994). Bone marrow appears in the clavicle in the second month of gestation and develops sequentially in all skeletal bones (Fliedner 1993). By week 20 haematopoiesis is firmly established in the bone marrow while hepatic haematopoiesis gradually wanes until only a small amount of erythropoiesis (~10%) remains (Babior & Stossel 1994, Pallister 1994).

Bone marrow

At birth haematopoietic cells occupy all the bone marrow space – a volume so large that it is nearly equivalent to the marrow space occupied by haematopoietic cells in adults (Gluckman et al 1993). During childhood yellow, fatty marrow replaces approximately 50% of the available space until red marrow is confined to the pelvis, sternum, ribs, vertebrae and cranium. However, the absolute amount of haematopoietic tissue is constant in both adult and child (Babior & Stossel 1994). If the need for haematopoiesis increases, marrow throughout the body can become reactivated. This gives a potential haematopoietic reserve of about six times normal capacity (Pallister 1994).

The bone marrow constitutes about 4–6% of total body weight and occupies about 4000 ml

in adulthood (Eastham & Slade 1992). The marrow is perfused with blood every 6 minutes and 5% of the cardiac output circulates directly there. This ensures an adequate supply of nutrients and oxygen and the removal of mitotic metabolites (Emerson 1992).

STEM CELLS

A stem cell is identified by its capacity to generate the entire haematopoietic and immunologic cellular repertoire of the host (including myeloid and lymphoid cell lineages) and it should be able to do so in a manner that is self-sustaining and durable
Demetri & Elias 1994

Haematopoietic tissue can be broadly divided into three cell populations: stem cells, committed progenitor cells and maturing/mature cells (Wright & Lord 1992). Stem cells comprise approximately 4% of the total number of haematopoietic cells, while committed progenitors account for 3% and maturing cells for 95% (Lord & Testa 1988). Haematopoiesis is a hierarchical system and the pluripotent stem cells are the origin of all mature myeloid and lymphoid cells. These cells are ultimately responsible for the maintenance of haematopoiesis, although their number relative to the total marrow cellularity is very small (Gordon 1993). Stem cells comprise between 0.01 and 0.05% of the total marrow population, and cannot be identified morphologically. As a result the stem cell is usually evaluated by the number and quality of its offspring (Babior & Stossel 1994). Recent attempts to measure actual numbers have focused on measuring a membrane glycoprotein of unknown function – cluster of differentiation 34 or CD34. CD34+ expression is highest in early progenitors and progressively reduces with maturation (Craig et al 1992). Using monoclonal anti-CD34+ antibodies, CD34+ cells can be identified using cytofluorimetric analysis (Wunder & Henon 1993).

Haematopoietic stem cells possess two features which make them unique:

- self-renewal
- differentiation (Dexter 1990).

Self-replication is necessary to maintain the stem cell pool and differentiation gives rise to the wide variety of blood cells which the body requires (Robinson 1993). The regulation of the balance between self-renewal and lineage commitment is an issue central to the understanding of haematopoiesis (Molineux & Dexter 1994). Overall, 50% of stem cell divisions produce daughter stem cells and 50% produce cells that are destined to differentiate, a process which has been termed 'quantal mitosis' (Emerson 1992, Gordon 1993). Deviation from this balance would result in marrow aplasia or marrow hypercellularity.

For all practical purposes stem cells can be considered immortal and appear to have a life-span which far exceeds the human biological life-span (Dexter 1990). They give rise to multiple lines of progeny in an ordered, structured manner. The pluripotent stem cell gives rise to the myeloid stem cell, the CFU-GEMM (colony-forming unit – granulocyte, erythrocyte, monocyte, megakaryocyte) or to the lymphoid stem cell. Further differentiation produces a variety of progenitor cells, each committed to a single cell pathway. The exception to this rule is in the case of neutrophils and monocytes which share a progenitor cell – the CFU-GM (Fig. 1.1).

Committed progenitor cells have less capacity for self-replication but are normally in a state of cell division. They are primarily responsible for the generation of mature cells and their mitotic rate reflects the balance between replication, differentiation and cell death. True stem cells divide infrequently. In the clinical situation stem cells are ultimately responsible for regenerating haematopoiesis following severe damage while the developmentally restricted progenitor cells facilitate short-term recovery (Fig. 1.2) (Dexter 1990, Robinson 1993). Greater maturity leads to a loss of self-replication ability.

BONE MARROW MICRO-ENVIRONMENT

Stromal layer

Blood cells develop in sinuses and the bone marrow is a rich mixture of all types of cells at all stages of development (Babior & Stossel, 1994). Each lineage occupies a specific marrow location. Megakaryocytes develop next to the venous sinus with their cytoplasmic projections extending directly into the lumen. Budding platelets form at the tips of the projections and are 'washed away' into the circulation. Red cell precursors lie adjacent to the venous sinus in erythroblastic islands and each is associated with a macrophage (Clark et al 1992). Granulocyte and monocyte precursors lie deeper within the medullary cavity but become motile as they mature and are able to migrate towards the venous sinus to be released into the circulation (Pallister 1994).

The framework on which cells grow is the stromal layer and to maintain haematopoiesis close physical contact between the stem cells and the lining of the marrow is required (Dexter 1990). A number of cells make up a confluent stromal layer: endothelial cells, macrophages, fibroblasts, adventitial reticular cells, adipocytes and endosteum. These stromal cells induce locally the generation of a complex mesenchymal tissue including vessels and bone, which are required to support cell development (Zipori 1988, Charbord 1993, Hogge et al 1994).

Stromal cells provide a specialised adhesive microenvironment in which stem and progenitor cells are embedded (Fig. 1.3) (Clark et al 1992). If this contact is prevented, haematopoiesis rapidly declines. This suggests that the required stimuli for haematopoietic cell growth are primarily localised. Thus, within the marrow there are anatomically discrete environments where stem cells bind in a stage- and lineage-specific manner (Gordon 1993). In so doing, the appropriate endogenous growth factors can be presented to the appropriate immobilised target cells (Dexter et al 1977, Dexter 1990, Emerson 1992, Testa et al 1993).

Intrinsic haematopoietic growth factors

Intricate cytokine interactions are employed in haematopoietic cell growth, differentiation and maturation (Mazanet & Griffin 1992). Studies in the 1960s demonstrated that the production of colonies of mature blood cells in vitro rested

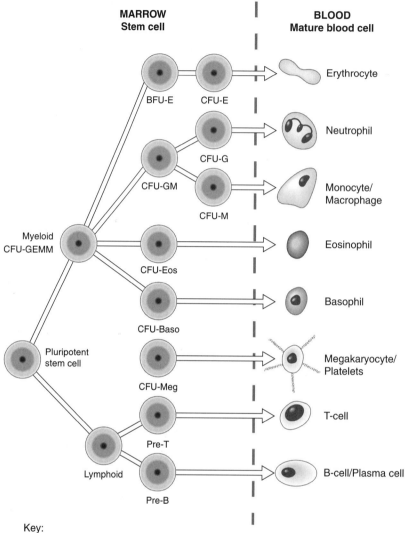

MARROW
Stem cell

BLOOD
Mature blood cell

Erythrocyte

BFU-E   CFU-E

Neutrophil

CFU-G

Monocyte/
Macrophage

CFU-GM

CFU-M

Myeloid
CFU-GEMM

Eosinophil

CFU-Eos

Basophil

CFU-Baso

Pluripotent
stem cell

Megakaryocyte/
Platelets

CFU-Meg

T-cell

Pre-T

Lymphoid

B-cell/Plasma cell

Pre-B

Figure 1.1
Haematopoietic
stem cells

Key:
CFU-GEMM: colony forming unit — granulocyte, erythrocyte, monocyte, megakaryocyte
BFU-E: burst forming unit — erythroid
CFU-GM: colony forming unit — granulocyte, monocyte
CFU-Eos: colony forming unit — eosinophil
CFU-Baso: colony forming unit — basophil
CFU-Meg: colony forming unit — megakaryocyte
Pre-T: pre-T-cell
Pre-B: pre-B-cell
CFU-E: colony forming unit — erythroid
CFU-G: colony forming unit — granulocyte
CFU-M: colony forming unit — monocyte

absolutely with the availability of haematopoi-etic growth factors. Growth factors are a family of glycoproteins which play a pivotal, but complex, role in controlling haematopoiesis and overlapping combinations regulate the growth and differentiation of progenitor cells. However, growth factors alone are insufficient. In the absence of direct homotypic (cell-to-cell) contact with a stromal layer, even large concentrations of growth factors will result in only

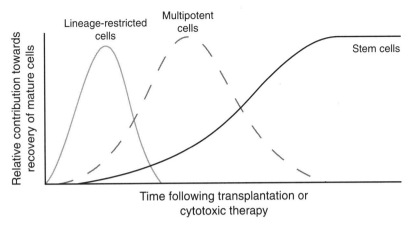

Figure 1.2 Relative contribution of progenitor cells towards the recovery of mature blood cells (from Dexter 1990, with permission)

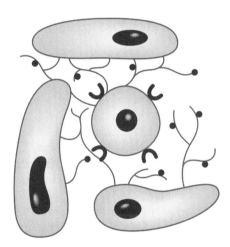

Figure 1.3 Stromal layer

three–four cell divisions (Emerson 1992, Wright & Lord 1992).

The major stimuli for growth factor secretion by stromal accessory cells are the products of inflammation or infection: interleukin-1α or β, tumour necrosis factor-α and interferon-γ. Detecting secretions of endogenous growth factors in the absence of inflammatory stimuli is possible, although difficult. Low levels of granulocyte–colony-stimulating factor (G-CSF) can be detected and higher circulating levels have been demonstrated following an insult to the bone marrow as in the case of cytotoxic therapy (Emerson 1992).

The factors which determine whether pluripotent stem cells differentiate or self-replicate remain relatively unclear and stem cell factor is one of the proteins involved (Zsebo et al 1990). Regulation of the later stages of mature cell development is better understood with factors such as G-CSF and erythropoietin stimulating more mature, committed precursor cells, neutrophils and erythrocytes, respectively (Robinson 1993, Molineux & Dexter 1994). The regulation of thrombopoiesis is less clear and platelet growth factors (thrombopoietins) have been elusive. Recently, however, some light was shed on thrombopoiesis when in-vitro studies showed that CD34+ cells incubated with a megakaryocyte growth and development factor for 8–12 days produced normal megakaryocytes capable of forming long cytoplasmic projections and, ultimately, platelets (Hunt 1995).

Growth factors exert their cellular activities by attaching themselves to distinct high-affinity receptor sites (Mazanet & Griffin 1992). Receptor expression is generally (but not exclusively) restricted to the particular cell lineage. As a growth factor binds to its receptor it becomes internalised, triggering the expression of cellular genes. This initiates cell cycling and shortens the G1 stage of the cell cycle (see Ch. 8). The production of mature cells and the time required for that production are both influenced by the concentration of growth factor available to the dividing progenitor (Metcalf 1990).

STEM CELL CIRCULATION

While the normal stem cell 'home' is the marrow space, small numbers can be found in the peripheral blood where they circulate in the mononuclear cell fraction (Kessinger 1990). In normal individuals steady-state peripheral blood contains approximately $0.2 \pm 0.1\%$ CD34+ cells.

In fetal life this balance is dramatically different. There is a very high concentration of stem cells in embryonic blood (>20 000 CFU-GM per ml in the 22nd week) as haematopoietic and lymphopoietic tissue is established (Fliedner 1993). The stem cells seen in neonate cord blood seem to be the tail end of this dramatic stem cell mobility and studies have demonstrated that the number of cells which can be obtained are large enough for transplant engraftment (Gluckman et al 1993). Stem cell movement continues throughout life and allows the bone marrow to act as one unique organ system although distributed through many bones of the skeleton. Circulating progenitors form part of haematopoietic cell renewal systems and depleted bone marrow sites are repopulated by endogenous stem cell seeding. Thus, circulation of stem cells can be considered as an ongoing, natural process which is used day-to-day to ensure haematopoietic functional integrity (Fliedner 1993).

Babior & Stossel (1994) suggest that stem cells may sense the environmental demands for differentiation and replication while circulating. This provides supplementary information to the humoral signals received in the bone marrow. Blood-derived stem cells are thus not useless overspills from overproduction within the marrow but a significant element of the dynamics of haematopoietic renewal and regulation (Fliedner 1993, Gordon et al 1992). Recognition of this natural phenomenon has led to developments in transplant medicine.

Many factors can increase the level of circulating stem cells. In normal individuals a diurnal variation in circulating CFU-GM levels has been noted, with increasing numbers in the morning (Ross et al 1980). Levels can increase between two- and four-fold following exercise, hydrocortisone, adrenocorticotropic hormone, antibiotics, vaccines and endotoxin (Gordon et al 1992). In certain myeloproliferative disorders, such as chronic myeloid leukaemia (CML), greatly increased numbers of circulating stem cells are found (McCarthy 1993). This might also explain how leukaemic and other malignant cells are almost invariably found throughout the marrow at the outset of clinical disease (Babior & Stossel 1994).

MATURE BLOOD CELLS

Megakaryocytes/platelets

The marrow precursor for platelets is the colony-forming unit – megakaryocyte (CFU-Meg). From this cell thrombopoiesis proceeds to give rise to the megakaryoblast, a cell that is difficult to detect morphologically but which can be detected by staining. The megakaryoblast gives rise to the megakaryocyte, a large distinctive cell and the source of platelets (Fig. 1.4). The megakaryocyte develops long cytoplasmic projections and platelets form at the tips. Each megakaryocyte can produce between 1000 and 8000 platelets. Platelets are disc-shaped anucleated fragments which survive approximately 7–10 days in the peripheral circulation (Babior & Stossel 1994) and account for less than 1% of the total blood volume. Approximately 30% of the platelet population is sequestered in the spleen, which acts as a reservoir pool (Robinson 1993).

The usual platelet count is between 150 and 400×10^9/L, and may be slightly higher in women than in men. More than 40 minutes of sudden exercise will increase platelet counts by about 25% due to release from the splenic pool. Ovulation can increase platelet counts and menstruation causes a slight lowering. Peripheral blood megakaryocyte counts show a diurnal variation and are highest in the evening (Eastham & Slade 1992).

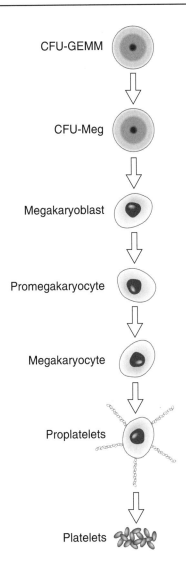

CFU-GEMM

CFU-Meg

Megakaryoblast

Promegakaryocyte

Megakaryocyte

Proplatelets

Platelets

Key:
CFU-GEMM: colony forming unit — granulocyte,
erythrocyte, monocyte, megakaryocyte
CFU-Meg: colony forming unit — megakaryocyte

Figure 1.4 Thrombopoiesis

Platelets are essential in preventing haemorrhage by adhering to injured blood vessel walls and aggregating to form a platelet plug. They form an integral part of haemostasis by maintaining the competence of the vascular endothelium. In cases of thrombocytopenia, fine blood vessels lose their competence, leading to haemorrhage.

Erythrocytes

Erythrocytes account for approximately 45% of total blood volume and their function is oxygen/carbon dioxide exchange. This exchange is made possible by the presence of haemoglobin and the biconcave shape of the erythrocyte, which increases O_2/CO_2 efficiency by making the interior of the cell more accessible. Red blood cells, like platelets, function entirely within the blood stream and normally live for around 120 days.

Erythropoiesis (Fig. 1.5) is stimulated in response to the degree of oxygen perfusion. When blood oxygenation decreases, the level of erythropoietin in plasma rises, accelerating the commitment of pluripotent stem cells into erythroid development (Babior & Stossel 1994). The first identifiable erythroid progenitor cell is the burst-forming unit – erythroid (BFU-E), from which the colony-forming unit – erythroid (CFU-E) develops. This further matures into the pronormoblast, where it develops increasing amounts of haemoglobin. As further differentiation into the normoblast takes place, the nucleus is lost and the cell reaches the reticulocyte stage. Reticulocytes remain in the bone marrow for about 2 days as they accumulate haemoglobin and lose some of their ribonucleic acid (RNA). They subsequently enter the circulation where, after a further day, any residual RNA is lost and they become adult erythrocytes. The transit time from the pronormoblast to the reticulocyte entering the peripheral blood is approximately 5 days. Increased numbers of circulating reticulocytes is indicative of increased erythropoiesis (Robinson 1993).

Leucocytes

The primary function of the white blood system is host defence. Leucocytes function extravascularly and the blood vessels merely serve as avenues which a white cell uses to get from one place to another (Babior & Stossel 1994). Within the leucocyte family are subpopulations of cells, each of which has a distinct but related function (Table 1.1). The adult

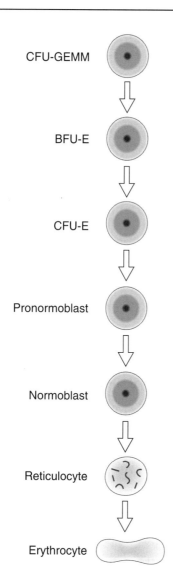

CFU-GEMM

BFU-E

CFU-E

Pronormoblast

Normoblast

Reticulocyte

Erythrocyte

Key:
CFU-GEMM: colony forming unit — granulocyte,
erythrocyte, monocyte, megakaryocyte
BFU-E: burst forming unit — erythroid
CFU-E: colony forming unit — erythroid

Figure 1.5 Erythropoiesis

monocyte progenitor cells, respectively. The myeloblast is the earliest recognisable granulocyte precursor. It is a large cell with a high ratio of nucleus to cytoplasm. Over a series of cell divisions from promyelocyte, to myelocyte, to metamyelocyte, the cytoplasm is lost, the nucleus attenuates and the neutrophilic granules develop. As the nucleus becomes kidney-shaped the cell is called a 'band' (Robinson 1993).

The nucleus of the neutrophil gradually segments into a varying number of lobes, which are joined by a thin chromatin strand (Pallister 1994). Segmentation is indicative of a fully mature cell. The majority of mature neutrophils have a three-lobed nucleus: 20–40% have a two-lobed nucleus (termed a 'shift to the left'). This is seen in infections, toxaemias, haemorrhage and childhood chronic neutropenia. The development of a four-lobed nucleus is termed a 'shift to the right' and where ⩾5% of neutrophils have a five-lobed nucleus this is indicative of incipient megaloblastic anaemia (Eastham & Slade 1992).

Neutrophils have a limited life-span and thus put a continuous replacement demand on the marrow. The marrow holds approximately 11 days' supply of banded and segmented neutrophils in a large storage pool to ensure that a reserve of cells is available. Release of neutrophils from the marrow is a function of their rate of loss from the blood and there is an inverse relationship between the percentage of progenitors in S phase of the cell cycle and the peripheral blood neutrophil count (Eastham & Slade 1992).

On entering the blood, neutrophils divide equally into circulating and marginated pools. This maintains a further reserve of neutrophils ready to migrate into the tissues in response to infection or inflammation (Kanwar & Cairo 1993). The mature neutrophil circulates for approximately 7–10 hours before entering the tissues where it may survive for another 2 days (Robinson 1993).

Neutrophils are small, highly phagocytic, granulocytes which play a vital role in host defence mechanisms. They become motile in response to a variety of chemotactic factors derived from bacteria, damaged tissues and the

differential count balance is reached around the age of puberty (Eastham & Slade 1992).

Neutrophils develop from the CFU-GM – a common committed progenitor cell which they share with the monocyte line (Fig. 1.6). Derived from the CFU-GEMM, the CFU-GM gives rise to the CFU-G and the CFU-M – granulocyte and

Table 1.1 Leucocytes

	Classification	$\times 10^9$/L	Per cent total WBC
Neutrophil	Granulocytes	2.5–7.5	40–75%
Eosinophil	Granulocytes	0.015–0.1	1–6%
Basophil	Granulocytes	0.04–0.44	<1%
Monocyte	Mononuclear cells	0.2–0.8	2–10%
Lymphocyte	Mononuclear cells	1.5–3.5	20–50%

C5, C6 and C7 parts of complement. Chemotaxis helps them to locate and move towards a site of infection. Following phagocytosis, neutrophils degranulate and hydrogen peroxide is produced by glucose oxidation, playing an important part in bacterial killing.

The neutrophil count can be influenced by exercise, emotion, the external temperature and food intake. Steroids can increase neutrophil counts by increasing the inflow of neutrophils and decreasing the rate of egress from the circulation (Eastham & Slade 1992). Decreased margination is seen in acute and chronic myeloid leukaemia and after exercise, adrenaline or alcohol.

Eosinophils

Eosinophils descend from the eosinophil committed progenitor cell, the CFU-Eos, which matures into the first recognisable cell – the eosinophilic myeloblast. This differentiates into the eosinophilic promyelocyte and from there through the stages of myelocyte and metamyelocyte, finally becoming a mature cell. Eosinophils are distinguishable morphologically by their large cytoplasmic granules, which stain reddish-orange. Once released into the blood, less than 1% of eosinophils circulate.

Approximately one-half are marginated and the remainder migrate to areas exposed to the external environment:

- skin epithelium
- bronchial mucosa
- gastrointestinal tract
- vaginal and uterine walls
- lactating mammary gland.

Their life-span in the tissues is approximately 12 days.

Eosinophils have a variety of roles. They participate in modulating and regulating the inflammatory response. By degranulation they release factors which degrade the vasoactive amines released by basophils and mast cells (Workman et al 1993). They can neutralise histamine and hydroxytryptamine. Eosinophils play an important role in defending against parasitic infections and are able to phagocytose, although their ability to do so is much less than that of neutrophils or macrophages. Eosinophils also carry profibrinogen from the bone marrow to other parts of the body (Eastham & Slade 1992).

Eosinophils have a diurnal variation. They are highest at night during sleep, lowest in the morning and begin to rise again by mid-afternoon. This is consistent, but reversed, in night workers (Eastham & Slade 1992). Eosinophil numbers are increased in CML although the existence of a pure eosinophil cell leukaemia is considered doubtful. Counts are also elevated in atopic individuals. Some families carry familial eosinophilia, which is a benign, hereditary autosomal dominant condition (Eastham & Slade 1992).

Basophils

Basophils, the least common of the granulocytes, descend from the committed progenitor cell CFU-Baso. This matures into the first recognisable cell – the basophilic myeloblast. Further differentiation leads to the basophilic promyelocyte, the myelocyte, the metamyelocyte and finally to a mature cell. Basophils are distinguishable morphologically by their large blue cytoplasmic granules.

Basophils carry all the blood histamine as well as a heparin-like substance and differ from other granulocytes in that they have no ability to phagocytose (Workman et al 1993). Basophil degranulation is stimulated primarily by the binding of IgE to the basophil cell surface. This may be localised to the skin or lungs (as in asthma) or it may be widespread and severe as in anaphylactic shock.

Basophils have a life-span of a few days in the circulation and can be recruited into the tissues during immune or inflammatory responses. Occasionally in CML up to 80% of the white cell count may be basophils, although the existence of a pure basophil cell leukaemia is also considered doubtful. A decrease in the number of basophils is associated with stress, thyrotoxicosis, steroid therapy and urticaria (Eastham & Slade 1992).

Monocytes/macrophages

Monocytes/macrophages also arise from the CFU-GM (see Fig. 1.6), which gives rise to the CFU-M – the monocyte precursor cell. The first recognisable cell in the bone marrow is the monoblast. This differentiates into the promonocyte and finally to the monocyte. Monocytes account for between 2 and 10% of leucocyte numbers and range from 0.2 to 0.8×10^9/L of cells in peripheral blood. They are the largest circulatory cells and have a blood transit time of some 14 hours.

Monocytes, however, are still immature cells and mature further in the tissues to become macrophages (Robinson 1993). Macrophages are long-lived phagocytic cells which have some capacity for cell division. Thus the macrophage, like the lymphocyte, may be able to act as its own stem cell (Robinson 1993). Macrophages may be wandering or fixed in strategic locations:

- lungs – alveolar macrophages
- liver – Kupffer cells
- kidneys – glomerulus mesangial cells
- brain – microglia

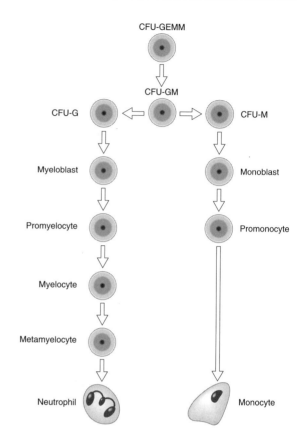

Key:
CFU-GEMM: colony forming unit — granulocyte, erythrocyte, monocyte, megakaryocyte
CFU-GM: colony forming unit — granulocyte, monocyte
CFU-G: colony forming unit — granulocyte
CFU-M: colony forming unit — monocyte

Figure 1.6 Neutrophil and monocyte development

- bone – osteoclasts
- spleen – sinusoids
- lymph nodes – medullary sinuses.

Macrophages provide non-specific immune defence and play a crucial role in initiating and regulating the immune response. Macrophages trap and concentrate antigens ready for presentation to T lymphocytes in association with class I major histocompatibility complex (MHC) molecules and they trap antigen–antibody complexes to stimulate B cell memory. They can also secrete an array of powerful chemical substances – monokines – including interferon and interleukin-1. Monocyte adherence leads to the development of procoagulant activity and may be a contributory factor in the development of disseminated intravascular coagulation (Eastham & Slade 1992).

DOWN REGULATION OF HAEMATOPOIESIS

It would be logical to maintain a population of early progenitors in a quiescent state during normal haematopoiesis to preserve resources and prevent marrow 'wear out'; thus, both positive and negative regulatory factors are required to maintain haemostasis. While the positive stimulation of growth factor proteins has been widely evaluated, Herrmann et al (1992) suggest a number of factors which may help to down regulate haematopoiesis. These include:

- macrophage inflammatory protein-1α (MIP-1α)
- interleukin-10 (IL-10)
- transforming growth factor-β (TGF-β)
- tumour necrosis factor-α (TNF-α).

MIP-1α reversibly inhibits the cell cycling of early progenitor cell populations and thus the percentage of marrow cells in S phase. It also suppresses growth-factor-stimulated CFU-GEMM, BFU-E and CFU-GM proliferation (Bernstein et al 1992). This effect is observed in enriched progenitor cell populations, which suggests that this is a direct effect of MIP-1α. Negative regulatory factors maintain haematopoiesis at a constant size by inhibiting cells from undergoing mitosis and thereby preventing stem cell loss through apoptosis (programmed cell death) (Han & Caen 1994). In times of stress, perhaps in addition to the increases in positive growth factors (e.g. G-CSF), a decrease in negative growth factors would allow quiescent stem cells to enter the cycling pool and thus be recruited for a needed haematological response (Lord et al 1976, Testa et al 1993).

IMMUNITY

> ...all of those physiologic mechanisms that give man the capacity to recognize something as foreign to self and to neutralize, eliminate or metabolize it with or without damage to its own tissues.
>
> *Bellanti 1985*

The immune system is the body's natural defence and has three major functions:

1. defence against microbial attack
2. maintenance of haemostasis by removing used/damaged cells
3. immune surveillance to eliminate mutated/damaged cells (Trahan Reiger et al 1992).

Immune mechanisms can be grouped into acquired and innate. Acquired immunity usually requires prior exposure to a particular stimulus. For example, a vast range of antibodies can be made against a specific antigen, and memory B cells retain the ability to manufacture these same antibodies again should a future need arise.

Innate mechanisms are those which are present from birth. They are usually non-specific and include physical barriers, such as the skin and mucous membranes, and chemical barriers, such as the body secretions, e.g. gastric acid, saliva, proteolytic enzymes, etc. (Pallister 1994).

Paradoxically too, the colonisation of the body by commensal organisms forms part of the body's intrinsic immunity, helping to protect against colonisation by more virulent pathogens. If these defences are breached, the cells of the immune system and factors such as complement are activated.

Major histocompatibility complex/ human leucocyte antigen system

At the core of the system is the ability to distinguish between 'self' and 'non-self' and the mechanisms which control immunity are complex. Immune responses involve interactions between macrophages and lymphocytes, based on specific recognition of foreign antigens: the cells involved in immunity must be able to recognise not only foreign antigens but also each other. This recognition process is centred around the products of the MHC, which directs the synthesis of three different types of protein – MHC classes I, II and III. MHC III proteins are complement components, while the proteins of MHC classes I and II are designated as human leucocyte antigens (HLA) (Pallister 1994). Class I antigens (HLA-A, HLA-B and HLA-C) are expressed on the surface membrane of all nucleated cells of the body, and hence the term human leucocyte antigen is not strictly-speaking correct (Workman et al 1993). Class II antigens (HLA-D, HLA-Dr, HLA-Dp and HLA-Dq) are restricted to cells of the immune system and are thus only expressed on monocytes, macrophages, B cells and, under certain circumstances, activated T cells.

The immune system can deal with foreign antigens effectively and efficiently if they are presented in close association with an appropriate MHC molecule. The MHC/HLA system thus controls which antigens the individual can respond to and how potently (Woods Schindler 1990). Cytotoxic T cells recognise antigen in association with class I MHC molecules and have the potential to respond to any infected host cell. Helper T cells only recognise antigen in association with Class II MHC molecules, e.g. on macrophages (Donnelly et al 1985, Woods Schindler 1990).

The HLA/MHC system is important in marrow, stem cell and tissue transplantation and in transfusions of platelets and white cells. The MHC is controlled by genes on a region of chromosome 6. Each individual derives three genes from each parent and thus carries a total of six MHC antigens, a pair from each of HLA-A, HLA-B and HLA-C. These vary widely from one individual to the next, with the exception of identical twins, and this diversity will result in tissue rejection unless an 'identical' donor can be found.

The ABO blood group system is another MHC which must be matched. Red cells carry ABO antigens but not HLA antigens. Neutrophils carry HLA antigens and a neutrophil-specific antigen, while platelets carry HLA antigens and a platelet-specific antigen.

The complement cascade

The complement system is a family of plasma proteins which plays an important part in the inflammatory response and microbial killing. Complement proteins (C1–C9) are sequentially activated by the presence of specific antigens in the body and the formation of antigen–antibody complexes. Three groups of complement proteins are involved in

- antigen recognition: C1 and its subunits
- immune activation: C2–C4
- cell membrane lysis: C5–C9.

Complement can also be stimulated by a variety of substances present in microbial infection, e.g. bacterial endotoxin. A fragment of C5, known as C5a, is the most potent chemotactic factor for neutrophils and can also act as an anaphylotoxin, stimulating the release of histamine from tissue mast cells in anaphylaxis (Pallister 1994). For a fuller description of the intricacies of the complement cascade the reader is referred to Pallister (1994).

Lymphocytes

Cells of the lymphoid system start life in the bone marrow and are derived from the lymphoid stem cell. Like the CFU-GEMM, the lymphoid stem cell is multipotent. It can either self-replicate or differentiate to produce B or T lymphocytes. Lymphoid cells, unlike myeloid cells, do not necessarily follow a unidirectional development flow from mitotic stem cell to mature cell. They can oscillate between mitotic forms and dormant memory cells capable of recruitment into a mitotic pool on demand. Lymphocytes also migrate back and forth between the blood, lymphatic system and tissues (Babior & Stossel 1994).

Shortly after birth lymphocytes number approximately $3.5–8.5 \times 10^9$/L, while by the end of the first week of life they have increased to about 12×10^9/L. The normal adult range of $1.5–3.5 \times 10^9$/L is reached by about the age of 12 years. It is not possible to distinguish between B and T lymphocytes based on morphological characteristics only. Distinction between the two relies on cell membrane markers and gene rearrangements. Full blood counts, therefore, generally report a total lymphocyte count as part of a white cell differential. Lymphocytes display a diurnal variation. They are lowest at 9.00 am and highest at 9.00 pm which is the inverse of the plasma cortisol concentration (Eastham & Slade 1992).

T lymphocytes

T lymphocytes originate in the bone marrow from the PRE-T progenitor cell but migrate to the thymus gland where they are processed by thymosin and become immunologically competent. Cells pass through the developmental phases of prothymocyte and T lymphoblast into mature T cell. T lymphocytes make up approximately 40–80% of the lymphocyte population and can migrate rapidly in response to stimuli. They are responsible for cellular immunity, including resistance against intracellular organisms which evade humoral immunity (Donnelly et al 1985).

There are several subpopulations of T cell. Regulatory T cells orchestrate the immune system to ensure a consistent, coordinated response. Helper T cells assist B lymphocytes to differentiate into plasma cells and to produce IgG immunoglobulin (antibodies). Suppressor T cells turn off the immune system and suppress the responses of other lymphocytes. A number of effector T cells are also present. Cytotoxic T cells rid the body of infected or malignant cells but are also responsible for tissue rejection and organ graft failure. Natural killer (NK) cells are another form of T lymphocyte. They are called 'natural' killer cells because, unlike cytotoxic T cells, they do not need to recognise a specific antigen or MHC molecule before acting (Donnelly et al 1985).

Cytotoxic T cells and NK cells both kill on contact. When a T cell meets an antigen it undergoes blast transformation. Activated T lymphocytes are produced, which bind to the target cell and secrete a lethal burst of substances known as cytokines or, more specifically, lymphokines. Lymphokines, such as interleukin-2, are potent chemicals which can both attract macrophages and have a direct cytotoxic effect by causing cellular lysis.

T cells carry various different glycoproteins on their surface membrane. All mature peripheral blood T cells express T1 and T3 antigens. Helper T cells (about 65%) express T4. Cytotoxic and suppressor T cells (about 35%) express T8. However, the relationship between the presence of phenotypic markers and functional activities is not so clear cut. The defining characteristic of the T4 and T8 subpopulations is the nature of the MHC molecule with which they interact. T4 cells recognise antigen in association with class II MHC molecules (HLA-D, HLA-Dr), while T8 cells recognise antigen in association with class I MHC antigen (HLA-A, HLA-B or HLA-C) (Donnelly et al 1985).

B lymphocytes

The B cell population is a very heterogeneous pool of clonal cells, each of which displays antigen specificity and can produce only a single antibody. The B cells originate in the marrow and, unlike T cells, mature there too. They originate from the PRE-B progenitor cell, which passes through the developmental phases of prothymocyte and B lymphoblast into the mature B cell. B cells have surface immunoglobulin and complement receptors and are responsible for the mediation of humoral immunity and immune 'memory'. On exposure to foreign antigens they synthesise RNA and differentiate into plasma cells. Plasma cells manufacture and contain antibodies – IgG, IgA, IgM, IgE and IgD – but there is normally only one immunoglobulin in a cell. Antibodies can interact with foreign particles, such as toxins or bacteria, but are unable to penetrate living cells (Eastham & Slade 1992).

B cells make up about 10–30% of circulating lymphocytes and have a life-span of days to weeks. They too are migratory, which facilitates their meeting with antigens, but some leave the blood to reside in the lymphoid tissues:

- lymph nodes
- spleen
- appendix
- tonsils
- bone marrow.

GENETICS

The marrow has the most active cell division of any organ and, therefore, it is predictable that some genetic mutations will occur. Many mutated cells will undergo apoptosis, while others will develop into abnormal clones. Throughout the body it is estimated that some 100–1000 mutant cells are produced daily, although these are generally eliminated by the immune system (Roitt et al 1985).

Some of the genetic aberrations involve the translocation of chromosomal regions and result in the juxtaposition of genes which would normally be apart. This can activate cellular oncogenes – genes whose activation is associated with the initial and continuing conversion of normal cells to tumour cells – and may provide a growth stimulation to the abnormal clone (Eastham & Slade 1992). A number of genetic rearrangements are associated with marrow disease (Table 1.2).

The Philadelphia (Ph) chromosome, which is characteristic of CML and is seen in approximately 95% of cases, is a translocation between chromosomes 9 and 22. This brings together, on chromosome 22, the breakpoint cluster

Table 1.2 Genetic rearrangement in marrow disease (adapted from Eastham & Slade (1992) and Hoelzer & Seipelt (1994))

Disease	Genetic mutation	Comments
Pre-B acute leukaemia	t(1:19)	One-third of cases
B acute lymphoblastic leukaemia	t(8:14)	
T acute lymphoblastic leukaemia	t(4 : 11)	In older children
Chronic myeloid leukaemia	t(9:22)(q34:q11) bcr/abl oncogene	Philadelphia chromosome
M1 acute myeloblastic leukaemia	t(8:21) Monosomy 7 Monosomy 5 Trisomy 8	
M2 acute granulocytic leukaemia	t(8:21) Monosomy 7 Monosomy 5 Trisomy 8	Mainly younger patients
M3 acute promyelocytic leukaemia	t(15:17) HLA-Dr negative Trisomy 8	More than 90% of cases Mainly younger patients About one-third of cases
M4 acute myelomonoblastic leukaemia	Trisomy 8 Monosomy 7	
M4 (Eo) acute myelomonoblastic leukaemia with abnormal eosinophils	Inversion/deletion of chromosome 16 Trisomy 8	Inversion of chromosome 16 generally indicates a better prognosis
M5 monocytic leukaemia	Trisomy 8	
M5a poorly-differentiated monocytic leukaemia	t(9:11) (11q23)	About 50% of cases
Burkitt's lymphoma	t(8:14) c-myc oncogene	

region (bcr) gene and the cellular proto-onco-gene Abelson (c-abl) from chromosome 9. The newly-formed bcr/abl gene has tyrosine kinase activity which leads to an increase in granulopoiesis (Eastham & Slade 1992).

About 60% of individuals with acute myeloid leukaemia (AML) have some form of genetic defect, and some of these are specific for the French–American–British (FAB) leukaemia subtype (see Table 1.2). (For a fuller explanation of AML subtypes refer to Ch. 4.) Trisomy 8 (three copies of chromosome 8) is the most common change in AML and is seen in about 19% of cases, particularly as the lone change in M1, M4 and M5 and as an additional change in M3 (Eastham & Slade, 1992). Monosomy 7 (one copy of chromosome 7) is the second most common change in AML and is associated with previous exposure to chemotherapy or other toxic agents. It is the sole anomaly in about 4% of cases of M2 and M4 and is also seen in myelodysplastic syndrome, which is generally recognised as a pre-leukaemic state (Greenberg 1991). Chromosome 21 may also play a role in the genetic control of white cell production. Individuals with trisomy 21 have abnormally high white cell counts while, conversely, people who have an abnormally small chromosome 21 have low white cell counts (Eastham & Slade 1992).

The genetics of endogenous growth factors may also be influential. The chromosomal locations of the cytokine genes are clustered in the human genome. The gene for erythropoietin rests on chromosome 7(q11–22) (Coze 1994). The genes for interleukin-3 (IL-3), interleukin-4 (IL-4), interleukin 5 (IL-5), granulocyte, macrophage–colony-stimulating factor (GM-CSF) and macrophage–colony-stimulating factor (M-CSF) have all been located on the long arm of chromosome 5 and deletions involving chromosome 5 have been described in various haematopoietic diseases (Mazanet & Griffin, 1992). It has been suggested that the loss of the GM-CSF gene may be important in understanding the generation of M2 AML (Crosier & Clarke 1992). The G-CSF gene is located on the long arm of chromosome 17(q11.2–21) near the t(15:17) translocation break point which is characteristic of acute promyelocytic leukaemia (Mazanet & Griffin 1992). The stem cell factor (SCF) gene is located on chromosome 12q22–24 (Coze 1994).

Growth factor receptors may be important too. The human GM-CSF receptor is located on the X–Y pseudoautosomal region. Loss or inactivation of the receptor could result in relatively immature cells, which are incapable of differentiation in response to endogenous GM-CSF. Thus, the GM-CSF receptor may function as a recessive oncogene and it has been reported that 25% of the M2 subtype of AML have lost either the X or the Y chromosome (Gasson 1991).

CONCLUSION

Haematopoiesis is a complex hierarchical system. The immune and blood systems both develop from a single common pluripotent stem cell. This stem cell divides infrequently but gives rise to the myeloid and lymphoid progenitor cells from which mature cells are derived. Endogenous regulatory factors – both positive and negative – ensure a balanced system which is neither over- nor under-productive. In any cell undergoing multiple mitoses the potential for genetic aberrations exists. A number of these are associated with myeloid and lymphoid disease.

DISCUSSION QUESTIONS

1. What is the importance of stem cell self-replication in haematopoiesis?
2. What role do growth factors play in haematopoiesis?
3. What is the role of apoptosis in the maintenance of blood cell numbers?
4. Each of the leucocytes has a distinct but different function. What are their different functions?
5. What is the importance of the HLA system in bone marrow transplantation and blood transfusion?
6. What are the most well-documented genetic abnormalities in haemato-oncology?

ACKNOWLEDGEMENT

The author is deeply indebted to Mrs Debbie Lorimer for her original illustrations.

References

Babior B M, Stossel T P 1994 Hematology. A pathophysiological approach, 3rd edn. Churchill Livingstone, New York

Bellanti J 1985 Immunology, basic processes. W B Saunders, Philadelphia

Bernstein S H, Kufe D W 1992 Future of basic/clinical hematopoietic research in the era of hematopoietic growth factor availability. Seminars in Oncology 19(4): 441–448

Burton R 1628. In: Babior B M, Stossel T P 1994 Hematology. A pathophysiological approach, 3rd edn. Churchill Livingstone, New York

Charbord P 1993 Stroma and hematopoiesis. In: Wunder E W, Henon P R (eds) Peripheral blood stem cell autografts. Springer-Verlag, Berlin, pp 35–46

Clark B R, Gallagher J T, Dexter T M 1992 Cell adhesion in the stromal regulation of haemopoiesis. In: Lord B I, Dexter T M (eds) Clinical Haematology. Growth Factors in Haemopoiesis 5(3): 619–652. Baillière Tindall, London

Coze C M 1994 Glossary of cytokines. In: Brenner M (ed) Clinical Haematology. Cytokines and Growth Factors 7(1): 1–15. Baillière Tindall, London

Craig J, Turner M, Parker A 1992 Peripheral blood stem cell transplantation. Blood Reviews 6: 59–67

Crosier P, Clark S 1992 Basic biology of the hematopoietic growth factors. Seminars in Oncology 19(4): 349–361

Demetri G D, Elias A D 1994 Current understanding of PBPCs and hematopoietic growth factors. Advances in Oncology 10(1): 11–19

Dexter T M, 1990 Haematopoietic growth factors. Review of biology and clinical potential. Gardiner-Caldwell Communications Ltd, Macclesfield, UK

Dexter T M, Allen T D, Lajtha L 1977 Conditions controlling the proliferation of hematopoietic stem cells in vitro. Journal of Cell Physiology 91: 335–344

Donnelly P, Irving W, Starke I 1985 Infection and the immunocompromised patient. Current Medical Literature Ltd, London

Eastham R D, Slade R R 1992 Clinical haematology, 7th edn. Butterworth-Heinemann, Oxford

Emerson S G 1992 The Hematopoietic microenvironment. In: Armitage J O, Antman K H (eds) High-dose cancer therapy. Pharmacology, hematopoietins, stem cells. Williams and Wilkins, Baltimore, pp 143–150

Fliedner T M 1993 Foreword. In: Wunder E W, Henon P R (eds) Peripheral blood stem cell autografts. Springer-Verlag, Berlin, pp v–vi

Gasson JC 1991 Molecular physiology of granulocyte-macrophage colony-stimulating factor. Blood 77: 1131–1145

Gluckman E, Thierry D, Brossard Y et al 1993 Stem cell harvesting from umbilical cord blood: a new perspective. In: Wunder E W, Henon P R (eds) Peripheral blood stem cell autografts. Springer-Verlag, Berlin, pp 262–267

Gordon M Y 1993 Biology of haematopoietic stem cells. In: Wunder E W, Henon P R (eds) Peripheral blood stem cell autografts. Springer-Verlag, Berlin, pp 26–34

Gordon M Y, Healy L E, Craddock C F, Apperley J F 1992 Experimental models for peripheral blood stem cell autografting. International Journal of Cell Cloning 10, Suppl 1: 2–5

Greenberg P L 1991 Treatment of myelodysplastic syndromes. Blood Reviews 5: 42–50

Han Z C, Caen J P 1994 Cytokines acting on committed haematopoietic progenitors. In: Brenner M (ed) Clinical Haematology. Cytokines and Growth Factors 7(1): 65–89. Baillière Tindall, London

Herrmann F, Brugger W, Kanz L, Mertlesmann R 1992 In vivo biology and therapeutic potential of hematopoietic growth factors and circulating progenitor cells. Seminars in Oncology 19(4): 422–431

Hoelzer D, Seipelt G 1994 Acute leukaemias and myelodysplastic syndromes, 2nd edn. Gardiner-Caldwell Communications Ltd, Macclesfield, UK

Hogge D E, Sutherland H J, Cashman J D, Lansdorp P M, Humphries R K, Eaves C J 1994 Cytokines acting early in human haematopoiesis. In: Brenner M (ed) Clinical Haematology. Cytokines and Growth Factors 7(1): 49–63. Baillière Tindall, London

Hunt P 1995 Megakaryocyte growth and development factor. Helix IV(3): 32–33

Kanwar V S, Cairo M S 1993 Neonatal neutrophil maturation, kinetics, and function. In: Abramson J S, Wheeler J G (eds) The natural immune system. The neutrophil. IRL Press, Oxford, pp 1–21

Kessinger A 1990 Autologous transplantation with peripheral blood stem cells: a review of clinical results. Journal of Clinical Apheresis 5: 97–99

Lord B, I Testa N G 1988 The hemopoietic system. Structure and regulation. In: Testa N G, Gale R P (eds) Hematopoiesis. Marcel Dekker, New York, pp 1–26

Lord B I, Mori K S, Wright E G 1976 An inhibitor of stem cell proliferation in normal bone marrow. British Journal of Haematology 34: 441–445

Mazanet R, Griffin J D 1992 Hematopoietic growth factors. In: Armitage J O, Antman K H (eds) High-dose cancer therapy. Pharmacology, hematopoietins, stem cells. Williams and Wilkins, Baltimore, pp 289–313

McCarthy D M 1993 Peripheral blood stem cells: 1909 to the nineties. In: Wunder E W, Henon P R (eds) Peripheral blood stem cell autografts. Springer-Verlag, Berlin, pp 3–15

Metcalf D 1990 The colony stimulating factors: Discovery, development and clinical applications. Cancer 65(10): 2185–2195

Molineux G, Dexter T M 1994 Biology of G-CSF. In: Morstyn G, Dexter T M (eds) Filgrastim in clinical practice. Marcel Dekker, New York, pp 1–21

Pallister C 1994 Blood. Physiology and pathophysiology. Butterworth-Heinemann, Oxford

Robinson S H 1993 Physiology of hematopoiesis. In: Robinson S H, Reich P R (eds) Hematology. Pathological basis for clinical practice, 3rd edn. Little, Brown and Company, Boston, pp 1–13

Roitt I, Broff J, Male D 1985 Immunology. Mosby, St. Louis

Ross D D, Poliak A, Ackman S A, Bachur N R 1980 Diurnal variation of circulating human myeloid progenitor cells. Experimental Hematology 8: 954

Testa N G, Coutinho L H, Radford J A, Will A 1993 Growth factors and the microenvironment. In: van Furth R (ed) Hemopoietic growth factors and mononuclear phagocytes. Karger, Basle, pp 36–43

Trahan Reiger P, Harle M, Rumsey K A 1992 The immune system. In: Rumsey K A, Trahan Reiger P (eds) Biological response modifiers. A self instruction manual for health professionals. Precept Press Inc, Chicago, pp 4–34

Woods Schindler L 1990 Understanding the immune system. US Department of Health and Human Services. NIH Publication No. 90–529

Workman M L, Ellerhorst-Ryan J, Hargreave-Koertge V 1993 Nursing care of the immunocompromised patient. W B Saunders, Philadelphia

Wright E G, Lord B I 1992 Haemopoietic tissue. In: Lord B I, Dexter T M (eds) Clinical Haematology. Growth Factors in Haemopoiesis 5(3): 499–507. Baillière Tindall, London

Wunder E W, Henon P R 1993 Preface. In: Wunder E W, Henon P R (eds) Peripheral blood stem cell autografts. Springer-Verlag, Berlin, pp vii–viii

Zipori D 1988 Hemopoietic microenvironments. In: Testa N G, Gale R P (eds) Hematopoiesis. Marcel Dekker, New York, pp 27–62

Zsebo K, Martin F, Suggs S et al 1990 Biological characterisation of a unique early acting hematopoietic growth factor. Experimental Hematology 18: 703 (abstr)

Further reading

The following further reading provides a more in-depth review of cytokines and haematopoietic growth factors.

Brenner M (ed) (1994) Clinical Haematology. Cytokines and Growth Factors 7(1). Baillière Tindall, London

Lord B I, Dexter T M (eds) (1992) Clinical Haematology. Growth Factors in haemopoiesis 5(3). Baillière Tindall, London

Rumsey K A, Trahan Reiger P (eds) (1992) Biological response modifiers. A self instruction manual for health professionals. Precept Press Inc, Chicago

Testa N G, Gale R P (eds) (1998) Hematopoiesis. Marcel Dekker, New York

2 | *Myelodysplastic syndromes*

TRACEY BURGOYNE AND ALISON KNIGHT

> **Key points**
> - The myelodysplastic syndromes are a group of disorders
> - Myelodysplasia is primarily a disease of the elderly
> - Treatment for myelodysplasia is mainly supportive
> - Bone marrow transplant is the treatment of choice for younger individuals

INTRODUCTION

The myelodysplastic syndromes are haematological disorders characterised by abnormalities in the maturation and effectiveness of blood cells. Abnormalities are attributed to an abnormal clone of the myeloid stem cell which differentiates ineffectively halting blood cell maturation at differing stages of development. The number, structure and functional ability of all blood cells may be abnormal, resulting in anaemia, leucopenia and thrombocytopenia.

Myelodysplastic syndromes (MDS) or myelodysplasia have the potential to develop into acute myeloid leukaemia (AML) and have previously been known as pre-leukaemia, smouldering acute leukaemia or oligoblastic leukaemia. However, not all individuals with MDS develop acute leukaemia and these titles have now fallen into disuse. This chapter examines MDS, classification, treatment options and specific nursing issues.

THE DISEASE

MDS usually arises as a primary condition (de novo) and is an idiopathic disease, but may also be secondary to treatment with chemotherapy and/or radiotherapy for other diseases. Exposure to benzene has also been associated with the development of MDS. Accurate estimation of the incidence of MDS is difficult, as it may be asymptomatic and therefore go undetected for many years. MDS is more common in males and is primarily a disease of the elderly, mainly affecting those over the age of 60 and being rare below the age of 30. However, patients as young as 2 years have been reported. The incidence of secondary MDS in those under the age of 60 may increase in future years as increased numbers of individuals survive cancer and its treatment.

The clinical course and prognosis of MDS is variable; the disease may remain stable for many years or progress rapidly to AML. Survival after diagnosis varies, but the majority of patients die within 2 years due to either complications of pancytopenia or transformation to acute leukaemia (de Witte et al 1990). However, some individuals with stable disease may survive as long as 10 years. Prognosis is directly related to the number of bone marrow blast cells and degree of blood cell cytopenias. Secondary MDS usually has a poorer prognosis than de novo MDS.

The incidence of AML transformation varies, depending on the classification of MDS (see Table 2.1). It is estimated that between 10 and 40% of individuals with MDS will develop AML

(Ganser & Karthaus 1997). Once leukaemic transformation occurs it is less responsive to anti-leukaemic treatment than de novo AML, with individuals often only surviving for a few months (Ahmad et al 1995).

Diagnosis

Many individuals present with symptoms of one or more cytopenias, such as fatigue, infection or bleeding, although MDS may be detected accidentally through a blood test taken for other reasons.

MDS is diagnosed by bone marrow aspirate, trephine biopsy, peripheral blood and chromosomal studies. Abnormalities of haematopoiesis vary according to the different classifications of disease within this group. Characteristically, bone marrow and blood cell morphology are abnormal, being normocellular or hypercellular with peripheral blood cytopenias, although occasionally hypocellularity may be noted (Whittaker & Judge 1990). Abnormalities may affect one or more of the three myeloid blood cell lines and symptoms are related to the particular cells involved. Manifestations of anaemia, neutropenia or thrombocytopenia do not necessarily correlate with the blood cell count as ineffective function may increase the risk of infection or bleeding (Hoffbrand & Pettit 1993).

Megaloblastic erythroid hyperplasia with macrocytic anaemia is common early in the disease process. Vitamin B_{12} and folate levels should be normal and are estimated, to exclude any deficiencies which would affect the blood picture. Abnormal myeloid progenitors (blast cells) and ringed sideroblasts may be identified in the marrow, in varying percentages, depending on the disease classification (see Table 2.1). Granulocytopenia is common with functional abnormalities and hypogranular appearance. The acquired Pelger–Huët abnormality (single or bilobed nuclei) may be seen in neutrophils, and abnormalities in the number and function of monocytes may occur (Hoffbrand & Pettit 1993, Prodan et al 1995). Leucocytosis may be present in the chronic myelomonocytic leukaemia (CMML) sub-type of MDS.

Thrombocytopenia is common and micromegakaryocytes may be seen in the bone marrow and giant platelets in the peripheral blood. Platelets may also have functional abnormalities. Furthermore, chromosomal abnormalities affecting chromosomes 5, 7, 8, 11, 12, 14, 17 and 20 have been identified in the various subtypes of MDS (Jacobs 1997). Approximately 10% of patients will also have splenomegaly. This is particularly common in those with CMML (Oscier 1997).

As the disease progresses there is a gradual increase in abnormal cells and normal haematopoiesis is reduced. Blast cells within the bone marrow increase and pancytopenia occurs. This results in an increased incidence of infection and bleeding episodes, which are often resistant to supportive therapy (Belcher 1993).

Classification of the disease

MDS has been subdivided into five categories according to the abnormalities within the bone marrow and peripheral blood (Bennett et al 1982). The French–American–British (FAB) classification system is used as a prognostic indicator, based on the percentage of blast cells, ringed sideroblasts, monocytes and the presence of Auer rods. The system has been criticised as there are instances where it is difficult to categorise the disease accurately (Verhoef et al 1995). However, it is currently the most widely accepted MDS classification system (Table 2.1).

RA and RARS have the longest median survival times of approximately 50 months with less risk of leukaemic transformation (Verhoef et al 1995). The remaining three FAB subtypes are estimated as having an approximate survival time of 15 months (Jacobs 1997), although different studies show differing length of survival.

However, survival times and the course of the disease vary tremendously, even within the same subgroup, and a number of other methods have been developed as a means of predicting leukaemic transformation and length of survival. The most recent of these methods is the International Prognostic Scoring System (Greenberg et al 1997), which incorporates the number and degree of cytopenias at diagnosis, percentage of blast cells in the bone marrow and cytogenetic abnormalities, age

Table 2.1   French–American–British (FAB) classification of myelodysplastic syndromes

FAB type	Percentage of blasts in bone marrow	Percentage of blasts in peripheral blood
Refractory anaemia (RA) is an anaemia which will not respond to therapy with blood products and requires constant transfusion therapy	<5	<1
Refractory anaemia with ringed sideroblasts (RARS) is an unresponsive anaemia with sideroblasts (erythroid precursors with deposits of iron in the mitochondria around the nucleus) seen on the marrow film	<5 Ringed sideroblasts >15% of total erythroblasts	<1
Refractory anaemia with excess blasts (RAEB) is an unresponsive anaemia with the presence of immature cells (nucleated precursor cells) on the marrow or blood film	5–20	<5
Refractory anaemia with excess blasts in transformation (RAEB-t) is an unresponsive anaemia with a large amount of immature cells (nucleated precursor cells) in the marrow or blood film	20–30 or presence of Auer rods	>5
Chronic myelomonocytic leukaemia (CMML) is characterised by monocytosis in peripheral blood with features of both MDS and myeloproliferative disease	5–20 Monocyte count $>1.0 \times 10^9/l$	<5

and gender. Cytogenetic abnormalities are categorised as

■ good (normal karyotype or absent Y chromosome, deletion of long arm of chromosomes 5 or 20)
■ intermediate (other abnormalities)
■ poor (complex abnormalities, ≥3 abnormalities or chromosome 7 anomalies).

This system identifies four categories of risk:

■ low
■ intermediate risk 1
■ intermediate risk 2
■ high.

In those over the age of 60 greatly reduced survival times are associated with low and intermediate risk 1 groups. However, age is not

Reflection point

The unpredictable nature of MDS results in uncertainty about the future. Consider what psychological support may be needed to help individuals and their families adapt and cope with the disease.

associated with survival rates in the other groups. Women are also associated with slightly longer survival than men.

TREATMENT

There is no consistently effective treatment that provides prolonged improvement in haematopoiesis. Therefore treatment decisions tend to depend largely on the severity of the presenting disease, age and general physical status of the individual (Cain et al 1991).

Supportive therapy

Supportive therapy remains the treatment of choice for the majority of patients. As many individuals with MDS are elderly, they are more likely to have additional coexisting medical conditions and may be unable to withstand aggressive treatment with chemotherapy or bone marrow transplant (BMT). Supportive treatment aims to minimise the risk of life-threatening complications associated with anaemia, leucopenia and thrombocytopenia and maintain quality of life.

Risk of infection is high for individuals with leucopenia. It is essential that signs of infection are detected early and close observation of the individual is necessary. Education of the individual and their relatives to enable them to both minimise the risk of infection and recognise signs of infection is also an important nursing role (see Ch. 13). If infection does occur, prompt treatment with an appropriate antimicrobial agent is vital to prevent the occurrence of septicaemia.

Thrombocytopenia is treated with platelet transfusions prophylactically or when spontaneous bleeding occurs (see Ch. 11). Individuals with MDS need educating to avoid trauma and recognise bleeding: again, an important role for nurses (see Ch. 14).

Anaemia may cause fatigue and breathlessness, which interferes with an individual's ability to undertake normal daily activities and affects the quality of life. Treatment consists of regular red cell transfusions, as required. Regular blood transfusions may lead to a progressive increase in body iron stores and iron overload, as the body has no means of increasing iron excretion (Hughes-Jones & Wickramasinghe 1996). If iron stores become greatly increased, organ damage may occur, with the heart, liver and endocrine organs being most susceptible. Desferrioxamine, an iron-chelating agent administered subcutaneously with blood transfusions, is used to prevent iron overload or reduce serum iron levels. Prevention of iron overload is especially important in younger individuals to reduce risk of organ damage and associated complications. In younger patients, desferrioxamine treatment has also been shown to improve granulocyte and platelet counts and thereby reduce transfusion requirements and the risk of infection (Jensen et al 1992).

Colony-stimulating factors

Colony-stimulating factors (CSFs or growth factors) are cytokines, which promote the growth and differentiation of blood cells. Potentially CSFs may improve supportive treatment of MDS by reducing infection and bleeding associated with cytopenias and the blood component support required. They comprise the following:

- Granulocyte, macrophage–colony-stimulating factor (GM-CSF), which promotes the growth and differentiation of granulocyte and macrophage progenitors.
- Granulocyte–colony-stimulating factor (G-CSF), which stimulates neutrophil precursors to produce large amounts of circulating mature neutrophils.
- Erythropoietin, which promotes erythrocyte production.

G-CSF and GM-CSF increase the number of neutrophils in most people and enhance maturation of cells. Fewer infections have therefore been reported, but clinically effective stimulation of cells is infrequent (Hansen et al 1998). These agents also increase the number of blast cells in some individuals and this has led to speculation that they may promote transition of MDS to acute leukaemia in those with excess blast cells (Thompson et al 1989). However, data from phase I and II clinical trials indicate that G-CSF does not increase progression to AML (Forman 1996).

Used alone, erythropoietin only stimulates an erythroid response in a minority of individuals with MDS. A response has been noted when erythropoietin is used in conjunction with GM-CSF (Negrin et al 1996). However, those individuals with the greatest need for transfusion are least likely to respond to treatment with erythropoietin (Casadevall 1998).

It is suggested that, in combination, colony-stimulating factors may be of clinical benefit for some individuals with MDS, particularly those with repeated infections and neutropenia. However, the outcome remains unpredictable and their cost is high (Hansen et al 1998). Side-effects of colony-stimulating factors are shown in Box 2.1.

Box 2.1 Side-effects of colony-stimulating factors	
G-CSF	*GM-CSF*
Bone pain	Bone pain
Transient hypotension	Flu-like symptoms
Occasional fever	Transient
Disruption in serum	hypotension
liver function tests	Fatigue
Headache	Nausea and
Fatigue	vomiting
Nausea	Dyspnoea

Interleukin-3 (IL-3) in combination with low-dose cytosine arabinoside (cytarabine) has also been investigated. It is suggested that IL-3 may be able to stimulate normal haematopoiesis in MDS and may also sensitise leukaemic progenitor cells to S phase specific cytotoxic drugs such as cytarabine. An overall response rate of 42% and a median overall survival time of 18 months has been shown (Gerhartz et al 1996). However, further research is required to substantiate these findings and determine the role of IL-3 in the treatment of MDS.

Differentiation-inducing agents

Differentiation-inducing drugs encourage cell maturation. A number of agents, most notably retinoic acids and vitamin D analogues, have been studied in the treatment of MDS, both as single agents and in conjunction with colony-stimulating factors or cytotoxic drugs. However, research evidence to support use of these agents is currently inconclusive (Jacobs 1997).

Hormonal/steroid therapy

Androgens and corticosteroids have previously been recommended in the treatment of MDS. However, their use has been challenged as they increase infection risk and they are not currently advocated (Utley 1996, Jacobs 1997).

Biological therapy

Interferon-α and interferon-γ have both been studied as treatment for MDS. Interferons can induce cell differentiation and suppress myeloid proliferation (Belcher 1993). Responses in blood counts have been noted although these are usually temporary. Side-effects experienced with interferon-α and interferon-γ include nausea, fatigue, myelosuppression, flu-like symptoms and depression.

Cell suppression with chemotherapy

Both low-dose cytotoxic drug therapy and aggressive anti-leukaemic regimens have been used to treat MDS, with cytarabine being the most commonly studied drug.

Low-dose cytarabine subcutaneously has been shown to have some beneficial effect. However, a recent review of the literature suggests that complete remission rate is less than 20% and no survival benefit has been found (Cheson 1998). The use of other cytotoxic drugs such as 5-azacytidine and 6-thioguanine have also been studied but there is little evidence of prolonged survival. Agents such as hydroxyurea, etoposide or mercaptopurine may have a beneficial effect in CMML, RAEB or RAEB-t with high circulating white blood cell counts (Hoffbrand & Pettit 1993). Additionally, newer agents such as topotecan show promise in clinical trials (Cheson 1998). However, topotecan also has major toxicities and none of the current treatment strategies consistently improve the outcome for individuals with MDS.

Aggressive chemotherapy regimens may be contraindicated in many elderly individuals. However, protocols using aggressive anti-leukaemic chemotherapy can achieve a complete response, although a percentage of patients may die due to complications relating to marrow hypoplasia (Cheson 1990). Aggressive chemotherapy is less likely to induce complete remission in secondary AML than in treatment of de novo AML and generally does not prolong survival (Fenaux et al 1991). Some young patients with advanced MDS may achieve prolonged, disease-free survival when treated with intensive anti-leukaemic chemotherapy (Fenaux et al 1992). However, results are inconsistent and remissions may also be short.

Treatment with cytotoxic drugs enhances disease-induced cytopenias and these effects are discussed in Chapter 8.

Bone marrow transplantation

Bone marrow transplant offers the best chance of curative treatment for MDS, but is only suitable for the small proportion of individuals who are physically able to tolerate the treatment and have a histocompatible sibling or unrelated donor. In determining whether individuals are suitable for such 'aggressive' treatment their age, stage of the disease, remission state, general well being and past medical history including previous infections, response to antimicrobials, liver, lung, renal and cardiac function, availability of a suitable donor, psychological state and ability to cope with isolation procedures must all be considered (see Chs 10 and 19).

For individuals considered suitable, allogeneic BMT offers potentially long-term disease-free survival and is considered the treatment of choice. Furthermore, for those with secondary MDS, allogeneic BMT is the only available treatment with a realistic chance of achieving prolonged remission (Giles & Koeffler 1994).

Prognosis is better when individuals do not have excess blast cells and transplantation takes place early in the course of the disease. In a recent European study of 131 individuals, 5-year disease-free survival was 34% (Runde et al 1998).

Unrelated donor marrow transplants for MDS have demonstrated disease-free survival of 38%

and 28% (Anderson et al 1996, Arnold et al 1998). However, follow-up time post-transplant was much shorter at 2.4 and 2 years, respectively. Older age and longer disease duration were found to be significant factors in transplant-related mortality and the FAB classification influenced the relapse rate, with those having fewer blast cells having decreased risk of relapse (Arnold et al 1998).

Autologous peripheral blood stem cell transplant has also been investigated as a treatment modality for MDS (Carella et al 1996, Demuynck et al 1996). Some difficulties were experienced in collecting adequate numbers of stem cells and only small numbers of patients were included in these studies. Further research is required but results indicate that this is a possible future treatment strategy for some patients with high-risk MDS.

 Case study 2.1

A 36-year-old lady, married with two children, presented to her GP with weight loss, petechial haemorrhage on the skin, lethargy and an eruption of dark purple spots on her abdomen and chest. The GP performed a blood test, the results of which showed mild anaemia, thrombocytopenia and a large percentage of monocytes in the peripheral blood film. She was diagnosed as suffering with CMML.

Upon referral to the consultant haematologist a bone marrow aspirate and trephine biopsy were performed and showed 15% blast cells. The patient also had a pyrexia of 39°C.

Blood results showed a haemoglobin level of 10.5×10^9/L, which was untreated, platelets of 90×10^9/L and a white cell count of 1.2×10^9/L.

The patient was treated with supportive care and antibiotic therapy and, because of her age, she was considered a candidate for bone marrow transplant. Her two sisters were human leukocyte antigen (HLA) typed to assess if either would be suitable to donate bone marrow. One of the sisters was found to be compatible, resulting in an allogeneic bone marrow transplant being successfully performed.

SPECIFIC NURSING ISSUES

Nursing an individual with MDS requires specialised knowledge and experience. A sound understanding of the disease, its manifestations, the side-effects and adverse reactions of the differing treatment modalities is required. This knowledge enables the nurse to fully assess an individual, minimise the possibility of side-effects occurring and detect and manage side-effects if they do occur. Education of the patient and their family and provision of emotional support are also important nursing roles.

Many of the side-effects and reactions encountered are discussed in subsequent chapters and therefore only a brief outline is provided here.

Anaemia

■ observe for fatigue and shortness of breath
■ monitor haemoglobin levels
■ educate the individual to reduce activity and therefore reduce oxygen requirements.

Encouraging individuals to prioritise the most important activities in their daily routines and to conserve their energy to enable them to undertake these tasks can help in reducing fatigue and maintaining their quality of life. (Care of the individual receiving blood component support is discussed in Ch. 12.)

Thrombocytopenia

Nursing management of thrombocytopenia is discussed in Chapter 14.

Reflection point

Reflect on the main factors which may affect an individual's quality of life and consider how you could help someone with MDS to maintain their quality of life.

Neutropenia

Prevention of infection is discussed in Chapter 13.

Education

The role of the nurse as an educator is of paramount importance. Facilitating the individual and their families to have a good understanding of the disease and its manifestations should help the individual to reduce hospital admissions and improve quality of life. The side-effects and adverse reactions resulting from the different treatment modalities are often acute in onset and very distressing. Patients should receive information about the potential side-effects associated with the particular treatment they are receiving. Education may help promote compliance with treatment and allow the individual to retain some 'control' over their treatment regimen. Education requirements are illustrated in Box 2.2.

Box 2.2 Education requirements for individuals with MDS

Purpose of red and white blood cells and platelets
Need for regular blood sampling to detect cytopenias

Anaemia
Explanation of symptoms such as fatigue and shortness of breath
Need for prioritising activities to conserve energy
Maintaining a balance between rest and activity
Procedure for administering red cell transfusion
Possible reactions to red cell transfusions

Thrombocytopenia
Procedure for administering a platelet transfusion
Possible reaction to platelet transfusions
Protection from injury/trauma
Recognising bleeding, e.g. petechiae/bruising
First aid measures to stem bleeding, e.g. nose bleed
Importance of reporting bleeding to a doctor immediately
Avoidance of intramuscular injections
Continued

Box 2.2 Continued

Neutropenia
Importance of minimising risk of infection
Ways of avoiding infection
Recognising infection
Temperature monitoring
Need for antimicrobial agents

Treatment modalities
Purpose of individual therapy/treatment schedule
Possible side-effects
How side-effects will be reduced
Leaflet/booklet to back up verbal information.

Treatment for MDS entails frequent hospital visits, and nurses have many opportunities to forge strong links with the individuals and their families, providing an ideal situation for teaching and emotional support.

CONCLUSION

There are many physiological and social problems associated with suffering from MDS, primarily due to the poor prognosis and few positive treatment alternatives. Therefore, all members of the multidisciplinary team have a role in the care of these individuals.

Together with the medical team the nurse will plan, implement and evaluate care, and the expert nurse has an important role in the management of individuals with MDS.

DISCUSSION QUESTIONS

1. What are the presenting features of myelodysplasia?
2. What are the informational and educational needs of the individual with MDS and their family?
3. Does high-dose chemotherapy have a role in the treatment of MDS?
4. MDS is mainly a disease of the elderly. Should aggressive treatment with high-dose chemotherapy be an option?

References

Ahmad Y H, Kiehl R, Papac R J 1995 Myelodysplasia, the clinical spectrum of 51 patients. Cancer 76: 869–874

Anderson J E, Anasetti C, Appelbaum F R et al 1996 Unrelated donor marrow transplantation for myelodysplasia (MDS) and MDS-related acute myeloid leukaemia. British Journal of Haematology 93(5): 9–67

Arnold R, de Witte T, van Biezen A et al 1998 for the Chronic Leukaemia Working Party of the European Blood and Marrow Transplantation Group 1998 Unrelated bone marrow transplantation in patients with myelodysplastic syndromes and secondary acute myeloid leukemia:

An EBMT survey. Bone Marrow Transplantation 21: 1213–1216

Belcher A 1993 Blood disorders, Mosby's Clinical Nursing Series. Mosby, St. Louis.

Bennett J M, Catovsky D, Daniel M T et al 1982 Proposals for the classification of the myelodysplastic syndromes. British Journal of Haematology 51: 189–199

Cain J, Hood-Barnes H, Spangler H 1991 Myelodysplastic syndromes: a review for nurses. Oncology Nursing Forum 18(1): 113–117

Carella A M, Dejana A, Lerma E et al 1996 In vivo mobilization of karyotypically

normal peripheral blood progenitor cells in high-risk MDS secondary or therapy-related acute myelogenous leukaemia. British Journal of Haematology 95: 127–130

Casadevall N 1998 Update on the role of epoetin alfa in hematologic malignancies and myelodysplastic syndromes. Seminars in Oncology 25(3) Suppl. 7: 12–18

Cheson B D 1990 The myelodysplastic syndromes: current approaches to therapy. Annual International Medicine 122: 939

Cheson B D 1998 Standard and low dose chemotherapy for the treatment of myelodysplastic syndromes. Leukaemia Research 22, Suppl 1: S17–S21

Demuynck H, Delforge M, Verhoef G E G et al 1996 Feasibility of peripheral blood progenitor cell harvest and transplantation in patients with poor-risk myelodysplastic syndromes. British Journal of Haematology 92: 351–359

De Witte T, Zwann F, Hermans H et al 1990 Allogeneic bone marrow transplantation for secondary leukaemia and myelodysplastic syndrome: a survey by the Leukaemia Working Party of the European Bone Marrow Transplant Group. British Journal of Haematology 74(2): 151–155

Fenaux P, Morel P, Rose C et al 1991 Prognostic factors in adult de novo myelodysplastic syndromes treated by intensive chemotherapy. British Journal of Haematology 77: 497–501

Fenaux P, Preudhomme C, Hebba M 1992 The role of chemotherapy in myelodysplastic syndromes. Leukaemia 8: 43–49

Forman S 1996 Myelodysplastic syndrome. Current Opinion in Haematology 3: 297–302

Ganser A, Karthaus M 1997 Clinical use of hematopoietic growth factors in the myelodysplastic syndromes. Leukemia and Lymphoma 26, Suppl. 1: 13–27

Gerhartz H H, Zwierzina H, Walther J et al 1996 Interleukin-3 plus low-dose cytosine arabinoside for advanced myelodysplasia: A pilot study. Cancer Investigation 14(4): 299–306

Giles F J, Koeffler H P 1994 Secondary myelodysplastic syndromes and leukaemia. Current Opinion in Haematology 1: 256–260

Greenberg P, Cox C, LeBeau M et al 1997 International scoring system for evaluating prognosis in myelodysplastic syndromes. Blood 89(6): 2079–2088

Hansen P B, Penkowa M, Johnsen H E 1998 Hematopoietic growth factors for the treatment of myelodysplastic syndromes. Leukemia and Lymphoma 28(5–6): 491–500

Hoffbrand A V, Pettit J E 1993 Essential haematology, 3rd edn. Blackwell Science, Oxford

Hughes-Jones N C, Wickramasinghe E 1996 Lecture notes on haematology, 6th edn. Blackwell Science, London

Jacobs P 1997 The myelodysplastic syndromes. Disease a Month 43(8): 532–546

Jensen P D, Jensen I M, Ellegard J 1992 Desferrioxamine treatment reduces blood transfusion requirements in patients with myelodysplastic syndrome. British Journal of Haematology 80(1): 121–124

Negrin R S, Stein R, Doherty K et al 1996 Maintenance treatment of the anemia of myelodysplastic syndromes with recombinant human granulocyte colony-stimulating factor and erythropoietin: evidence for in vivo synergy. Blood 87: 4076–4081

Oscier D G 1997 ABC of haematology, the myelodysplastic syndromes. British Journal of Medicine 314: 883–886

Prodan M, Tulissi P, Perticarari G, Franzin F, Pussini E, Pozzato G 1995 Flow cytometry assay for the evaluation of phagocytosis and oxidative burst of polymorphonuclear leukocytes and monocytes in myelodysplastic disorders. Haematologica 80(3): 212–218

Runde V, de Witte T, Arnold R et al on behalf of the Chronic Leukaemia Working Party of the European Blood and Marrow Transplantation (EBMT) Group 1998 Bone marrow transplantation from HLA-identical siblings as first line treatment in patients with myelodysplastic syndromes: early transplantation is associated with improved outcomes. Bone Marrow Transplantation 21: 255–261

Thompson M K, Lee D, Kidd P et al 1989 Subcutaneous granulocyte–macrophage colony-stimulating factor in patients with myelodysplastic syndrome – toxicity, pharmacokinetics and haematological effects. Journal of Clinical Oncology 7(5): 629–637

Utley S 1996 Myelodysplastic syndromes. Seminars in Oncology Nursing 12(1): 51–58

Verhoef G E G, Pittaluga S, de Wolf-Peeters Boogaerts M A 1995 FAB classification of myelodysplastic syndromes: merits and controversies. Annals of Haematology 71: 3–11

Whittaker J A, Judge M 1990 Myelodysplastic syndromes. In: Ludlam C A (ed) Clinical haematology. Churchill Livingstone, Edinburgh, 247–253

Further reading

Thomas M L 1998 Quality of life and psychosocial adjustment in patients with myelodysplastic syndromes. Leukaemia **Research 1001: S41–S47** This interesting article, which examines quality-of-life issues in myelodysplasia, includes good sections on the elderly, fatigue, uncertainty and lack of understanding.

3 Aplastic anaemia

EVELYN DANNIE

Key points
- Aplastic anaemia is a frequently fatal disease
- Aplastic anaemia may be inherited or acquired
- Treatment options include supportive care, bone marrow transplant and immunosuppressive therapy

INTRODUCTION

Aplastic anaemia (AA) was first described by Paul Ehrlich in 1888 in a pregnant young woman who died following a short illness consisting of severe anaemia, bleeding and a high fever. At postmortem, nucleated red cells were absent from the bone marrow, having been replaced by fat cells (Plates 1 and 2).

Today AA is still frequently fatal and although certain subsets of AA are curable it remains a disease of poor prognosis. Aplastic anaemia can be divided into two main groups: 'inherited' and 'acquired'. The pathophysiology and treatment options for both groups of the disease will be reviewed within this chapter. Patient education strategies and specific nursing issues will also be addressed.

THE DISEASE

Definition of aplastic anaemia

Aplastic anaemia is characterised by pancytopenia (reduced red cells, white cells and platelets) associated with a 'hypocellular' bone marrow in which haemopoietic cells are replaced by fat cells. The prognosis of the disease is directly related to the severity of bone marrow depression (Gordon-Smith 1989). Severe aplastic anaemia (SAA) is defined by the Camitta criteria with two out of three of the following criteria being present:

- neutrophils $< 0.5 \times 10^9$/L
- platelets $< 20 \times 10^9$/L
- reticulocytes $< 40 \times 10^9$/L ($< 1\%$).

In SAA the marrow shows severe hypocellularity, with $< 25\%$ of the marrow being normal or populated by cells (Lewis 1965, Camitta et al 1975).

Epidemiology

The incidence of aplastic anaemia in developed countries is probably in the order of 3–6 per million of the population per year (Szklo et al 1985). These data are only estimates and there is substantial geographic variation in incidence with up to 30 cases per million in some parts of Asia. In the Far East the incidence appears to be higher than in the West. This may be due in part to the high incidence of hepatitis, the widespread use of chloramphenicol as an effective and cheap antibiotic, and the extensive use and exposure to insecticides (Young & Issaragrasil 1986).

There is a male predominance in aplastic anaemia, with two peaks in age distribution between the ages of 10 and 25 and over 60 years. However, the incidence in old age can be confused with the myelodysplastic syndromes and the small peak in childhood is due to the inclusion of inherited cases such as Fanconi's anaemia (FA).

The majority of patients belong to the acquired category of aplastic anaemia. Occasionally in acquired aplastic anaemia it is possible to identify a factor which may have

Table 3.1 Classification of the aplastic anaemias

Inherited	Acquired		
	Idiopathic	Secondary to other diseases	Inevitable
Fanconi's anaemia	Drug induced	Systemic lupus erythematosus (SLE)	Ionising radiation
Dyskeratosis congenita	Viral	Acute lymphoblastic leukaemia	Cytotoxic drugs
Others	Toxins		

acted as a trigger to initiation of the disease. However, in the majority of cases (approx 70%) there is no obvious aetiological factor and the disease is referred to as idiopathic (Table 3.1).

Acquired aplastic anaemia

Pathophysiology

The pathophysiology of acquired aplastic anaemia is poorly understood. Sufficient evidence exists to suggest abnormalities in the haematopoietic stem cell, although precise aetiology remains unknown. Immunological abnormalities in AA combined with the response of the majority of cases to immunotherapy suggests that abnormalities in immune function must play a role in its pathophysiology. These abnormalities include cytotoxic T-lymphocyte activation and increased interferon-γ expression. However, it is likely that the primary triggers of these abnormalities are diverse and may include drugs, chemicals and viruses which may act as non-specific trigger factors although in the majority of cases the primary aetiology is unclear (Knospe & Crosby 1971, Kurtzman & Young 1989, Nissen-Druey 1989, Dokal 1996b).

Triggers of acquired aplastic anaemia

Drugs and chemicals

A wide variety of drugs have been implicated as causative agents in aplastic anaemia (Heimpel & Heit 1980). In most instances the risk of developing aplastic anaemia is small (International Agranulocytosis and Aplastic Anaemia Study 1986). Chloramphenicol is perhaps the best documented and most notorious of all drugs with

the potential to cause aplastic anaemia. It produces what is termed an idiosyncratic response with aplastic anaemia occurring weeks or months after discontinuation of the drug. Chloramphenicol contains a nitrobenzene ring and is similar to amidopyrine, a drug known to cause agranulocytosis. Toxicity is dose-related and has been ascribed to mitochondrial damage inhibiting the growth of both granulocyte, macrophage colony-forming units (GM-CFU) and erythrocyte colony-forming units (E-CFU) (see Ch. 1) (Yunis et al 1980, Alter & Young 1993). It has also been shown to induce an autoimmune reaction (Nagro & Maver 1969). A variety of other drugs have the potential to cause aplastic anaemia and are detailed in Box 3.1.

Box 3.1 Trigger factors associated with aplastic anaemia

Drugs
Antibiotics (e.g. chloramphenicol)
Anti-inflammatory (e.g. phenylbutazone indomethacin, gold)
Antithyroid (e.g. carbimazole)
Antimalarial (e.g. amodiaquine)
Anticonvulsant (e.g. phenytoin)

Infective agents
Viruses (e.g. hepatitis A, B and C)
Bacterial (e.g. mycobacteria)

Toxins
Commercial solvents
Insecticides

Systemic disease
Systemic lupus erythematosus

Idiosyncratic aplastic anaemia has also been associated with a number of chemicals (Jick 1977). In particular, the effects of benzene, commonly found in organic solvents, coal tar derivatives and petroleum products are well studied. Long-term exposure to benzene leads to decreased blood cell progenitors and DNA damage. Other chemicals associated with aplastic anaemia include insecticides and pesticides, toluene and acetanilide. These substances have been shown to inhibit haematopoietic colony formation (Gallicchio et al 1987). Marrow aplasia may also result following exposure to radiation. Bone marrow cells are affected by high-energy rays, with the greatest damage being to the actively dividing pool of blood cell precursor and progenitor cells (Kirshbaum & Matsuo 1971, Gale 1987).

Viruses and infection

Some viruses are well-documented trigger factors, with aplastic anaemia often occurring during or early after viral hepatitis (both A and B and non A and B) or exposure to other viruses such as Epstein–Barr, B19 Parvovirus and retroviruses such as the human immunodeficiency virus (HIV). No single pathological phenomenon explains aplastic anaemia.

Bacterial and fungal infections depress bone marrow function (Alter & Young 1993). These infections are often treated by antibiotics and it is often unclear whether an ensuing AA is caused by the infection, the drug or a combination of both, or whether the infection is a result of the illness and not the cause of the AA.

Only a minority of infected patients develop bone marrow failure, and infection appears to act as a trigger rather than the cause of AA. It is conceivable that an immune imbalance of any origin can act as a trigger to AA (Kutzman & Young 1989). Viral infections and drugs can act synergistically, increasing their potential as risk factors, and the incidence of AA rises sharply after exposure to a virus such as hepatitis and a drug such as chloramphenicol (Hagler et al 1975).

Clinical features

Clinical manifestations are related to the severity of the disease. Reduction of platelets leads to bruising and bleeding from mucous membranes. Neutropenia and red cell depletion tend to occur later in the disease trajectory, resulting in susceptibility to infection and anaemia. The bone marrow shows hypoplasia with loss of haematopoietic tissue and marked decreases in all cell lines (Gordon-Smith 1989, Hoffbrand & Pettit 1993).

Reflection point

Fatigue is a common experience for patients with SAA. There are a number of reasons for this but a low haemoglobin level is a major contributing factor. The sheer frustration of not being able to pursue a normal lifestyle can cause individuals added anxiety.

Identify strategies which could be developed through participative nurse/patient relationships to help individuals minimise the effects of fatigue on their life.

TREATMENT

The main aim of treatment is to improve blood counts to prevent dependency on transfusions of blood and blood products and reduce the risk from opportunist infections and haemorrhage (Gordon-Smith 1989). The pathophysiology of the disease suggests two approaches to treatment: (a) replacement of the deficient stem cells by bone marrow transplantation (BMT), or (b) immunosuppressive therapy to stop the immunological process (Young & Barrett 1995).

In both cases a relatively long period of intensive supportive treatment is necessary until the choice of specific therapy is made and during treatment until self-supporting peripheral blood counts are obtained. Figure 3.1 outlines treatment options.

Supportive care

Blood and blood components

The major supportive measures are the provision of blood components and both prophylactic

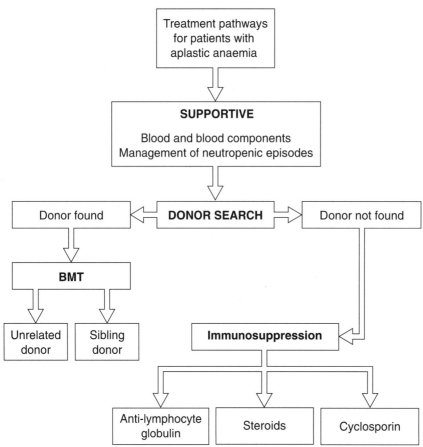

Figure 3.1 Treatment options for patients with severe aplastic anaemia and inherited aplastic anaemia

and therapeutic antibiotic therapy. One of the first treatment decisions is eligibility for BMT. Blood components must be used sparingly if the individual is eligible for BMT and blood components from family members must be avoided to minimise sensitisation (see Ch. 11). Blood component support consists mainly of packed red cells and platelet transfusions and is based on clinical need. In non-bleeding patients 3–4 units of red cells are transfused every 3–4 weeks. In SAA, prophylactic platelet transfusions should be given to reduce the risk of fatal haemorrhage (Gordon-Smith & Lewis 1990).

Infection

Patients with AA are at risk from infections, which progress rapidly in the presence of neutropenia, and protective measures are designed

to avoid acquired bacterial or fungal infections (see Ch. 13).

Bone marrow transplantation

Irrespective of the underlying pathophysiology, BMT has become the treatment of choice for the young person with SAA when an identical human lymphocyte antigen (HLA) donor is available (Storb et al 1974, Dokal 1996b). BMT is fully discussed in Chapter 10, but a brief discussion is included here in relation to the management of AA.

BMT has been shown to have a clear survival advantage over no treatment or other treatment options (Camitta et al 1982). Long-term survival is projected at 60–70% for most patients and above 80% in certain groups (Sullivan & Witherspoon 1988). Improved survival has been attributed to many factors, including intensified conditioning regimens to prevent graft rejection, the use of cyclosporin to prevent graft rejection and graft versus host disease (GVHD), better blood product preparation to reduce allosensitisation and prompt use of antimicrobials. However, graft rejection, GVHD and infection remain the limiting factors to the success of BMT (Young & Barrett 1995).

The indication for BMT is considered in two parts: first, relating to the disease; and, secondly, to the transplant itself. In the first instance, concerns may arise as to whether the disease can be treated successfully with alternative therapy, and in the second considerations relate to the recipient's age, general health and the availability of a suitable donor.

The main conditioning regimen used includes cyclophosphamide 200 mg/kg with cyclosporin and methotrexate for GVHD prophylaxis. Conditioning regimens including cyclophosphamide and antithymocyte globulin (ATG) appear to have a higher survival rate for sibling donors, 90% at 3 years, compared with regimens employing irradiation programmes, 60–70% at 3 years (Paquetto et al 1995).

A recent analysis of 993 evaluable BMT patients (Hows et al 1996) showed that actual survival after sibling BMT was 65% at 10 years compared with only 20% transplanted from partially mismatched family donors and HLA-matched unrelated donors.

Immunosuppressive therapy

Antilymphocyte globulin and antithymocyte globulin

The use of antilymphocyte globulin (ALG) and ATG as immunosuppressive therapy has become an accepted form of treatment in AA (Bacigalupo 1989). ALG and ATG are the sera produced by the immunisation of horses or rabbits with human thymocytes (ATG) or thoracic duct lymphocytes (ALG). They are lymphotoxic reagents with activity against all blood and marrow cells, including progenitors, and are used to decrease rejection of transplanted HLA-matched bone marrow.

The mechanism of action of ALG is almost certainly immunosuppressive: it is cytolytic of

T cells and inhibits T-cell function. ALG rapidly reduces circulating lymphocytes, usually to less than 10% of starting values, and when total blood counts return to pre-treatment values months later, activated lymphocyte numbers in recovered patients remain decreased (Lopez-Karpovitch et al 1989).

A review of the results in the 1980s suggested that about 45% of patients with SAA responded to ALG (Young & Speck 1984). Early protocols used 10–28 daily intravenous infusions but a short course of 40 mg/kg/day for 4 days is effective and less toxic, especially for induction of serum sickness (Bielory et al 1988). ALG has not proved very useful in children with AA or in patients with severe neutropenia (Locasciulli et al 1990). Immediate allergic reactions are rare but a test dose is recommended. Serum sickness due to immune complex deposition is seen in all patients. This is manifested in a number of distressing symptoms, which can be treated effectively with corticosteroids.

Manifestation of serum sickness following ALG and ATG

- fever
- rash
- joint pains
- arthralgia
- myalgia
- lassitude
- renal toxicity.

Response to ALG and ATG is usually seen within 3–6 months after treatment. If no response is observed after 6 months, a second dose from a different source may be given. Approximately 50–60% of patients will respond to ALG. The marrow does not return entirely to normal and some degree of cytopenia may persist for several years without requiring support. Relapse occurs in 10–15% of responders. There is no criteria for determining response to ALG and it is recommended as a first-line treatment for candidates ineligible for BMT (Marsh & Gordon-Smith 1988, Gordon-Smith & Lewis 1990, Alter & Young 1993).

Case study 3.1

In February 1984, Kathleen, aged 23, was found to be anaemic when volunteering to donate blood. Her GP prescribed iron supplements. She noticed her motions were black, she bruised easily, suffered nose bleeds and was always tired. In July she presented with symptoms of anaemia and being generally unwell.

On examination, Kathleen was pale, with clinical symptoms of anaemia, no lymphadeno-pathy or hepato-splenomegaly. Her blood count was as follows: Hb 4.6 g/L, WCC 2×10^9/L, platelets 13×10^9/L. All other indices were within normal limits. A bone marrow examination showed hypoplasia with markedly decreased erythropoiesis. She was supported with blood, platelets and antimicrobials. Her siblings were HLA typed and her older sister was a perfect match. As Kathleen was well, immunosuppressive therapy using ALG was proposed. She received two courses (November 1984 and February 1985) and responded well, maintaining her blood counts with no support. She remained reasonably well until July 1991, when her blood counts began a downward trend with marrow hypocellularity. The decision to treat her by allogeneic BMT was made and this was planned for November 1991.

Her conditioning regimen was cyclophosphamide and total body irradiation, and GVHD prophylaxis consisted of cyclosporin and methotrexate. She received healthy marrow from her sister following her conditioning and made a fairly uneventful recovery with minimal GVHD. Kathleen has recovered well and continues to be followed up at yearly intervals with minimal problems. Her current medications are Prempack C, penicillin and thyroxine.

Corticosteroids

Very high doses of corticosteroids have been used as an alternative to ALG. They are administered intravenously, with a starting dose of 20 mg/kg/day for 3 days, gradually reducing over the next month. The response rate of corticosteroids has been reported to be similar to ALG, and combination therapy using prednisolone and cyclosporin have produced responses in patients. However, toxicity is high. Commonly observed toxicities include hypertension, hyperglycaemia, fluid retention and aseptic necrosis of the femur or humerus. The period of hospitalisation for patients receiving corticosteroids is often longer, due to masking of fevers and increased episodes of fungal infections (Bitencourt et al 1995, Young & Barrett 1995, Dokal 1996b).

Cyclosporin

Cyclosporin is an effective immunosuppressive agent used both as a first-line treatment of AA and as GVHD prophylaxis in BMT. It is a specific T-cell inhibitor that prevents the production of interleukin-2 and interferon while continuing to allow production of colony-stimulating factors (Kahan 1989). Initial reports of its use in the treatment of AA have suggested a 50% response rate in individuals refractory to ALG (Hinterberger-Fischer et al 1989). The recommended oral dose is 12 mg/kg/day in adults and 15 mg/kg/day in children, in order to maintain adequate blood levels (Alter & Young 1993). These regimens require regular monitoring of blood levels. Toxicities are not insignificant, and are mostly dose-related (Young & Barrett 1995).

Commonly reported side-effects associated with cyclosporin

- hypertension
- seizures
- hirsutism
- immunodeficiency
- raised creatinine levels
- *Pneumocystis carinii* pneumonia.

Recently, combination therapy consisting of ALG, ATG and cyclosporin has been shown to produce useful haematological response in 75% of cases (Rosenfeld et al 1995). This response is enhanced if G-CSF is added to the above combination, with 82% of patients showing haematological reconstitution of the three main blood cell lines. This appears to be an alternative treatment for patients with SAA who lack an HLA identical donor (Bacigalupo et al 1995).

INHERITED OR FAMILIAL APLASTIC ANAEMIA

A number of inherited disorders are associated with aplastic anaemia. Among these, Fanconi's anaemia (FA) and Dyskeratosis congenita (DC) are the most common (Young & Alter 1994, Dokal 1996a,b).

Fanconi's anaemia

Fanconi's anaemia was first described in 1927 in a family in which three brothers developed aplastic anaemia. The brothers also had microencephaly, abnormal skin pigmentation, internal strabismus and genital hypoplasia. Further families and cases were described and it was later suggested that the condition be named Fanconi's anaemia. Since 1982 more than 700 cases have been reported, in varying detail, to the International Fanconi Anaemia Registry (IFAR) at the Rockefeller Institute in the USA with males more commonly affected than females (ratio 2:1) (Auerbach et al 1989, Auerbach & Allen, 1991).

Pathophysiology

Fanconi's anaemia is inherited as a recessive trait (e.g. resulting from the marrying of first cousins) and is often associated with other congenital abnormalities. Cells from patients with FA characteristically show a high frequency of chromosomal breakage. These increased chromosomal abnormalities have been taken to indicate a defect in DNA repair and to underline the increased malignancies seen in these patients (Gordon-Smith & Rutherford 1989, Dokal 1996b).

The underlying defect in FA is unknown and the relationship between birth defects, haematopoietic failure, chromosomal breakages and malignancy is elusive. The variability in expression of the disease makes firm diagnosis of FA on clinical grounds almost impossible and cytogenetic analysis is necessary to confirm diagnosis. The haematopoietic defect in FA is evident at the progenitor cell level: colonies derived from bone marrow GM-CFU, E-CFU, E-BFU as well as blood E-BFU are all decreased in FA patients with AA (Alter & Young 1993).

Clinical features

The typical clinical features of FA are characteristic but are not expressed in all patients. Children are usually of low birth weight at term and do not grow normally. Microcephaly, microphthalmia, broad nasal base and a small mouth and jaw give a classical appearance. The skin shows a general hyperpigmentation with increased patches of pigment (café-au-lait patches) and other areas of depigmentation. Internal strabismus is common. Males often have undescended testes and horse shoe or pelvic kidney are common. Skeletal abnormalities with hypoplastic veins may be present. (Gordon-Smith & Rutherford 1989, Gordon-Smith & Lewis 1990).

The blood count is usually normal at birth and common features such as anaemia, bruising or nose bleeds associated with bone marrow failure do not present until age 5–10 years. A low platelet count is usually the most common presenting haematological finding; anaemia then becomes apparent, granulocytes being the last affected cell line. In typical cases the bone marrow becomes hypoplastic with replacement of haematopoietic tissue by fat cells. There is progressive bone marrow failure, probably due to chromosomal instability, leading to progressive depletion of stem cells. Reduction in CFU-GM and BFU-E is evident prior to the occurrence of pancytopenia and there is a high incidence of acute leukaemic transformation in these children (Gordon-Smith & Lewis 1990, Alter & Young 1993, Young & Alter 1994). Presentation is usually in the first decade of life and patients die young from complications of bone marrow failure or leukaemia (Smith et al 1989, Dokal 1996b).

Treatment of Fanconi's anaemia

The treatment of FA remains the same as for acquired aplastic anaemia (see Fig 3.1). Specific treatment usually consists of blood and blood product support; anabolic steroids, which are known to cause a number of side-effects (Young and Barrett 1994); and BMT, which is now a well-established treatment for inherited AA and offers the only possibility of a cure (Gluckman et al 1995, Davis et al 1996). Treatment options in familial AA are shown in Figure 3.2.

Dyskeratosis congenita

Dyskeratosis congenita is a rare inherited disorder characterised by reticulate skin pigmentation, mucosal leucoplakia and nail dystrophy. Aplasia occurs in 50% of cases. The disease presents usually within the first 10 years of life, and has a predisposition to malignancy (Drachtman & Alter 1992). Most patients die from complications of aplastic anaemia, pulmonary disease and malignancy (Sirinavin & Trowbridge 1975, Alter & Young 1993, Dokal 1996a). In the majority of families the pattern of inheritance is compatible to an X-linked recessive trait and approximately 85% out of 200 published cases are male. DC shares many features with FA: for example, bone marrow failure, a predisposition to malignancy and

chromosomal instability. In DC the precise pathophysiology of the bone marrow remains unclear but it is possible that the chromosomal instability leads to progressive depletion of the stem cell pool, which manifests as pancytopenia towards the first decade of life or mid-teens (March et al 1992, Dokal 1996a).

Clinical features

In DC, cutaneous features are the most common clinical feature. The reticulated skin pigmentation involves the face, neck, shoulders and trunk. Nail dystrophy (Plate 3) involves both hands and feet, and nail plates are small with longitudinal ridging. Leucoplakia involves the oral mucosa, but is also seen in the conjunctiva, anal, urethral and genital mucosa (Alter & Young 1993, Dokal 1996a). Characteristically, a number of other important features are also observed: these are shown in Box 3.2 (Chambers & Salinas 1982, Kelly & Stelling 1982, Brown et al 1993).

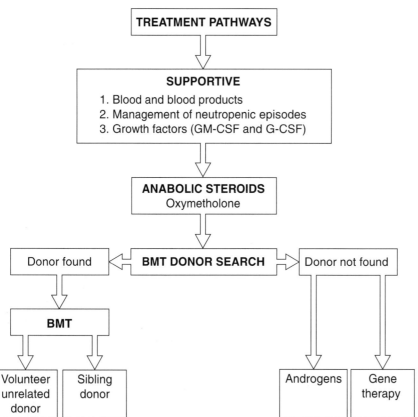

Figure 3.2 Treatment options in familial aplastic anaemia (Fanconi's anaemia and Dyskeratosis congenita)

Box 3.2   Abnormalities seen in Dyskeratosis congenita (adapted from Drachtman & Alter 1995)

Part of body affected	Abnormality
Skin	Pigmentation of face, neck, shoulders and trunk
Nails	Dystrophy involving hands and feet
Eyes	Conjunctivitis, blepharitis, glaucoma, cataracts, strabismus, loss of eyelashes, optic nerve dystrophy
Teeth	Dental decay, early loss of teeth
Tongue	Leucoplakia
Hair	Early hair loss
Skeleton	Osteoporosis, fractures, aseptic necrosis, scoliosis and mandibular hypoplasia, short stature
Genitourinary tract	Hypoplastic testes, phimosis, urethral stenosis, and horseshoe kidney
Gastrointestinal tract	Oesophageal strictures, hepatomegaly, cirrhosis of liver

---

Clinical manifestations often occur during childhood; skin and nail changes usually appear by the age of 10 years, mucosal leucoplakia later, and by mid-teens serious progressive bone marrow failure is seen in 50% of affected individuals and 10% develop a malignancy. Seventy per cent of deaths are related to bone marrow failure and 30% are due to bleeding or opportunist infections such as cytomegalovirus. Mean age at death is approximately 30 years (Forni et al 1993, Dokal 1996a).

TREATMENT FOR DC

Treatment for patients with DC is similar to that in FA and is currently unsatisfactory. For those presenting with bone marrow failure, anabolic steroids and growth factors (GM-CSF, G-CSF) may provide transient improvement in marrow function (Oehler et al 1994). BMT has been used successfully in only a few children with DC. Unfortunately, there is a high incidence of early and late fatality, mainly due to interstitial pulmonary complications (Dokal 1996a). Therefore, even with an identical HLA-matched

sibling donor, the results are poor; thus, there is a great need to develop alternative treatment strategies such as gene therapy. DC patients may be good candidates for gene therapy, as it is a single-gene disorder and the main cause of mortality relates to bone marrow failure with no satisfactory treatment (Dokal 1996b).

SPECIFIC NURSING ISSUES

Nursing management of patients with AA requires expert skills and knowledge. The nurse plays an active role by providing appropriate therapeutic and supportive care. Treatment is usually delivered in specialist centres and nurses must be well versed in potential and expected complications such as life-threatening infections and haemorrhage (British Committee for Standards in Haematology 1995).

While the development of day care units and high-quality outpatient services enables supportive treatment to be administered, hospitalisation becomes necessary in neutropenic episodes, when ALG is initiated and for BMT.

Information, education and support of the patient and family are important aspects of care (Walker et al 1994, Whedon & Wujcik 1997): they should be ongoing from diagnosis and be encompassed in the care plan. Equally important is nurse education, with emphasis on research-based practice, to deliver quality care to this group of patients.

Reflection point

Nursing challenges in this field are numerous and offer a wide range of issues for nursing research. Consider the importance of research-based practice. What areas would you like to see further researched? Consider how you and your colleagues could undertake a research project.

CONCLUSION

In spite of improved means of support and treatment and advances in nursing care, aplastic anaemia remains a devastating and frustrating disease from which a proportion of patients still die. For patients with SAA, BMT from a sibling donor is the treatment of choice. For patients lacking donors, treatment is still unsatisfactory. Despite years of research the primary pathology remains unclear, highlighting the need for new research strategies. However, as acquired AA and FA have several features in common, new research findings may indicate gene therapy as a viable treatment option for AA, and further studies may lead to a better understanding of the pathophysiology of acquired AA and the possibility of new treatment options.

DISCUSSION QUESTIONS

1. How would you explain the main criticisms, difficulties and limitations of the differing treatment approaches to a more junior nurse?
2. Assess critically your current patient education programme. Are there any improvements which could be made to this programme?
3. What physical, emotional and psychosocial problems may the individual with aplastic anaemia and their significant others experience?
4. What support services available both within and outwith your own organisation could be employed to minimise distress and enhance individuals' coping mechanisms?

References

Alter B P, Young N S 1993 The bone marrow failure syndromes. In: Nathan D G, Oski F A (eds) Bone marrow failures in infancy and childhood. W B Saunders, Philadelphia, pp 216–316

Auerbach A D, Allen R G 1991 Leukaemia and preleukaemia in Fanconi anaemia patients: a review of the literature and report of the International Fanconi Registry. Cancer Genet Cytogenet 51: 1–12

Auerbach A D, Rogatko A, Schroeder-Kurth T M 1989 International Fanconi Register First Report. In: Schroeder-Kurth T M, Auerbach A D, Obe G (eds)

Fanconi's anaemia clinical, cytogenetic and experimental aspects. Springer-Verlag, Heildelberg

Bacigalupo A 1989 Treatment of severe aplastic anaemia. Baillière's Clinical Haematology, 2(1): 19–35 Baillière Tindall, London

Bacigalupo A, Brocoiag Acress W, Caroluneto M et al 1995 Antilymphocyte globulin, cyclosporin granulocyte colony stimulating factor in patients with acquired aplastic anaemia. A pilot study of the EBMT SAA Working Party. Blood 85: 1348–1353

Bielory L, Gascon P, Lawlet T, Nienhuis A W, Young N S, Frank M 1988 Human serum sickness. A prospective clinical analysis of 35 patients treated with equine antithymocyte globulin for bone marrow failure. Medicine 67: 40–57

Bitencourt M A, Medeiroe C R, Zanis-Neto J et al 1995 Prednisolone and cyclosporin for severe acquired aplastic anaemia. 101 cases treated in a single institution. Blood 86, Suppl. 1: 476a (abstr).

British Committee for Standards In Haematology Clinical Haematology Task Force 1995 Guidelines on the provision of facilities for care of adult patients with haematological malignancies (including leukaemia and lymphoma and severe bone marrow failure). Clinical Laboratory Haematology 17(1): 3–10

Brown K E, Kelly T E, Myers B M (1993) Gastro-intestinal involvement in a woman with dyskeratosis congenita. Digestive Diseases and Sciences 38: 181–184

Camitta B M, Rapeport J M, Parkman R, Nathan D G 1975 Selection of patients for bone marrow transplantation in severe aplastic anaemia. Blood 45: 355–363

Camitta B M, Storb R, Thomas E D 1982 Aplastic anaemia: pathogenesis, diagnosis, treatment and progress. New England Journal of Medicine 306: 645–652

Chambers J K, Salinas C F (1982) Ocular findings in dyskeratosis congenita. Birth Defects 18: 167–174

Davis S M, Khan S, Wagner J E et al 1996 Unrelated bone marrow transplantation for Fanconi's anaemia. Bone Marrow Transplantation 17: 43–47

Dokal I 1996a Dyskeratosis congenita: an inherited bone marrow failure syndrome. British Journal of Haematology 92: 775–779

Dokal I 1996b Severe aplastic anaemia including Fanconi's anaemia and Dyskeratosis congenita. Current Opinion in Haematology 3: 453–460

`Drachtman R A, Alter B P 1992 Dyskeratosis congenita clinical and genetic heterogeneity. American Journal of Paediatric Haematology/Oncology 14: 297–304

Drachtman R A, Alter B P 1995 Dyskeratosis congenita. Dermatol Clin 13: 33–39

Ehrlich P I 1888 In: Nathan D G, Oski F A (eds) 1993 Bone marrow failures in infancy and childhood. W B Saunders, Philadelphia

Forni G L, Melevendi C, Jappelli S, Rasore-Quadino A 1993 Dyskeratosis congenita unusual presenting features within a kindred. Paediatric Haematology and Oncology 10: 145–149

Gale R P 1987 The role of bone marrow transplantation following nuclear accidents. Bone Marrow Transplantation 2: 1–6

Gallicchio V S, Casale G P, Watts T 1987 T inhibition of human bone marrow-derived stem cell colony formation (CFU-E, BFU-E and CFU-GM) following in vitro exposure to organophosphates. Experimental Haematology 15: 1099–2007

Gordon-Smith EC 1989 Aplastic anaemia aetiology and clinical features. Baillière's Clinical Haematology, 2(1), Chapter 1. Baillière Tindall, London

Gordon-Smith E C, Lewis S M 1990 Aplastic anaemia and other types of bone marrow failure. In: Hoffbrand V V, Lewis S M (eds) Post-graduate haematology. Heinemann Medical Books, London, Chapter 4, pp 83–120

Gordon-Smith E G, Rutherford T R 1989 Fanconi's anaemia constitutional familial aplastic anaemia. Baillière's Clinical Haematology, 2(1), Chapter 8, Baillière Tindall, London

Gluckman E, Auerbach A D, Horwitz M M et al 1995 Bone marrow transplantation for Fanconi's anaemia. Blood 96: 2856–2862

Hagler L, Pastore B, Bergin J J, Wresch M R 1975 Aplastic anaemia

following viral hepatitis. Reports of two fatal cases and literature review. Medicine Baltimore 54: 139–163

Heimpel H, Heit W 1980 Drug-induced aplastic anaemia clinical aspects. Clinics in Haematology 9: 641–662

Hinterberger-Fischer F M, Hocker P, Lechner K, Seewann H, Hinterberger W 1989 Oral cyclosporin A is effective treatment for untreated and also for previous immunosuppressed patients with severe bone marrow failure. European Journal of Haematology 43: 136–142

Hoffbrand V V, Pettit J E 1993 Essential haematology, 3rd edn. Blackwell Scientific Publications, Oxford

Hows J, Bacigalupo A, Downis T, Brand R 1996 Alternative donor (ALT/BMT) for SAA in Europe. Blood 86, Suppl. 1: 290A

International Agranulocytosis And Aplastic Anaemia Study 1986 Risks of aplastic anaemia. A first report of their relation to drug use with special reference to analgesics. Journal of the American Medical Association 256: 1749–1759

Jick H 1977 The discovery of drug-induced illness. New England Journal of Medicine 296: 481–485

Kahan B D 1989 Cyclosporin. New England Journal of Medicine 321: 1725–1738

Kelly T E, Stelling CB (1982) Dyskeratosis congenita: radiological features. Paediatric Radiology 12: 31–36

Kirshbaum J D, Matsuo T, Sato K, Ichimura M, Tsuchimoto T, Ishimura T 1971 A study of aplastic anaemia. In: An autopsy series with special reference to atomic bomb survivors in Hiroshima and Nagasaki. Blood 38(1): 17–26

Knospe Y M, Crosby Y M 1971 A disorder of the bone marrow sinusoidal microcirculation rather than stem cell failure. Lancet 1: 20–25

Kurtzman G, Young N 1989 Viruses and bone marrow failure. Baillère's Clinical Haematology 2(1), Chapter 4, pp 51–67. Baillière Tindall, London

Lewis S M 1965 Course and prognosis in aplastic anaemia. British Medical Journal 1: 1027–1030

Locasciulli A, Vant Veer L, Bacigalupo A et al 1990 Treatment with marrow transplantation or immunosuppression of childhood acquired aplastic anaemia. A report from the EBMT SAA Working Party. Bone Marrow Transplant 6: 211–217

Lopez-Karpovitch X, Zarzosa M E, Cardenas M R, Piedras J 1989 Changes in peripheral blood mononuclear cell subpopulations during antithymocyte globulin therapy in aplastic anaemia. Acta Haematol 81: 176–180

March C W, Will A J, Hows J H et al 1992 Stem cell origin of the haematopoietic defect in dyskeratosis congenita. Blood 79: 3138–3144

Marsh J C, Gordon-Smith E C 1988 The role of antilymphocyte globulin in the treatment of chronic acquired bone marrow failure. Blood Reviews 2(4): 141–148

Nagro T, Maver A M 1969 Concordance for drug-induced aplastic anaemia in identical twins. New England Journal of Medicine 281: 11–17

Nissen-Druey C 1989 Pathophysiology of aplastic anaemia. Baillière's Clinical Haematology, 2(1), Chapter 3. Baillière Tindall, London

Oehler L, Reiter E, Freidl J et al 1994 Effective stimulation of neutrophils with RH G-CSF in dyskeratosis congenita. Annals of Haematology 69: 325–327

Paquetto A T, Tobynl N, Frane M et al 1995 Long-term outcome of aplastic anaemia in adults treated with antilymphocyte globulin comparison with bone marrow transplantation. Blood 85: 283–290

Rosenfeld S J, Kimball J, Vining D, Young N S 1995 Intensive immunosuppression with antithymocyte globulin and cyclosporin as treatment for severe aplastic anaemia. Blood 85: 3058–3065

Sirinavin C, Trowbridge A A 1975 Dyskeratosis congenita, clinical features and genetic aspects. Report of a family and review of the literature. Journal of Medical Genetics 12: 339–354

Smith S, Marx N W, Jordon C J, Van Niekerk C H 1989 Clinical aspects of a cluster of 42 patients in South Africa with Fanconi's anaemia. In: Schreoder-Kurth T M, Auerbach A, Obe G (eds) Fanconi anaemia clinical, cytogenetic and experimental aspects. Springer-Verlag, Heidelberg.

Storb R, Thomas E D, Weiden P L et al 1974 Allogeneic marrow grafting for treatment of aplastic anaemia. Blood 43: 157–180.

Sullivan K M, Witherspoon R P 1988 Long-term results of allogeneic bone marrow

transplantation. Transplant Proc. 21: 2926–2928

Szklo M, Sensenbrenner L, Markowitz J, Weida S, Warm S, Linett M 1985 Incidence of aplastic anaemia in metropolitan Baltimore, a population based study. Blood 66: 115–119

Walker F, Roethke S K, Martin G 1994 An overview of the rationale, process and nursing implications of peripheral blood stem cell transplantation. Cancer Nursing 17(2): 141–148

Whedon M B, Wujcik D 1997 Blood and marrow stem cell transplantation. Principles, practice and nursing insights, 2nd edn. Jones and Bartlett, Boston

Young N, Barrett J A 1995 The treatment of severe acquired aplastic anaemia. Blood 85 (12): 3367–3377

Young N S, Alter B P 1994 Aplastic-anaemia, acquired and inherited. W B Saunders, Philadelphia

Young N S, Issaragrasil S 1986 Aplastic anaemia in the orient. British Journal of Haematology 62: 1–6

Young N S, Speck B 1984 Antithymocyte and antilymphocyte globulins: clinical trials and mechanism of action. In: Young N S, Levine A, Humpheries R K (eds) Aplastic anaemia stem cell biology and advances in treatment. Alan R Liss, New York, pp 221–226

Yunis A A, Miller A M, Salem Z, Arimura G K 1980 Chloramphenicol toxicity, pathogenic mechanisms and the role of p-NO2 in aplastic anaemia. Clinical Toxicology 17(3): 359–373

Further reading

Treleaven J A, Barrett J A 1992 Bone marrow transplantation in practice. Churchill Livingstone, London
This book is written by British haematologists and gives the British perspective on BMT for both red and white cell disorders. Well worth reading.

Gordon-Smith E C (ed) 1989 Aplastic anaemia. Baillière's Clinical Haematology 2(1) Baillière Tindall, London.
Several chapters in this book are written by the editor who is a leader in the field of AA. A very well-written book with short concise chapters covering all aspects of aplastic anaemia with contributions by different professionals. A small, easily read and understood book.

Nathan D G, Oski F A (eds) 1993 Bone marrow failure syndromes in infancy and childhood. W B Saunders, Philadelphia
An excellent haematology book, though highly scientific. It covers all aspects of haematology including BMT. Chapter 7 covers bone marrow failure syndromes in great depth and examines causes, treatment and outcome of AA in both adults and children, including some nursing aspects.

Young N S, Alter B P 1994 Aplastic anaemia acquired and inherited. W B Saunders, Philadelphia
An excellent reference text covering all aspects of AA, including epidemiological aspects. Well worth reading.

4 *The leukaemias*

ROSLYNE BRATT-WYTON

Key points

■ Leukaemia is a neoplastic
   proliferation of cells of haematopoietic origin
■ Leukaemia is classified as chronic or acute
■ Clinical manifestations of leukaemia are due
   either directly or indirectly to the proliferation of
   leukaemic cells and their infiltration into
   normal tissues
■ The primary treatment for leukaemia is
   chemotherapy
■ The nursing role has a great impact on the
   patient's quality of life

INTRODUCTION

In 1847 the German pathologist Rudolf Virchow first described leukaemia, simply as 'white blood'. Microscopically, there were very few red blood corpuscles. The relationship between red and colourless corpuscles was the reverse of the normal; hence the term 'white blood'.

Leukaemia is a neoplastic proliferation of cells of haematopoietic origin which arises following somatic mutation in a single haematopoietic cell, the progeny of which form a clone of leukaemic cells (see Ch. 1). Often a series of events rather than a single genetic alteration is required to convert a normal cell into a neoplastic one (Maur 1990). The cell in which the leukaemic transformation occurs may be of lymphoid, erythroid or myeloid origin or a cell maturer, which is capable of differentiation into any of the cell lines. The clinical manifestations of the leukaemias are due directly or indirectly to the proliferation of leukaemic cells and their infiltration into normal tissues. Increased cell proliferation has metabolic consequences and infiltrating cells also disturb tissue function. Anaemia, neutropenia and thrombocytopenia are important consequences of infiltration of the bone marrow, which can lead to infection and haemorrhage (Dexter 1977).

The four most common types of leukaemia are

■ acute myeloid leukaemia (AML)
■ acute lymphoblastic leukaemia (ALL)
■ chronic myeloid leukaemia (CML)
■ chronic lymphoblastic leukaemia (CLL).

THE DISEASE

Classification of leukaemia

Chronic leukaemias

Leukaemia is classified as chronic or acute. In chronic leukaemia the predominant cell appears mature, although function is usually abnormal. Typically, the disease has a gradual onset, with a prolonged clinical course. Chronic leukaemia is divided into two categories – CML and CLL. In 90–95% of patients with CML there is a replacement of normal bone marrow by cells with an abnormal chromosome – the Philadelphia (Ph) chromosome.

Other rarer disorders grouped under the broad heading of CML include:

■ chronic granulocytic leukaemia (CGL) (Ph −)
■ eosinophilic leukaemia
■ chronic myelomonocytic leukaemia
■ atypical CML.

The Ph chromosome is not present in any of these other variants.

There are two main types of chronic lymphocytic leukaemia: B cell and T cell. In 95% of individuals, CLL originates from a clone of B lymphocytes, while 5% show a T-lymphocyte origin. Other chronic lymphoid leukaemias include prolymphocytic and hairy cell leukaemias (HCLs).

Prolymphocytic leukaemia (B-PLL) is an entity distinct from CLL and is characterised by bone marrow and splenic infiltration by cells with prolymphocytic morphology. The prognosis of B-PLL is much worse than that for CLL.

HCL is a syndrome that consists of cytopenia and splenomegaly. Microscopic examination shows proliferation of cells with an irregular cytoplasmic outline ('hairy'), a type of B lymphocyte, in the peripheral blood, bone marrow and some organs.

Acute leukaemias

In acute leukaemia the predominant cell is immature (undifferentiated), usually a 'blast cell'. The disease has a sudden onset, with rapid progression.

AML develops from abnormalities in maturation and proliferation of the pluripotent myeloid stem cell.

ALL develops from abnormalities in maturation and proliferation of the lymphoid series. The lymphoid stem cell matures to form plasma cells, T cells and B cells (see Ch. 1).

A classification of acute leukaemias known as the FAB system (from the French, American and British nationalities of the haematologists involved) has been devised (Table 4.1).

This system subdivides ALL into three subtypes (L1–L3) and AML into eight subtypes (M0–M7). Leukaemia is further defined by the use of monoclonal antibodies against tissue markers (Bain 1990). This is important for lymphoid malignancies, and all cases of lymphoid malignancy are defined according to the presence of T- or B-cell markers.

The FAB system is of considerable clinical importance because some forms of therapy are only effective against specific subtypes of leukaemia, confirming that the categories indicate genuine differences in a group of related diseases.

Originally, the FAB classification was based entirely on morphological appearances (such as cell size, nuclear chromatin and shape, nucleoli, amount and basophilia of cytoplasm, vacuolation, granulation, nucleocytoplasmic ratio, etc.) of bone marrow and peripheral blood films, supplemented by certain cytochemical reactions (Sudan black B and myeloperoxidase for identification of granulocytic variants and non-specific esterase for monocytic differentiation). Revisions of the classification were published in 1985 (Coasgeun & Bennett 1993) to include the identification of surface markers and cytogenetics, which provide important therapeutic and prognostic information.

Epidemiology

Leukaemia is no respecter of age, gender or ethnicity and represents approximately 30% of cancer incidence internationally, although

Table 4.1 The FAB classification of acute leukaemia

Acute myeloid leukaemia		Acute lymphoblastic leukaemia	
M0	Undifferentiated myeloblastic	L1	T-cell and B-cell (childhood)
M1	Myeloblastic without maturation	L2	T-cell and B-cell (adult)
M2	Myeloblastic with granulocytic maturation	L3	B-cell (Burkitt-cell type)
M3	Promyelocytic		
M4	Myelomonocytic		
M4e0	Myelomonocytic with eosinophilia		
M5a	Monoblastic		
M5b	Differentiated monocytic		
M6	Erythroleukaemia		
M7	Megakaryoblastic		

published incidence rates vary widely (Muir & Waterhouse 1987).

Acute myeloid leukaemia represents the majority of acute leukaemias in adults in England and Wales with incidence increasing with age. AML rates vary worldwide, with the highest rates recorded in Western countries and the lowest in Asia (International Agency for Research on Cancer 1987, Cartwright et al 1990).

Acute lymphoblastic leukaemia is most common in childhood, with the peak of incidence being from 2 to 7 years (Leukaemia Research Fund 1997). Incidence then decreases as age increases. However, there is a secondary rise in incidence after the age of 40 years (Liesner & Goldstone 1997). As with AML, ALL rates vary worldwide, with the highest incidence occurring in Costa Rica and the lowest incidences in Nigeria.

Chronic myeloid leukaemia tends to be the disease of middle life, with a slowly increasing age trend. Peak incidence for CML is between the ages of 40 to 60.

Chronic lymphocytic leukaemia is the commonest form of leukaemia seen in the Western world, accounting for 25% of all leukaemias. CLL is rare before the age of 40, with peak incidence between 60 and 80 years at diagnosis and only 6% of cases being below the age of 50 years. It is more common in men.

Prolymphocytic leukaemia affects mainly elderly men.

Hairy cell leukaemia is a rare disease; HCL accounts for only 2–4% of all leukaemias, predominantly in men between 40 and 60 years old.

The incidence of leukaemia worldwide continues to increase steadily. This may be due to improved diagnostic procedures and reporting or to the influence of occupational and environmental exposure and an ageing population (Sandler 1987).

Aetiological factors

The cause of most types of leukaemia is unknown. The aetiological factors most commonly considered are

- familial
- radiation
- chemicals
- drugs
- viruses
- genetic predisposition.

Familial

Research by the Leukaemia Research Fund (McKinney et al 1990) on childhood leukaemia has found no evidence that leukaemia is inherited. The medical records of 788 survivors of childhood leukaemia born between 1940 and 1969 were examined and none of the 382 children born to them have developed leukaemia.

In adult ALL, an unusual family history of cancer has been reported (McKinney et al 1990), with evidence of an increased risk in individuals with a family member diagnosed with leukaemia. Incidence is also higher in monozygous twins (Miller 1968, Rosner & Lee 1972).

Radiation

Exposure to ionising radiation is the most conclusively identified aetiological factor, with an increased incidence among early radiologists, and Japanese atomic bomb and Chernobyl survivors. However, controversy remains about the leukaemogenic nature of low levels of radiation.

Radiation used in the treatment for other diseases was first identified as a cause of secondary leukaemia by Court-Brown & Doll (1965), who reported a higher incidence of AML in patients irradiated for ankylosing spondylitis. An excess of AML has also been shown in patients previously treated with radiation for breast cancer and Hodgkin's disease (Bolvern et al 1986, Kaldor et al 1990).

Epidemiological studies continue to investigate leukaemia in the population surrounding nuclear power stations and other areas where a high incidence 'cluster of leukaemia' has been reported (Leukaemia Research Fund 1990). For example, distinct clusters of childhood leukaemia have been reported in the village of Seascale close to the Sellafield nuclear plant (Drapper et al 1993). However, the link between nuclear power plants and the incidence of leukaemia remains inconclusive.

Occupational radiation exposure and paternal preconceptual radiation exposure in nuclear power stations have also been implicated in the development of leukaemia, but the links remain unproven (Smith & Douglas 1986, Cragle et al 1988, Kinlen 1993, Kinlen et al 1993, Carpenter et al 1994).

Electromagnetic fields have also been implicated as a cause of leukaemia (Cartwright 1989). Again results remain inconclusive, but this remains an area of high research activity (Myers et al 1990, Savitz et al 1990, Washburn et al 1994, UK Childhood Cancer Study Investigators 1999).

Chemicals

Exposure to high levels of certain chemicals has been clearly proven to be leukaemogenic. The most significant chemical leukaemogen in Britain is probably cigarette smoke, estimated to cause as many as 25% of all cases of AML (Austin & Cole 1986, Kinlen & Roget 1988).

Other chemicals such as benzene, an aromatic hydrocarbon found in unleaded petrol, rubber, cement, and cleaning products and perchloroethylenes used in the dry-cleaning industry (Blair et al 1990) have also been associated with leukaemia.

Additionally, shoe workers in Istanbul have shown excesses of various types of AML, CLL and myelodysplastic states and those working with explosives, distilling, dyes and paints have been identified as being at risk (Rinsky & Young 1981, Wong 1987).

Agrichemical exposure has also been associated with HCL and CLL in farmers (Morrison et al 1992, Rask-Andersen et al 1995).

Drugs

Various drugs have been shown to have a relationship to leukaemia, including alkylating agents (Brenner & Carter 1984), chloramphenicol (Shu et al 1987), phenylbutazone (Friedman 1982) and growth hormone therapy in childhood leukaemia (Stahnke & Zisel 1989).

Generally, chemotherapy is the overwhelming source of risk, with a higher risk of leukaemia in patients treated with combination chemotherapy over the last 20 years (Chen et al 1989). The time of greatest risk of developing a secondary leukaemia appears to be the first 10 years post-treatment. Additionally, the combination of alkylating agents used in chemotherapy regimens and irradiation results in a higher incidence of 'secondary' leukaemia.

Viruses

The role of retroviruses in human leukaemia remains unclear (Lancet Editorial 1990). Human T-cell leukaemia virus (HTLV-1) has been associated with an acute T-cell leukaemia syndrome in adults of Caribbean or Japanese origin (Blattner 1989, Gerard et al 1995), whereas HTLV-II has been identified in a rare form of HCL in an intravenous drug addict (Wiktor & Blattner 1991).

Greaves (1989) suggests that the childhood peak in incidence in ALL may be a result of altered immune responses in the early years of life. Additionally, Kinlen (1988) suggests that the migration of populations and population intermixing can, in certain circumstances, lead to an excess of leukaemias in young people.

Genetic predisposition

An increased incidence of leukaemia has been associated with certain genetic disorders. Children with Down's syndrome (trisomy 21) have an approximate 20-fold increase in risk of leukaemia over background levels, 70% of cases being ALL and 30% AML (Rosner & Lee 1972).

Damaged or fragile chromosomes in some disorders increase the possibility of malignant change. Other syndromes that have demonstrated an increased incidence of leukaemia are Bloom's syndrome, Fanconi's anaemia, and diseases such as ataxia telangiectasia and congenital agammaglobulinaemia (Gunz 1983). Although these conditions account for only a small number of leukaemia cases, they can offer valuable insights into its pathophysiology.

Pathophysiology

An understanding of normal cell maturation (Ch. 1) is needed to understand the leukaemic disease process. Normal bone marrow regulating mechanisms ensure that cell proliferation and maturation are able to meet the body's needs. The mechanisms regulating this balance are not fully understood. However, it is known that the process involves intracellular communication through chemical messengers, surface markers that declare the type and maturity of cells, and genes that control cell growth, maturation and programmed cell death (apoptosis). Damage to, or interference with, the various components is of fundamental significance to the causes of leukaemia (Fig. 4.1).

Acute leukaemia cells have an average doubling time of 7 days, which is considerably slower than the average doubling time of 18 hours in normal haematopoietic cells. Thus, leukaemia is not caused by too rapid cell proliferation but rather is a disease of abnormal cellular development (Secker-Walker & Goldman 1989). Leukaemia cells are often unresponsive to growth factors that modulate growth and maturation of normal cells. After stem cells divide, daughter cells ordinarily go through a complex process of differentiation as they develop into mature blood cells. Many types of leukaemia occur when immature cells fail to mature, and are unable to assume their normal function yet continue dividing. Malignant stem cells typically produce a large number of abnormal daughter cells, so leukaemia is characterised by an overabundance of one or a few cell types in the blood (Lord & Testa 1988).

Arrested maturation produces crowding of the bone marrow, inhibiting growth and function of other cells. Individuals are at risk of infection, owing to decreased production of normal mature white cells. Anaemia and thrombocytopenia develop because of the reduced production of red blood cells and platelets and crowding of the bone marrow with immature white cells. Infiltration of lymph nodes, liver, spleen and brain with proliferating leucocytes may occur.

Diagnostic studies

Differentiating between AML and ALL is essential because treatment and prognosis differ.

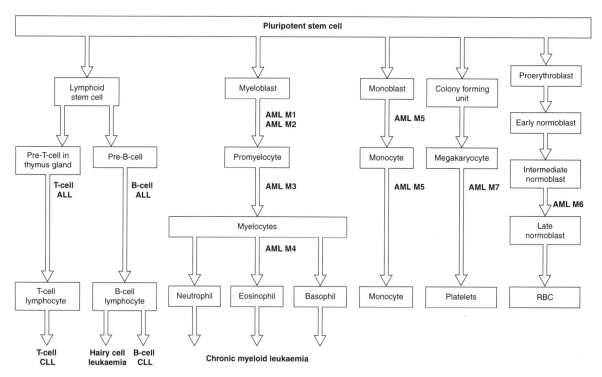

Figure 4.1 Diagrammatic representation of haematopoietic cascade with FAB classification

The FAB classification requires examination of peripheral blood (full blood count) and bone marrow films and differential counts. In the case of bone marrow, a 500-cell differential count is performed.

Peripheral blood film

In acute leukaemia:

- 90% of patients have blast cells in their peripheral blood. The FAB classification identifies two types of myeloblast.

   type 1 blasts lack granules, have uncondensed chromatin, a high nucleocytoplasmic ratio and prominent nucleoli

   type 2 blasts resemble type 1, except for the presence of a few acurophilia granules and a somewhat lower nucleocytoplasmic ratio
- white blood count can be low, or high
- platelet count can also be low (thrombocytopenia).

If AML M3 (acute hypergranular promyelocytic leukaemia, APL) is suspected, laboratory tests should include coagulation studies, as abnormalities of coagulation (disseminated intravascular coagulation (DIC)) are seen in this subgroup (see Ch. 14).

Bone marrow aspiration and trephine biopsy

Bone marrow aspiration enables subclassification, while a bone marrow trephine, especially if an aspirate fails (dry tap), enables diagnosis of AML M7. Appropriate cytochemistry, histological staining and cell surface immunological markers and cytogenetics are required for both aspiration and trephine to ensure clearer subclassification (Henderson & Afshani 1990).

Auer rods (needle-like, crystalline structures thought to be derived from primary granules by coalescence of the granules within autophage vacuoles) are diagnostic of AML together with cytochemical reactions of Sudan black and myeloperoxidase.

Cytogenetics can provide information confirming the diagnosis and specific classification of the leukaemia (Table 4.2). Specific aberrations are related to a favourable or unfavourable outcome.

Chromosome studies have become an integral part of the diagnostic approach to patients with leukaemia because of their diagnostic and prognostic significance. Some genetic aberrations involve translocation of chromosomal regions and result in juxtaposition of genes,

Table 4.2 Some consistent chromosome abnormalities associated with leukaemia

Chromosome abnormality[a]	Leukaemia	Possible oncogene
t(9;22) (q34;q11) (Philadelphia chromosome)	CML, ALL	bcr, c-abl
t(8;21) (q22;q22)	AML M2	?c-mos, ?c-myc
t(15;17) (q22;q12)	AML M3	RARα, PML
t or del (11) (q23)	AML M5, M4	Int-2
inv or del (16) (p13,q22)	AML M4 with eosinophilia	
t(4;11) (q21;q23)	ALL	Int-2
+12	CLL	
+8 −7 −7q −5q	AML CLL (secondary changes)	

[a] t = translocation.
Each chromosome has two arms: p, the short arm; and q, the long arm.
+ or − is put in front of the chromosome number if part of the chromosome is gained or lost.

that would normally be apart. This can activate cellular oncogenes associated with the development of neoplasia. A number of specific genetic rearrangements are associated with leukaemia (Brenner 1998) (Table 4.2): for example, the Philadelphia chromosome found in CML involving translocation of 22q and 9q. Identification of chromosomal abnormalities such as the retinoic acid (RARa) gene in AML M3 t(15;17) has also helped considerably in the development of treatment for leukaemia. Clinical trials using oral all-*trans*-retinoic acid (ATRA) have demonstrated that nearly all individuals with acute promyelocytic leukaemia (APL) will have a complete response, without the use of chemotherapy. In APL, leukaemic cells can mature to neutrophils under the influence of ATRA and this response correlates with the presence of an abnormal gene translocation (Nimmer 1995).

In CLL clonal chromosome abnormalities are found in 50% of patients; trisomy 12 or 14q+ translocation 11:14 are the most common chromosome findings (Hamblin & Oscier 1998). Other chromosomal defects, ranging from point mutations to chromosomal loss, are associated with leukaemogenesis.

Surface immunological markers can help distinguish myeloid and lymphoid cells and B-cell ALL and T-cell ALL. Other markers on blood cells uniquely define a specific stage in the maturation of a specific cell type. These markers are clusters of monoclonal antibodies termed 'clusters of differentiation' and are assigned different numbers. For example, an unusual feature in CLL is expression of the CD5 membrane antigen seen on mature T lymphocytes. In hairy cell leukaemia, cells express the B-cell markers CD19, CD20 and CD22, with the distinctive expression of the IL2 receptor CD25.

Acute leukaemia

Clinical features

Individuals usually present with a short clinical history of days or weeks. Presenting symptoms are commonly those of bone marrow failure. Individuals frequently visit their GP with a history of repeated infections, malaise, pallor, bruising and sometimes weight loss. Common

sites for recurrent infection are the upper respiratory tract, urinary tract, oral cavity and perianal tissue. Patients may have unexplained bleeding, bruising or petechiae (red or purple flat pinhead spots occurring on skin or mucous membranes caused by local haemorrhage) (Plate 11). Bleeding from the gums, heavy menses or midcycle bleeding are common. Patients may also complain of pain due to enlarged lymph nodes, spleen or liver and bone pain.

Treatment

AML and ALL are treated with different chemotherapy agents (see Ch. 8). The chemotherapeutic strategy is to achieve remission by eradicating leukaemic cells from the bone marrow and allowing normal marrow to regenerate. Remission is defined as less than 5% blasts in the bone marrow. Once remission is achieved, management includes consolidation and/or maintenance chemotherapy (Ch. 8).

Cytotoxic drugs interfere with various stages of DNA synthesis or function. There are several categories of drugs, which act at different stages of the cell cycle. The most effective way of causing damage to the leukaemic cell is to give drugs which belong to several categories together (combination chemotherapy) or in sequence. Combination drug therapies have improved remission rates and reduced the frequency of drug resistance. Protocols often administer the drugs in cyclical combinations with treatment-free intervals to allow the bone marrow to recover. This recovery depends upon the differential regrowth pattern of the normal haematopoietic and leukaemic cells (see Ch. 8 for a further discussion of chemotherapy).

Both AML and ALL are treated according to established protocols or current Medical Research Council trials. Typical treatment regimens are shown in Figs 4.2 and 4.3.

Cytotoxic drugs have many side-effects, but nausea, vomiting, bone marrow toxicity, infertility, mucositis, hair loss and skin sensitivity are the most common (see Ch. 8). Hyperkalaemia and hyperuricaemia may be caused by induction therapy (see Ch. 8) and allopurinol should always be prescribed before commencing treatment.

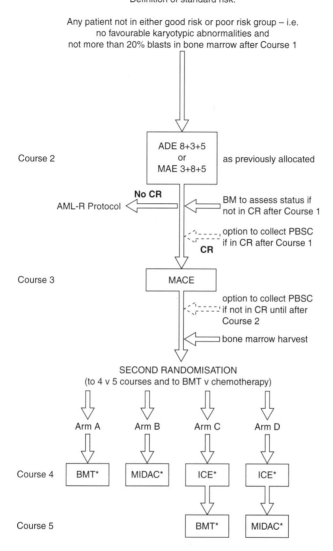

Definition of standard risk:

Any patient not in either good risk or poor risk group – i.e.
no favourable karyotypic abnormalities and
not more than 20% blasts in bone marrow after Course 1

Course 2 — ADE 8+3+5 or MAE 3+8+5 — as previously allocated

No CR

AML-R Protocol ← | BM to assess status if not in CR after Course 1

option to collect PBSC if in CR after Course 1

CR

Course 3 — MACE

option to collect PBSC if not in CR until after Course 2

bone marrow harvest

SECOND RANDOMISATION
(to 4 v 5 courses and to BMT v chemotherapy)

Arm A   Arm B   Arm C   Arm D

Course 4   BMT*   MIDAC*   ICE*   ICE*

Course 5   BMT*   MIDAC*

*PBSC augmentation optional (but not after allo-BMT)

BMT will be allogeneic if sibling donor available and patient considered suitable for the procedure,
otherwise it will be autologous

Figure 4.2 AML 12 protocol flow chart for standard risk patients (reproduced with permission)

In ALL, central nervous system (CNS) relapse occurs in the majority of patients unless prophylactic therapy is given. CNS prophylaxis is therefore administered to all patients with ALL. Traditionally, CNS prophylaxis has involved all patients receiving intrathecal methotrexate and cranial irradiation. However, the use of intrathecal treatment and high-dose systemic chemotherapy has been shown to be effective CNS prophylaxis in adults (Cortes & Kantarjian 1995). Some clinicians may therefore reserve prophylaxis with cranial irradiation for those individuals at high risk of CNS relapse.

CNS prophylaxis is not usually given in AML; a meningeal relapse occasionally occurs, especially in children and young adults with M4 or

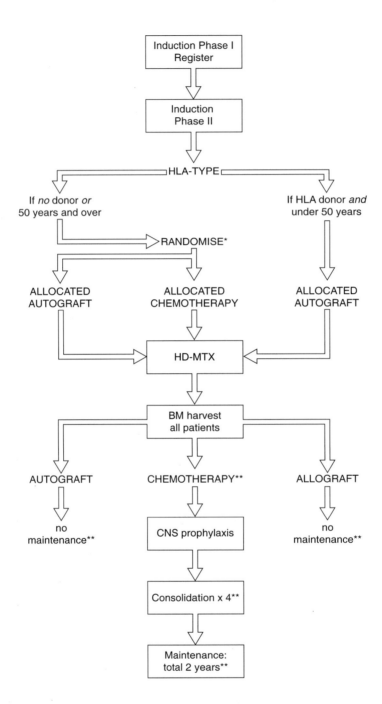

*   For Ph+ patients with no matched donor, a MUD transplant may be considered
** Ph+ patients receive α-interferon for 15 months after transplant or consolidation

Figure 4.3   UK ALL XII summary (reproduced with permission)

M5 disease; prophylactic CNS therapy may then be given.

The use of growth factors in acute leukaemia remains an area of debate; granulocyte–colony-stimulating factor (G-CSF) or granulocyte, macrophage–colony-stimulating factor (GM-CSF) are undergoing trials in the prevention of infection. Growth factors are often commenced 6–8 days after the end of chemotherapy and continue until the neutrophil count is greater than 1.0×10^9/L. Other growth factors are undergoing trials.

All units should have protocols in place for regularly checking:

- full blood count
- urea and electrolytes
- temperature and pulse rate
- ECG (electrocardiogram)
- fluid input and output
- coagulation studies
- condition of the oral cavity using an oral assessment tool (Ch. 16).

Fluid and nutritional intake should be monitored, with advice being sought from the nutritional nurse specialist or the dietician (Ch. 17). These protocols should be research based and aid audit and reflective practice.

All patients aged less than 50 years should be tissue typed and attempts made to identify a potential bone marrow donor for allogeneic bone marrow transplantation (BMT). Patients without a donor should be considered for autologous bone marrow transplantation (ABMT) or peripheral blood stem cell transplant (PBSCT) (see Ch. 10).

Patients with the diagnosis of AML M3 (APL) are treated with ATRA prior to chemotherapy.

AML treatment in the elderly depends on patients' age, their general health, presenting complications, rate of disease progression and their wish for treatment. Patients will have either supportive therapy, intensive chemotherapy or low-intensity chemotherapy. AML in the elderly is sometimes associated with a history of myelodysplasia (see Ch. 2).

Treatment of relapse

Patients who relapse after induction and post-induction chemotherapy have a 30–60%

Case study 4.1

Danny, a 25-year-old male with no relevant past medical history other than recurring tonsillitis presented in the Accident and Emergency Department following trauma while playing football. His initial symptoms were pleuritic-type chest pain and haemoptysis.

A ventilation/perfusion (VQ) scan confirmed multiple pulmonary emboli and he was anticoagulated. On admission he was neutropenic, with normal haemoglobin and platelet counts. A diagnosis of acute promyelocytic leukaemia was confirmed following a bone marrow trephine; cytogenetic analysis showed the presence of the t(15;17) translocation. He was then entered with his consent into the AML 12 trial and randomised to receive ADE (cytarabine, daunorubicin and etoposide) which was commenced in the first week of diagnosis. He was also prescribed ATRA.

Unfortunately Danny did not go into remission following the first course of chemotherapy but did so after the second course of therapy; however, the chromosome translocation was still detectable by polymerase chain reaction (PCR) and minimal residual disease was still detectable by bone marrow trephine.

Following successful completion of the planned five courses of intensive combination chemotherapy, a further bone marrow trephine confirmed a normal regenerating bone marrow with no evidence of disease. The PCR was negative. Twelve months later Danny played his first 90 minute football match and plans to get married next month.

likelihood of achieving a second remission (Gale & Foon 1987). Patients with early relapse or resistant leukaemia, are in the forefront of research where drugs are being tested to overcome multidrug resistance (MDR). MDR is the phenomenon by which a cancer becomes resistant to multiple drugs from different categories of cytotoxic agents that have different modes of action and chemical structure (Dalton & Miller 1991). MDR can be present in the cell from the beginning or can be acquired; it is associated with P-glycoprotein, a transmembrane protein that acts as a pump to transport drugs in and out of the cells. MDR is found in 10–20% of newly diagnosed AML and 50% of relapsed AML (see Ch. 8).

SPECIFIC NURSING ISSUES

The diagnosis of leukaemia is still viewed by many as a death sentence. Newly diagnosed patients are suddenly faced with the possibility that they may soon die. It is crucial that nurses help patients and their families with counselling at this time, as they need time to express their fears.

During diagnostic studies it is important to keep the patient and their family/carer informed at all times. This will facilitate cooperation and decrease anxiety, creating an ongoing atmosphere of confidence and trust.

Many patients with acute leukaemia (if they agree) are entered into clinical trials. Patients should be allowed to participate in treatment decisions, and offered information about the illness and its treatment: 'too little' information is a far more frequent complaint than 'too much'. Needless delays in passing on new information to the patient should be avoided, as emotional problems are minimised if the patient is kept informed. Written information should supplement verbal.

If possible, sperm banking should be carried out prior to the commencement of treatment in male patients. The storage of ova is also now being undertaken in some centres (see Ch. 18).

Patients undergoing intensive treatment require expert nursing care with an emphasis on infection control (Ch. 13). For patients with acute leukaemia, all courses of chemotherapy are given as inpatient treatment, and patients stay in hospital throughout the pancytopenic phase. Patients will therefore spend long periods of time in hospital during induction and maintenance therapy, and nurses and patients should build relationships based on trust, allowing for frank discussions to take place. The nursing role has a great impact on the patient's quality of life, as well as an indirect influence on prognosis through symptom management and support.

Patient survival can depend upon the supportive strategy they are taught and this is an important nursing role. The strategy should include:

- the importance of adequate fluid intake
- observing for signs of oedema
- taking their own temperature
- observing for signs and symptoms of infection
- caring for their skin
- diet and foods to avoid
- checking their body for signs of bruising or bleeding.

Patients and relatives should be given telephone numbers and names of who to contact if any of the above symptoms arise.

Multidisciplinary teams are involved in delivering all aspects of physical and psychological care to the patient. Most units operate an open door policy for patients and their carer/relative, ensuring that they do not feel isolated when at home. Survivorship, issues of employment, life insurance and mortgages are now a problem, especially for the younger adult (see Ch. 20).

Patients' disease status may change from curative to palliative care quickly, and death may occur within a short space of time; this may be due to overwhelming infection (septicaemia) or a decision by the haematologist that sustaining life is futile because of overwhelming disease. Patients and families will need support throughout such a decision-making process.

 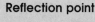

Reflection point

Individuals once diagnosed with acute leukaemia need to commence treatment almost immediately.

- Consider the implications of giving informed consent to treatment when individuals may be traumatised by their diagnosis and lack supportive confiding relationships with family and friends.
- Think about patient information and the types of information that are available to patients and their relatives in your workplace. Are individuals always given enough information?

Chronic leukaemia

The term 'chronic' was applied in the era prior to the development of chemotherapeutic agents as a result of the longer survival observed in patients with these conditions when compared with the survival of the patient with 'acute leukaemia' (Wujcik 1993). In common with the acute leukaemias the cells of the neoplastic clone retain the capacity to differentiate, resulting in the accumulation of cells with a mature appearance in the peripheral blood and bone marrow. However, the diseases are not similar in any other way.

Clinical features and treatment

Patients present with features of anaemia, pallor, dyspnoea and tachycardia, bruising, epistaxis, menorrhagia or haemorrhage from other sites due to abnormal platelet function. Symptoms related to hypermetabolism such as weight loss and night sweats, and gout or renal impairment due to hyperuricaemia from excessive purine breakdown may also be present. Bone pain or neurological symptoms may be caused by leucostasis. Splenomegaly is present in 90% of patients which may cause considerable pain, discomfort or indigestion.

CML is divided into phases: chronic and accelerated/transformation into acute leukaemia (terminal or blast phase).

Chronic phase
Treatment consisting of oral chemotherapy, busulphan, and a single alkylating agent is used to reduce the white cell count and consequently reduce symptoms. Regular blood counts allow the doses to be titrated in individuals. Long-term busulphan therapy may cause pulmonary fibrosis and an Addisonian syndrome; therefore, hydroxyurea has become the preferred treatment. It is given daily and regular blood profiles are needed to monitor the white cell count. Interferon is also used in early disease and to maintain the patient in the chronic phase. Average length of survival is 3–4 years.

In the quest to extend survival The Medical Research Council (MRC) are currently running two CML trials: CML IV and CML V. CML IV seeks to determine whether the survival advantage of using α-interferon (demonstrated

in CML III) can be increased by incorporating a cycle of high-dose chemotherapy and an autograft followed by maintenance interferon. Further trials are seeking to determine the advantages of using cytarabine and α-interferon.

CML V is examining whether there is a significant difference in survival, side-effects and patient tolerance between low- or high-dose maintenance interferon with or without hydroxyurea.

Currently, the only chance for cure of CML is with ablation of the Ph+ clone of cells. This occurs in 50–70% of patients aged under 55 years after chemotherapy followed by allogeneic BMT.

Accelerated phase
Acute transformation to acute leukaemia may occur rapidly over a few days or the individual may gradually fail to respond to treatment, becoming anaemic and thrombocytopenic. When blast transformation occurs, survival is usually 2–6 months, with survival over 1 year uncommon. Individuals with a leucocyte count previously controlled by busulphan entering an accelerated phase may respond, temporarily, to hydroxyurea and vice versa.

Prognosis is generally poor and historically there has been little benefit in treating these patients with conventional first-line regimens for AML or BMT due to the high mortality rates and relapse.

Responses can be achieved with chemotherapy agents such as mitozantrone and high-dose cytarabine but remission is usually brief and the incidence of prolonged pancytopenia and infective complications are high (Bain 1990).

In CLL the stage of the disease at presentation correlates with survival and the two most widely adopted staging systems were put forward by Rai et al (1977) and Binet et al (1981), respectively (Table 4.3). The Rai staging system correlates well with survival. Median survival for stage 0 is 12 years; for stages I and II, 7 years; and for stages III and IV, less than 12 months. The Binet staging system has only three groups (A, B and C), but is otherwise similar to the Rai system.

Individuals may live for up to 10 years after diagnosis, but this is dependent on staging.

Table 4.3 Clinical staging in CLL (modified Rai classification)

Clinical features	Risk		
	Low (stage 0)	Intermediate (stages I and II)	High (stages III and IV)
Lymphocytosis	Present	Present	Present
Lymphadenopathy/ splenomegaly	Absent	Present	May be present
Thrombocytopenia	Absent	Absent	Present
Anaemia	Absent	Absent	Present
Median survival (years)	>10	6–8	1–2

Typically, the white count gradually rises as the disease progresses. In the early stages, it is unnecessary to institute treatment immediately and patients may only need to be kept under observation.

The standard treatment of CLL is single alkylating agent chemotherapy with or without corticosteroids. Chlorambucil has long been the treatment of choice. Purine analogues, notably fludarabine and 2-chlorodeoxyadenosine, have been found to be effective agents in the treatment of patients with disease refractory to standard therapy or who subsequently relapse. Fludarabine in particular has been shown to have a high level of activity in these patients, with response rates of the order of 40–60%.

Complete remission for HCL patients is now obtained with purine analogues such as deoxycoformycin or chlorodeoxyadenosine. These treatments have replaced prolonged therapy with α-interferon as first-line therapy.

SPECIFIC NURSING ISSUES

For patients with chronic leukaemia there is usually more time to prepare patients and their families when the disease enters the terminal phase. Control of symptoms is paramount to allow patients quality time with their families. Each patient and family is unique in their coping mechanisms, and the aim of the multidisciplinary team is to recognise their needs and to be able to react to their individual needs.

CONCLUSION

Leukaemia, both acute and chronic, is a disease that affects all ages, gender and ethnic origin. Delivery of effective care requires an understanding of the disease process and the factors which contribute to the diagnosis of the disease, enabling the nurse to guide his/her patient throughout their haemato-oncology journey.

DISCUSSION QUESTIONS

1. How is the diagnosis of leukaemia made in your hospital?
2. In chronic myeloid leukaemia what is the most common chromosome change?
3. In acute myeloid leukaemia what are the FAB subtypes?
4. What are the clinical features of bone marrow failure?
5. What is the role of ATRA (all-*trans*-retinoic acid) in APL?
6. Is the prognosis for long-term survival more favourable for individuals with ALL than AML?

EDITOR'S NOTE

The World Health Organization Classification Steering Committee has recently produced a new classification for haematological neoplasms: Harris N L, Jaffe E S, Diebold J et al 1999 Special article. Journal of Clinical Oncology 17(12): 3835–3849

References

Austin H, Cole P 1986 Cigarette smoking and leukaemia. Journal of Chronic Diseases 39: 417–421

Bain B J 1990 Leukaemia diagnosis. Gower, London

Binet J L, Catovsky D, Chandra P 1981 Chronic lymphocytic leukaemia proposals for a revised prognostic staging system. British Journal of Haematology 48: 365–367

Blair A, Stewart P A, Tolbert P E 1990 Cancer and other causes of death among a cohort of dry cleaners. British Journal of Industrial Medicine 47: 162–168

Blattner W A 1989 Retroviruses. In: Evans A S (ed) Viral infections in humans, 2nd edn. Plenum, New York, pp 545–592

Bolvern J F, Hutchinson G B, Evans F B 1986 Leukaemia after radiotherapy for first primary cancers of various anatomic sites. American Journal of Epidemiology 1223: 993–1003

Brenner B, Carter A 1984 Acute leukaemia following chemotherapy and radiation therapy. Oncology 41: 83–87

Brenner M K 1998 Gene transfer in leukaemia and related disorders. In: Whittaker J A, Holmes J A (eds) Leukaemia and related disorders, 3rd edn. Blackwell Science, Oxford

Carpenter L, Higgins C, Douglas A, Fraser P, Beral V, Smith P 1994 Combined analysis of mortality in three United Kingdom nuclear industry workforces 1946–1988. Radiation Research 138: 224–238

Cartwright R A 1989 Low frequency alternating electromagnetic fields and leukaemia; the saga so far. British Journal of Cancer 60: 6499–6510

Cartwright R A, Alexander F E, McKinney P A 1990 Leukaemia – lymphoma, an atlas of distribution within areas of England & Wales 1984–1988. Leukaemia Research Fund, London

Chen S J, Chen Z, Dene J et al 1989 Are most secondary acute lymphoblastic leukaemias mixed acute leukaemias. Nouville Revue Francaise Haematologie 31: 17–22

Coasgeun J, Bennett J M 1993 The acute myeloid leukaemias, morphology and cytochemistry. In: Bick R, Bennett J M et al (eds) Haematology. Mosby, St. Louis

Cortes J, Kantarjian H M 1995 Acute lymphoblastic leukaemia: a comprehensive review with emphasis on biology and therapy. Cancer 76(12): 2392–2417

Court-Brown W M, Doll R 1965 Mortality from cancer and other causes after radiotherapy for ankylosing spondylitis. British Medical Journal 2: 1327–1332

Cragle D L, McLain R W, Qualters J R 1988 Mortality amongst workers at nuclear fuels production facility. American Journal of Industrial Medicine 14: 379–401

Dalton W S, Miller T P 1991 Multidrug resistance. PPO Updates 5(7): 1–13

Dexter T M 1977 Conditions controlling the proliferation of haematopoietic stem cells. Journal of Cell Physiology 91: 334–335

Drapper C J, Stiller C A, Cartwright R A, Croft A W, Vincent T J 1993 Cancer in Cumbria and in the vicinity of the Sellafield nuclear installation 1963–1990. British Medical Journal 306: 89–94

Friedman G B 1982 Phenylbutazone, musculoskeletal disease and leukaemia. Journal of Chronic Diseases 34: 233–243

Gale R P, Foon K A 1987 Therapy of acute myelogenous leukaemia. Seminar Haematology 24: 40–54

Gerard Y, Lepere J, Pradinaud R et al 1995 Clustering and clinical diversity of adult T-cell leukaemia/lymphoma associated with HTLV-I. International Journal of Cancer 60: 773–776

Greaves M F 1989 Etiology of childhood ALL. In: Gale R, Hoeizer D (eds) Acute lymphoblastic leukaemia. UCLA Symposium on Molecular & Cellular Biology. Academic Press New Series 108: 91–97. Wiley-Liss, New York

Gunz F W 1983 Genetic factors in human leukaemia, 4th edn. Grune-Stratton, New York, pp 313–328

Hamblin T J, Oscier D G 1998 Chronic lymphocytic leukaemia. In: Whittaker J A, Holmes I (eds) Leukaemia and related disorders, 3rd edn. Blackwell Science, Oxford, pp 105–135

Henderson E S, Afshani E 1990 Clinical manifestation and diagnosis. In: Henderson E S, Lister A (eds) Leukaemia, 5th edn. W B Saunders, Philadelphia

International Agency for Research on Cancer 1987 Cancer incidence in 5 continents, Vol. 5. IARC, Lyon, France

Kaldor J M, Day N E, Clarke E A 1990 Leukaemia following Hodgkin's disease. New England Journal of Medicine 13: 322–327

Kinlen L J, Roget E 1988 Leukaemia and smoking habits among United States Veterans. British Medical Journal 287: 657–659

Kinlen L J 1988 Evidence for an infective cause of childhood leukaemia. Lancet ii: 1323–1326

Kinlen L J 1993 Can paternal preconceptional radiation account for the increase of leukaemia and non-Hodgkin's lymphoma in Seascale? British Medical Journal 306: 1718–1721

Kinlen L J Clarke K, Balkwill A 1993 Paternal preconceptual radiation exposure in the nuclear industry and leukaemia and non-Hodgkin's lymphoma in young people in Scotland. British Medical Journal 306: 1153–1158

Lancet Editorial 1990 Childhood leukaemia an infectious disease? Lancet ii: 1477–1479

Leukaemia Research Fund 1990 Leukaemia and lymphoma atlas. Leukaemia Research Fund, University of Leeds

Leukaemia Research Fund 1997 The descriptive epidemiology of leukaemia and related conditions in parts of the United Kingdom 1984–1993. Leukaemia Research Fund, London

Liesner R J, Goldstone A H 1997 ABC of clinical haematology: the

acute leukaemias. British Medical Journal 314: 733–736

Lord B, Testa N 1988 The hemopoietic system. Structure and regulation. In: Testa N, Gale R P (eds) Hematopoiesis. Marcel Dekker, New York

McKinney P A, Alexander F E, Roberts B E 1990 Yorkshire case control study of leukaemia and lymphomas. Leukaemia & Lymphomas Leukaemia Research Fund, London

Maur A M 1990 Clinical features of human leukaemia. In: Maur A M (ed) The biology of human leukaemia. Johns Hopkins Press, Baltimore

Miller R W 1968 Relations between cancer and congenital defects. Journal of the National Cancer Institute 40: 1079–1080

Morrison H L, Wilkins K, Semenciw R, Mao Y, Wiggle D 1992 Herbicides and cancer. Journal of National Cancer Institute 84: 1866–1874

Muir C S, Waterhouse J 1987 Cancer incidence in five continents. Scientific Publication No. 88. Vol. 5. International Agency for Research on Cancer, Lyon, France

Myers A, Clayden D, Cartwright S C, Cartwright R A 1990 Childhood cancer and overhead power lines. British Journal of Cancer 62: 1008–1085

Nimmer S D 1995 Transcription factors and malignancy. In: Kurzrock R, Talpaz M (eds) Molecular biology in cancer medicine. Martin Dunitz, London

Rai K R, Sawitsky A, Cronkite E R 1977 Clinical staging of chronic lymphocytic leukaemia. Blood 46: 219–234

Rask-Andersen A, Hagberg H, Hardell L, Nordstrom M 1995 Is hairy cell leukaemia more common

among farmers – pilot study. Oncology Reports 2: 447–450

Rinsky R A, Young R J 1981 Leukaemia in benzene workers. American Journal of Industrial Medicine 2: 217–245

Rosner F, Lee S H 1972 Down's syndrome and acute leukaemia. American Journal of Medicine 53: 203–218

Sandler O P 1987 Epidemiology of acute myelogenous leukaemia. Seminars in Oncology 14: 359–364

Savitz D A, John E M, Kleckner R C 1990 Magnetic field exposure from electric appliances and childhood cancer. American Journal of Epidemiology 131: 763–773

Secker-Walker L M, Goldman J 1989 Cytogenetics and leukaemogenesis. In: Hoffbrand A (ed) Postgraduate haematology. Heinemann Press, London

Shu X O, Gao Y T, Linet M et al 1987 Chloramphenicol use in childhood leukaemia in Shanghai. Lancet ii: 934–937

Smith P G, Douglas A J 1986 Mortality of workers at the Sellafield Plant of British Nuclear Fuels. British Medical Journal 293: 8445–8540

Stahnke N, Zisel H 1989 Growth hormone therapy and leukaemia. European Journal of Paediatrics 148: 591–596

UK Childhood Cancer Study Investigators 1999 Exposure to power-frequency magnetic fields and the risk of childhood cancer. Lancet 354: 1925–1931

Washburn E P, Orza M J, Berlin J A et al 1994 Critique of studies of EMF exposure. Cancer Causes and Control 5: 299–309

Wiktor S, Blattner W 1991 Epidemiology of HTLV-I. In: Gallo R C, Jay G (eds) The human retrovirus. Academic Press, Orlando, pp 121–129

Wong O 1987 An industry wide mortality study of chemical workers occupationally exposed to benzene. British Journal of Industrial Medicine 44: 382–395

Wujcik D 1993 Leukaemia. In: Groenwald S L, Frogge M H, Goodman M, Yarbro C H Cancer nursing, 3rd edn. Jones and Bartlett, Boston, pp 1149–1173

Further reading

Hoelzer D 1995 Acute leukaemia in adults. In: Peckham M, Pinedo H M, Veronesi U (eds) Oxford textbook of oncology. Oxford Medical Publications, Oxford
Easy to read, with clear subheadings giving the reader a greater understanding of issues surrounding the diagnosis of acute leukaemia.

Hoffbrand A V, Pettit J E 1993 Essential haematology, 3rd edn. Blackwell Science, Oxford
Chapter 11, acute leukaemias, and Chapter 12, chronic leukaemias provide a clear picture of the pathogenesis of leukaemia and the clinical manifestations of the diseases. A very useful reference book.

Whittaker J A, Holmes J A 1998 Leukaemia and related disorders. Blackwell Science, Oxford
A comprehensive text for nurses working in this specialist field. Excellent reference book.

A wide variety of patient information literature is available and the following organisations provide booklets and information sheets (see Appendix: Useful Resources):

BACUP
Leukaemia Research Fund
Leukaemia Care
The Royal Marsden Hospital

5 *Myeloma*

MAURA DOWLING

Key points
- Myeloma is an incurable disease arising from uncontrolled growth of plasma cells
- Pain is the most frequent presenting symptom
- The goal of treatment is symptom control
- Symptom control is crucial in maintaining quality of life
- Nursing interventions are important in preventing and managing complications of the disease and its treatment

Reflection point

Pause for a few minutes to consider what you already know about this disease.

INTRODUCTION

This chapter reviews myeloma, a malignant disorder characterised by uncontrolled growth of plasma cells in the bone marrow. Management of myeloma is aimed at symptom control and improving quality of life because there is no known cure. This complex illness affects multiple body systems; therefore, informed nursing care requires a thorough knowledge of its pathophysiology.

THE DISEASE

Myeloma (also known as multiple myeloma, myelomatosis, plasma cell myeloma) is a disease that is often misunderstood and underestimated in its ability to debilitate. The incurable and systemic nature of this disease presents a great challenge to nurses in managing symptoms and improving the patient's quality of life.

Plasma cells are mature B lymphoctyes which normally constitute less than 5% of the cells in the bone marrow. Individuals with myeloma have uncontrolled growth of plasma cells and subsequently can have >10% plasma cells in their bone marrow (often over 90%) (International Myeloma Foundation 1994). Masses of plasma cells form plasmacytomas (plasma cell tumours), which can arise either in the intradural or extradural segments of bone (International Myeloma Foundation 1994). Plasma cells infiltrate the bone and the bone marrow in a patchy manner, presenting as a focal tumour mass. These tumours have osteolytic properties and eventually erode bone, resulting in skeletal abnormalities which are present in about two-thirds of individuals with myeloma. The mechanism of the development of these osteolytic lesions is not fully understood but osteoclast activating factors (OAF) produced by the myeloma cells are known to be involved in the process (Souhami & Tobias 1995). OAF have been found to be associated with the reabsorption of bone, local destruction and secondary hypercalcaemia in 20% of patients with myeloma (Mundy 1987). Any bone can be affected and common sites include vertebrae, pelvis, skull, ribs and proximal long bones (Souhami & Tobias 1995) (Fig. 5.1).

Normal plasma cells produce immunoglobulins (antibodies) which are the body's major defence against most bacterial and viral infections. Immunoglobulins consist of two heavy and two light polypeptide chains. There are 5 classes of heavy chains (IgA, IgG, IgD, IgM and

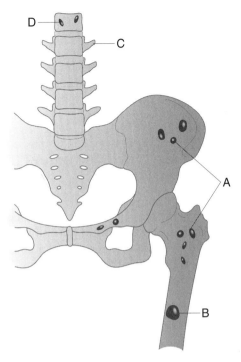

Key:

A The typical lesion is of multiple rounded
   translucencies without sclerosis
B Some lesions may be very large and fractures
   of long bones are frequent
C Vertebral osteoporosis and collapse is very
   common
D Loss of the vertebral pedicle is an easily
   missed sign of infiltration

Figure 5.1 Diagrammatic representation of bone
lesions in myeloma (from Souhami & Tobias 1995,
reproduced with permission)

IgE) and two classes of light chains (kappa (κ)
and lambda (λ)). In myeloma excessive
amounts of abnormal immunoglobulin are
secreted, with a reduction in the amount of
normal immunoglobulin produced. The abnormal immunoglobulin is referred to as a paraprotein. Myelomas are classified according to
which immunoglobulin is secreted and how it
affects the patient clinically. For instance, IgM
has a high molecular weight and hyperviscosity
syndrome may occur in IgM myeloma.
Furthermore, IgA molecules may polymerise in
the plasma, which also results in hyperviscosity.

Only a small percentage of myeloma patients
(approximately 5%) develop hyperviscosity
syndrome.

IgG myeloma represents 50–60% of all
myelomas and IgA represents 20%. The remaining types (IgM, IgD, IgE and non-secretory)
occur rarely (Foerster 1993). The excretion of
light chains only is known as Bence Jones
myeloma and accounts for approximately 20%
of all myeloma cases.

In myeloma normal bone marrow function is
inhibited largely due to infiltration of the bone
marrow by plasma cells. Many individuals present with anaemia and the severity of the
anaemia may be an indication of the severity of
the disease. Neutropenia is also common
because of marrow infiltration, especially in
the advanced stages of the disease. Platelet
counts can be normal but abnormal parapro-
teins may cause platelet and coagulation factor
dysfunction, which predisposes individuals to
bleeding. The more common sites of bleeding
tend to be the mucosal surfaces, such as those
of the nose and gastrointestinal tract.

Incidence

Multiple myeloma is more common in males
than in females and generally affects individuals from late middle age onwards, being rare
under the age of 40. The reported incidence of
multiple myeloma is 3 : 100 000 and, according
to figures from the USA, is more common
among Afro-Caribbeans than Whites (Bubley &
Schipper 1991). The exact cause of this disease
is unknown; however, there appears to be a
universal relationship between radiation exposure and subsequent progression of myeloma
(Souhami & Tobias 1995). Furthermore, occupational exposure to metal, rubber, wood, tex-
tile and petroleum have been associated with

 Reflection point

Pause and reflect on the need for nurses to
understand the pathophysiology of myeloma.

the development of myeloma, although their definite role in the progress of the disease remains ambiguous (Riedel & Pottern 1992).

Diagnosis

Multiple myeloma is normally a slow-growing neoplasm. It has been calculated from myeloma growth rates that the disease has frequently been present for several years before the tumour has grown adequately to cause symptoms (Velez et al 1982). The disease is therefore usually at an advanced stage at diagnosis. However, there is evidence available to indicate that multiple myeloma is being diagnosed earlier now than in the past (Riccardi et al 1991). Frequently, multiple diffuse tumours are present at diagnosis; hence, the use of the term 'multiple myeloma' which was first used by Rusitizy in 1873 (Salmon & Cassady 1989). Rarely, the disease presents as a solitary localised tumour known as a plasmacytoma and this is considered to be an indication of significant risk of eventually developing myeloma (International Myeloma Foundation 1994).

A diagnosis of multiple myeloma is usually reached when at least two of the criteria in Table 5.1 are found.

Clinical manifestations

Symptoms of the disease occur (a) directly from the excessive malignant plasma cell proliferation within the bone and (b) indirectly from the secreted products of the abnormal immunoglobulins throughout the body (Fig. 5.2).

Symptoms of skeletal involvement

Sixty-eight to eighty per cent of individuals will present with symptoms which are secondary to the inevitable bone destruction resulting from osteolytic lesions. Severe pain usually on movement and relieved on rest is frequently the presenting symptom. Other symptoms of skeletal involvement include:

- hypercalcaemia
- pathological fractures (especially of the ribs and clavicle)
- vertebral collapse with spinal cord compression.

Bone pain is typically dull or aching and is usually felt in the spine, ribs or pelvis and less frequently in the extremities. The pain is a

Table 5.1 Diagnostic criteria

Diagnostic test	Finding
Bone marrow aspirate/ biopsy	Shows an increase in abnormal, atypical or immature plasma cells in the bone marrow
Immunoelectrophoresis of urine	Presence of free light chains in the urine (Bence Jones protein – after Henry Bence Jones who described it in 1850)
Serum protein	The paraprotein produced by myeloma cells is found in the serum
Skeletal survey	X-rays show lytic lesions (punched out holes) where plasma cell tumours have eroded bone Lytic lesions are visible on X-ray when >30% of a bone has been destroyed (International Myeloma Foundation 1994) Approximately 70% of patients will have these X-ray findings at some stage of the disease (Alexanian 1985)

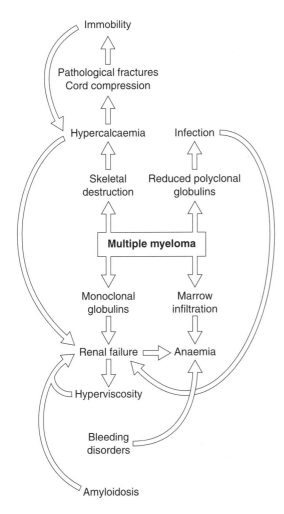

Figure 5.2 Complications of multiple myeloma (from Workman et al 1993, reproduced with permission)

result of the tumour pressing on the periosteum of the bone and also of bone demineralisation. In its end stages, multiple myeloma may be among the most painful of all cancers (Souhami & Tobias 1995).

Bone marrow involvement
Anaemia
Erythrocytes are the blood cells primarily affected in multiple myeloma; therefore, at the time of diagnosis 60% of all patients with myeloma will have anaemia (Riccardi et al 1991). The anaemia is usually accounted for by the presence of an intense plasma cell infiltration of the bone marrow and the decreased

production of erythrocytes. Renal failure is also a contributory factor, as are low endogenous erythropoietin levels (Thompson & Proctor 1985). Furthermore, myeloma proteins can coat erythrocytes in the peripheral circulation, causing stacking of erythrocytes, similar to a roll of coins (Rouleux formation), with resulting stagnation of erythrocytes in the capillary bed and erythrocyte destruction (Duffy 1992). Clinical features of anaemia include dyspnoea on exertion, fatigue and weakness.

Thrombocytopenia
Thrombocytopenia is not usually present until the later stages of the disease, and results largely from treatment or marrow replacement by myeloma cells (Thompson & Proctor 1985). Thrombocytopenia can contribute to an increased risk of bleeding, which further aggravates the individual's anaemia. Abnormal bleeding may occur in myeloma due to the paraprotein interfering with the normal function of platelets and coagulation factors.

Infection
Infection is the cause of death in at least 50% of myeloma patients (Oken 1984), pneumonia being a major risk. Many factors contribute to an increased risk of infection, including the neutropenia that may occur in advanced stages of the disease or secondary to chemotherapy. However, individuals with myeloma may contract infections with near normal neutrophil counts and both the decreased number of circulating immunoglobulins and the inability to generate antibodies are the most notable factors in the susceptibility to infection. It occurs most frequently and intensely in IgM myeloma, and to a lesser extent in cases producing Bence Jones proteins only (Souhami & Tobias 1995).

Hyperviscosity syndrome
Normal plasma viscosity is 1.8 centipoises (cP). If the viscosity exceeds 5 cP then the signs and symptoms of hyperviscosity syndrome are present (Thompson & Proctor 1985). Hyperviscosity syndrome results in circulatory impairment; for instance, intermittent claudication is a result of the occlusion of small blood vessels with M-protein. The M-protein also interferes

with circulation in the vessels of the retina, causing visual disturbances, retinal haemorrhages and papilloedema. Neurological symptoms may also occur due to circulatory impairment and include irritability, headache, drowsiness, confusion and even coma (Barton Cook 1990). Bleeding tendencies may result from hyperviscosity and are manifested by bruising, epistaxis, purpura and oozing from the mucosal surfaces (Bubley & Schipper 1991). Spontaneous haemorrhage may occur in the absence of hyperviscosity due to the M-protein coating the platelet and interfering with platelet aggregation. Additionally, IgM myeloma may cause cold precipitation, which results in vascular disturbances in the extremities due to intra-capillary agglutination of red cells in parts of the body exposed to cold (Souhami & Tobias 1995). Hyperviscosity may also cause renal failure, with clotting and bleeding within the renal vessels compromising renal function.

Renal failure

Renal insufficiency is common in individuals with myeloma and is one of the commonest causes of death. It is identified on routine serum chemistry (e.g. elevated blood urea nitrogen, creatinine and calcium levels) and may be present at diagnosis or develop at any stage in the disease (Sheridan 1996). However, its presence at diagnosis indicates a poor prognosis.

Other than hyperviscosity, causes of renal failure include hypercalcaemia and excretion of light-chain proteins (Alexanian et al 1990). In hypercalcaemia the destruction of bone frees excessive amounts of calcium which the renal tubules cannot filter. 'Myeloma kidney', an excess of light chains deposited in the renal tubules, may also contribute to renal failure (Souhami & Tobias 1995). In attempting to filtrate these proteins, increased demands are placed on the proximal tubules. Degeneration and atrophy of tubule cells result from the accumulation of large protein casts which cause obstruction, dilatation and fibrosis.

Other factors such as amyloid deposits and hyperuricaemia also contribute to the development of renal failure (Souhami & Tobias 1995). Amyloid is a deposition of a fibrillar substance, of which there are various varieties, and is largely due to abnormalities in protein metabolism. AL amyloid, also called primary amyloidosis, is derived from the light-chain immunoglobulin, and may occur with multiple myeloma. The amyloids are deposited in extracellular spaces of the kidneys, but may also be found in the blood vessels of other organs, and change the function of tissues and cells (Damjanov 1996). Amyloid deposition in the blood vessels of the glomerulus occurs in 10% of people with myeloma, especially among those who excrete light chains alone. Dehydration and infection can further impair renal excretion.

Hyperuricaemia may also result in renal failure, due to the precipitation of uric acid crystals in the renal tubules (Fig. 5.3).

Spinal cord compression

Spinal cord compression (SCC) may result directly from tumour growth and metastases and occurs when bony metastases in the epidural space encroach upon the spinal cord or caudal equina (Otto 1994). SCC is an oncological emergency and those with thoracic spine lesions are at greatest risk of developing this condition. Pain or sensorimotor impairment such as numbness and paraesthesia are indicative of SCC (Dahlstrom et al 1979).

Hypercalcaemia

Hypercalcaemia should be suspected in a patient with myeloma who has nausea, fatigue, vomiting, polyuria, constipation, lethargy, confusion or drowsiness. In myeloma, hypercalcaemia is chiefly attributable to the direct bony destruction caused by osteoclastic activity resulting in the release of calcium from the bone into the blood. The tumour itself may also produce the highly potent OAF, which enhances osteoclastic activity.

TREATMENT

Currently, patients with asymptomatic disease are not usually treated until they become symptomatic. However, systemic antineoplastic

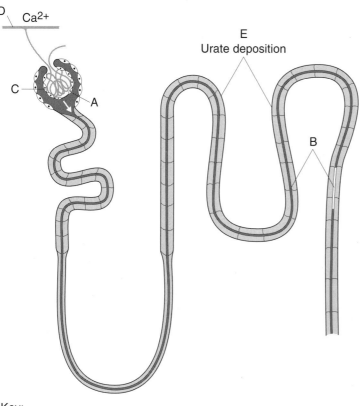

Figure 5.3 Renal damage in myeloma (Souhami & Tobias 1995, reproduced with permission)

Key:
A   Free light chains cross the glomerular basement membrane
B   Free light chains are deposited in cells of the distal tubule and
    collecting system and fill the collecting tubule causing obstruction
C   Amyloid is deposited in the glomerulus
D   Hypercalcaemia reduces glomerular filtration rate
E   Hyperuricaemia leads to distal tubular and interstitial urate deposition

therapy and more intensive treatments are resulting in longer remissions. Symptom control remains the main goal of therapy, aiming to optimise survival times and improve individual quality of life.

Chemotherapy

The alkylating agents, most commonly, melphalan and cyclophosphamide, have been used to treat multiple myeloma since the 1960s. These drugs may be used alone or in combination with prednisolone (often given in enteric-coated form as the doses tend to be high) (Souhami & Tobias 1995). Prednisolone potentiates the action of alkylating agents and their combined use has improved the remission rate (Souhami & Tobias 1995). It is believed that prednisolone affects the disease by inducing a hypercatabolism of proteins, which results in a negative nitrogen balance and a decrease in serum protein concentrations (Bergsagel & Rider 1985). Melphalan and prednisolone remain the 'gold standard' for initial treatment, as this combination produces a 50–60% response rate with a median survival of 2 to 3 years (Alexanian & Dimopoulos 1995).

Approximately 75% of persons with myeloma will respond to oral chemotherapy, showing improvements in symptoms, particularly pain and hypercalcaemia (Souhami & Tobias 1995). However, most individuals will experience progression of the disease as responses are generally short term. It is rarely considered necessary to continue initial treatment, beyond 6–9 courses for those individuals who respond to treatment, as a 'plateau' phase is reached and little further can be gained (Souhami & Tobias 1995).

Individuals receiving the 'gold standard' combination of melphalan and prednisolone require close monitoring of their renal function, and the dose of melphalan should be reduced if renal insufficiency occurs (Sheridan 1996). Allopurinol is usually administered with chemotherapy to reduce the potential for renal failure from the precipitation of uric acid crystals and the breakdown products of tumour cells lysed by chemotherapy (Barton Cook 1990).

Other treatments

More recently, high-dose chemotherapy followed by bone marrow transplant or autologous peripheral blood stem cell transplantation has shown encouraging results for younger patients (Anderson 1993).

Interferon-α has also been used to treat myeloma, particularly for prolonging the plateau phase achieved by chemotherapy (Anderson 1993). However, interferon is associated with significant side-effects: fatigue, flu-like syndrome, thrombocytopenia and neurological toxicity. Furthermore, a review of current research findings indicates that it has not shown significant impact in overall survival and is not currently recommended for either induction or maintenance therapy (Sheridan 1996).

Radiotherapy

Palliative radiotherapy is particularly useful in cases of skeletal destruction and lesions causing spinal cord or nerve root compression. Multiple myeloma is highly radio-responsive and large doses are infrequently necessary (Souhami & Tobias 1995). Severe and exhausting bone pain can be rapidly relieved by radiotherapy (Barton Cook 1990).

Pathological fractures may also be treated with radiotherapy. In some cases surgical internal fixation may be performed as a prophylactic measure to reduce the possibility of fracture before radiotherapy. If a fracture does occur in an area of diseased bone, internal fixation is required, as bone invaded by myeloma cells will not heal.

Emergency radiotherapy combined with high-dose steroid therapy is also used in the treatment of spinal cord compression and usually results in a significant improvement in symptoms. However, if paralysis has already occurred, emergency treatment will usually only prevent further worsening of the patient's disability (Salmon & Cassady 1989).

Treatment of pain

Severe bone pain is reported as the most distressing symptom experienced with this illness (Megliola 1980). Pain management is therefore a priority and a variety of methods are used, including opiates, non-steroidal anti-inflammatory drugs, chemotherapy and radiotherapy.

Non-steroidal anti-inflammatory drugs are often more effective for bony pain than opiates; however, their use has been associated with renal failure in individuals with myeloma and renal function requires close observation (Rota et al 1987).

Chemotherapy may also alleviate pain. Some individuals respond within days of commencing chemotherapy; whereas others may take 2–3 months to respond (Megliola 1980). Radiotherapy is extremely useful in controlling bone pain due to localised areas of bone disease (Barton Cook 1990).

Treatment of hypercalcaemia

Bisphosphonates such as pamidronate are now the drugs of choice in the treatment of hypercalcaemia. They are extremely effective in reducing calcium levels, as they inhibit bone reabsorption by osteoclasts (Dibbs & McIntyre 1994). Additionally, urinary excretion of calcium is encouraged through administration of intravenous fluids and the administration of frusemide prevents reabsorption of calcium by the kidneys (Hays & Rafferty 1982). Corticosteroids may also be administered and act by blocking the action of OAFs.

Plasmapheresis

Plasmapheresis may be necessary for the treatment of hyperviscosity syndrome. This is a process where plasma is removed from the blood by centrifugation and the cellular elements are transfused back into the patient (see Ch. 11). Plasmapheresis results in a reduced serum viscosity and subsequent reduction in vascular sludging, thereby reducing the possibility of thrombosis or vascular occlusion.

 Reflection point

Consider how comprehensive the assessment of individuals with myeloma must be in order to plan appropriate nursing care.

SPECIFIC NURSING ISSUES

Multiple myeloma is a chronic disease with no known cure and development of life-threatening complications is a constant risk. A sound knowledge of the disease process is therefore vital for effective nursing management. Major goals are:

1. Preventing life-threatening disruption to body chemistry and the immune system.
2. Relief of pain and discomfort and reduction in the severity of symptoms in an attempt to increase normal function and activities.

The disease process and its treatment results in chronic and acute symptomatic episodes. Nursing management is therefore challenging and nursing goals may vary and change over time, which requires ongoing assessment, evaluation and review (Sheridan 1996).

Management of pain

Successful management of pain, like any other symptom of disease, must begin with an accurate assessment, and this assessment should be ongoing (Ferrell & Ferrell 1995). The utilisation of a pain-assessment tool assists in achieving an accurate and objective assessment. A large number of pain-assessment tools have been developed to measure the multidimensional components of pain. However, many of these instruments are primarily intended to be used in research (Paice 1996); therefore their use in nursing practice is limited. The simplest unidimensional pain-assessment instrument requires the individual to rate their pain from 0 'no pain', to 10 'the worst pain imaginable' (Numeric Pain Intensity Scale). Because pain *intensity* is such an important aspect of pain, this scale is an excellent means of evaluating the success of specific interventions for pain (McGuire & Sheidler 1997). However, it is also important to measure pain *distress*, as pain is an individual experience, and a patient reporting mild to moderate pain intensity may report a great deal of pain distress (Ferrell & Ferrell 1995). Furthermore, it is important to evaluate the effectiveness of pain relief by employing a pain relief score on a 0–100% scale (Paice 1996).

The management of pain is a multidisciplinary team effort, and nurses must collaborate with medical colleagues in sharing information about individuals' responses to medication, thus ensuring that they receive appropriate medication, at the optimal dosages, with minimal side-effects (Rose 1997).

Non-pharmacological interventions, such as relaxation, guided imagery, distraction, transcutaneous electrical nerve stimulation (TENS), and other similar interventions, are also useful for pain management in cancer. Evidence of their value is largely anecdotal, so it is hard to generalise about their benefits (Rose 1997). However, cancer patients have reported their acceptance and desire for more complementary therapy (Burke & Sikora 1992). Furthermore, any measure which creates a sense of well-being in the individual with myeloma is welcome. Non-pharmacological interventions should be employed in conjunction with, rather than as a replacement for, pharmacological therapies (Paice 1996). These techniques should be taught early in the illness, as practice is required and may not be possible when fatigue becomes a problem.

Reflection point

What are the potential difficulties in pain management for an individual with myeloma?

Case study 5.1

Angela O'Neill is 42 years old and was diagnosed with multiple myeloma almost 3 years ago, 18 months after the birth of her first child. She believes that she developed myeloma as a result of chronic exposure to mercury and radiation in her many years as a dental nurse. She was very ill at diagnosis, requiring urgent treatment for severe anaemia, renal failure and cardiomyopathy. Angela is extremely well-informed on myeloma and actively seeks information. She accessed the case histories of other people with myeloma via the International Myeloma Foundation on the Internet and found this most helpful in making her decision on treatments.

Angela describes her experience of the disease as a 'lonely journey'. She failed to respond to two chemotherapy regimens – vincristine, busulphan, melphalan, cyclophosphamide and prednisolone (VBMCP) and vincristine, etoposide and dexamethasone (VED) – but did eventually respond well to autologous peripheral stem cell transplantation performed early in 1996. Her monoclonal band (the myeloma protein produced from a single form which shows up as a sharp spike in the serum electrophoresis test), reduced and she enjoyed 9 months of what she described as relatively good quality of life. However, Angela's monoclonal band has been steadily increasing over the past year, despite receiving another three cycles of VBMCP.

Continued

Case study 5.1 *Continued*

Angela was readmitted to hospital last week complaining of severe back pain. Initial investigation suggests that the cause is not her myeloma, but perhaps an existing lumbar disc injury. (However, the back pain was subsequently found to be due to bone destruction from the myeloma.) Pain control has been a difficult process. Angela cannot receive non-steroidal anti-inflammatory drugs due to her history of renal failure and low platelet count (WBC – 2.7×10^9/L; Hb – 10.1g/dl; platelets – 24×10^9/L), and morphine has not been useful in controlling her pain. After 4 days of intervention, the introduction of diazepam and TENS (transcutaneous electrical nerve stimulation) has brought some control over her pain.

Angela has described this admission as offering her a chance for some 'time out'. Since her main concern now is to have her pain managed she does not have to make a decision about having more chemotherapy. However, she finds that the feelings of uncertainty for her future are never far away, and it is this uncertainty that she finds the most difficult to bear.

Prevention of pathological fractures

Once pain control has been established, patients should be encouraged to mobilise, as mobilisation decreases calcium reabsorption from the bone and increases skeletal strength (Megliola 1980). However, mobilisation is frequently difficult, as activity may result in a worsening of existing pain and/or pathological fracture (Megliola 1980). Education of the patient and their family in providing a safe environment and removal of any obstacles that might interfere with mobilisation is important. Additionally, aids to mobilisation such as walking sticks may be helpful.

Prevention of renal failure

A high fluid intake is essential to reduce precipitation of uric acid crystals, calcium and Bence Jones proteins and the associated potential for renal failure (Barton Cook 1990). If renal failure does develop, it can also be reversed if fluid intake is increased (Alexanian et al 1990). The importance of a daily fluid intake of at least 2 to 3 litres should be explained to the patient and their family.

Consistent daily monitoring of fluid intake and output is essential, particularly if renal incompetence is already evident. Intravenous fluids should be given in preparation for any diagnostic testing requiring nil by mouth.

Prevention of infection

See Chapter 13.

Prevention of cardiovascular problems

This is managed mainly by correcting anaemia (see Ch. 11).

Prevention of hypercalcaemia

Hypercalcaemia (normal calcium = 2.3–2.6 mmol/L) is a common complication of multiple myeloma, especially in those experiencing increased bone destruction, and has a profound negative effect on quality of life (MacConnachie 1997). Nursing care is aimed at early detection and support through treatment (Otto 1994). A thorough nursing assessment should include a history of the patient's myeloma and its treatment and an investigation of all medications, since certain drugs such as thiazide diuretics may cause or potentiate hypercalcaemia (Otto 1994).

Renal excretion of calcium is enhanced by a high fluid intake and an intake of 3 litres daily will help reduce the potential for hypercalcaemia. Individuals should also be encouraged to be physically active, as this reduces release of calcium from bone. Weight-bearing through standing and ambulating produces physical stress at the ends of long bones, resulting in osteoblastic activity. Osteoblasts synthesise the collagen and glycoproteins that form the bone matrix. Wherever possible, less mobile individuals should be helped to stand at the bedside for short periods (several minutes, four to six times a day) (Otto 1994).

Hypercalcaemia often reoccurs and can herald the end stages of myeloma (Clayton 1997). It is an oncological emergency and prompt recognition is of vital importance. The individual with myeloma and their relatives must be educated in preventing hypercalcaemia and prompt recognition of its warning signs.

Prevention of constipation

Opioid therapy and the metabolic changes that accompany hypercalcaemia both contribute to the development of constipation in the individual with myeloma. It is vital that constipation is anticipated and adequately managed in order to avoid an unnecessary cause of discomfort and pain. Prevention and early detection of constipation is the goal. Elimination should be monitored daily with the goal of having a soft bowel motion daily, or less often if consistent with the individual's usual pattern of elimination (Curtiss 1996).

Assessment of constipation should be ongoing and necessitates an attentive history and physical examination. Assessment may be assisted by the use of the Constipation Assessment Scale (Macmillan & Williams 1989), which is easy to use and empirically tested for reliability and validity.

The usual measures to prevent and treat constipation are not always appropriate with myeloma. Increasing dietary fluid and fibre may not be tolerated due to other symptoms such as fatigue and reduced appetite, and may not be sufficient to prevent constipation (Curtiss 1996). Furthermore, exercise may be difficult. Therefore, daily stool softeners and peristaltic stimulators are both often required, especially for individuals receiving opioid analgesia (Curtiss 1996).

Spinal cord compression

Early recognition and treatment of SCC are imperative in preventing progression of this condition. Effects of SCC are irreversible and individuals may suffer paralysis if treatment is not initiated at an early stage. Recognition of the clinical manifestations of SCC is therefore an important part of the nurse's role. Patient teaching is of great importance to ensure patients notify staff immediately of any changes in their mobility or pain. Careful monitoring and assessment of patients is essential and if cord compression is suspected, appropriate treatment must be commenced immediately to prevent permanent damage.

CONCLUSION

Through vigilant monitoring, support and teaching, nurses can assist persons with myeloma to maximise their quality of living. Nursing care should strive to maintain a hopeful, caring environment. Quality of life, provision of support and fostering hope are considered to be key aspects of nursing (Barton Cook 1990, O'Berle & Davies 1992). Prompt recognition and identification of complications is essential in prolonging life and maintaining quality of life, and ongoing assessment and

evaluation of the patient, the effectiveness of treatment and nursing interventions is vital.

Education of the patient and their families is an important nursing role, and includes assisting the patient and their family to make treatment choices. It is crucial that the nurse acts as advocate so that the individual with myeloma can make informed decisions on treatment (Sheridan 1996).

DISCUSSION QUESTIONS

1. How do you view the advocate role of the nurse in caring for individuals with myeloma?
2. What information do individuals with myeloma require for decision making on treatment choices?
3. What are the treatment choices for the individual with myeloma?

References

Alexanian R 1985 Diagnosis and management of multiple myeloma. In: Wiernik P, Dutcher J, Kyle R, Cannelos G (eds) Neoplastic diseases of the blood. Churchill Livingstone, Edinburgh

Alexanian R, Dimopoulos M A 1995 Management of multiple myeloma. Seminars in Haematology 32: 20–30

Alexanian R, Barlogic B, Dixon D 1990 Renal failure in patients with multiple myeloma: pathogenesis and prognostic implications. Archives of Internal Medicine 150(8): 1693–1695

Anderson K 1993 Plasma cell tumours. In: Holland J, Frei E, Blast R (eds) Cancer medicine. Lea and Febiger, Philadelphia

Barton Cook M 1990 Multiple myeloma. In: Groenwald S, Hansen Frogge M, Goodman M, Henke Yarbo C (eds) Cancer

nursing, 3rd edn. Jones and Bartlett, Boston

Bergsagel D, Rider W 1985 Plasma cell neoplasms. In: DeVita V, Helman S, Rosenberg S (eds) Cancer: principles and practice of oncology, 2nd edn. J B Lippincott, Philadelphia

Bubley G, Schipper LE 1991 Multiple myeloma. In: Holleb A (ed) Textbook of clinical oncology. American Cancer Society, Atlanta

Burke C, Sikora K 1992 Cancer – the dual approach. Nursing Times 88(38): 62–66

Clayton K 1997 Cancer-related hypercalcaemia: how to spot it, how to manage it. American Journal of Nursing 97(5): 42–49

Curtiss C 1996 Constipation. In: Groenwald S, Hansen Frogge M, Goodman M, Henke Yarbo C (eds) Cancer symptom management,

4th edn. Jones and Bartlett, Boston

Dahlstrom U, Jarpe S, Lindstrom F 1979 Paraplegia in myelomatosis: a study of 20 cases. Acta Medico Scandinavica 205: 173–178

Damjanov I 1996 Pathology for health-related professionals, W B Saunders, Philadelphia

Dibbs C, McIntyre R 1994 Endocrine and metabolic disorders. In: Alexander M, Fawcett J, Runciman P (eds) Nursing practice: hospital and home – the adult. Churchill Livingstone, Edinburgh

Duffy T P 1992 The many pitfalls of diagnosis of myeloma. New England Journal of Medicine 326: 394–396.

Ferrell B R, Ferrell B 1995 Pain in elderly patients. In: McGuire D, Henke Yarbo C, Ferrell B R (eds) Cancer pain

management, 2nd edn. Jones and
Bartlett, Boston

Foerster J 1993 Multiple myeloma.
In: Lee R, Bithell T, Foerster J et al
(eds) Wintrobe's clinical
haematology, Vol. 2. Lea and
Febiger, Philadelphia

Hays, K, Rafferty D 1982 Care of
the patient with multiple myeloma.
Nursing Clinics of North America
17(4): 677–695

International Myeloma Foundation
1994 Myeloma Today 1 (6,7):
spring/summer

MacConnachie A M 1997
Pamidronate (Aredia, Ciba) in
malignant hypercalcaemia.
Intensive and Critical Care Nursing
13(1): 58–59

McGuire D B, Sheidler V R 1997
Pain. In: Groenwald S, Hansen
Frogge M, Goodman M, Henke
Yarbo C (eds) Cancer nursing,
4th edn. Jones and Bartlett,
Boston

Macmillan S C, Williams F A 1989
Validity and reliability of the
Constipation Assessment Scale.
Cancer Nursing 12: 183–188.

Megliola B 1980 Multiple myeloma.
Cancer Nursing 3(3): 209–218

Mundy G R 1987 Bone
reabsorption and turnover in health
and disease. Bone 8, Suppl. 1: 9

O'Berle K, Davies B 1992 Support
and caring: exploring the concepts.
Oncology Nursing Forum 19(5):
763–767

Oken M 1984 Multiple myeloma.
Medical Clinics of North America
68: 757–787

Otto S 1994 Oncology nursing.
Mosby, St Louis

Paice J 1996 Pain. In: Groenwald S,
Hansen Frogge M, Goodman M,
Henke Yarbo C (eds)
Cancer symptom management,
4th edn. Jones and Bartlett,
Boston

Riccardi A, Gobbi P G, Ucci G
et al 1991 Changing clinical
presentation of multiple myeloma.
European Journal of Cancer 27:
1401–1405

Riedel D A, Pottern L M 1992 The
epidemiology of multiple myeloma.
Haematology Oncology Clinics of
North America 6: 225–247

Rose K 1997 Pain management in
advanced cancer. Nursing Standard
15(11): 49–52

Rota S, Moungenot B, Baundovin B
et al 1987 Multiple myeloma and
severe renal failure: a clinico-
pathologic study of outcome and
prognosis in 34 patients. Medicine
66: 126–137

Salmon S, Cassady J 1989 Plasma
cell neoplasms. In: DeVita V,
Helman S, Rosenberg S (eds)
Cancer: principles and practice of
oncology, 3rd edn. J B Lippincott,
Philadelphia

Sheridan C 1996 Multiple myeloma.
Seminars in Oncology Nursing
12(1): 59–69

Souhami R, Tobias S 1995 Cancer
and its management, 2nd edn.
Blackwell Science, Oxford

Thompson R B, Proctor S J 1985 A
short textbook of haematology, 6th
edn. Pitman, London

Velez R, Beral V, Cuzick J 1982
Increasing trends of multiple
myeloma mortality in England &
Wales 1950–1979: are the changes
real? Journal of National Cancer
Institute 69: 387–392

Workman M, Ellerhurst-Ryan J,
Hargrave-Koetse V 1993 Nursing
care of the immunocompromised
patient. W B Saunders,
Philadelphia

Further reading

**Alexanian R, Dimopoulos M
1994 Drug therapy: the treatment of multiple myeloma.
New England Journal of
Medicine 330(7): 484–489**
A clearly written and comprehensive review of drug therapy for
myeloma.

**Belcher A 1993 Blood disorders.
Mosby, St Louis**
This colourful book has a chapter
outlining the care planning
process for myeloma patients.

6 *The lymphomas*

MAGGIE GRUNDY

> **Key points**
> - The lymphomas are a diverse group of diseases arising from lymphoid tissue
> - Lymphomas comprise two distinct groups: Hodgkin's disease and non-Hodgkin's lymphoma
> - Accurate classification and staging of the disease are important in ensuring optimum treatment and management
> - Many lymphomas are potentially curable

INTRODUCTION

The lymphomas are a diverse group of malignant diseases arising from lymphoid tissue. First described by Thomas Hodgkin in 1832 they were originally thought to be of an infectious rather than a malignant nature. The lymphomas can be divided into two distinct groups: Hodgkin's disease (HD), characterised by the large nucleated Reed–Sternberg cell, and non-Hodgkin's lymphoma (NHL), which encompasses all other types of lymphoma. Both these groups contain a number of subtypes of lymphoma and accurate identification of the specific subtype is important in determining prognosis and the most effective treatment and management. This chapter intends to illustrate the similarities and differences between HD and NHL and to outline their treatment and specific nursing management.

THE DISEASES

Incidence

The incidence of HD in the UK is approximately 2.4 per 100 000 a year, with between 1000–1500 new cases diagnosed annually. Two age-related peaks in incidence are apparent, the first in young adults between the ages of 15 and 25 years and the second in those over 65 years of age (Sweetenham 1998).

NHL occurs mainly in the elderly. It is the seventh most common cancer in the UK, accounting for 3% of all new cases. The incidence is approximately 11 per 100 000 a year, with between 7000–7500 new cases diagnosed annually (Cancer Research Campaign 1998). The incidence of NHL has increased dramatically worldwide in the last 20 years by approximately 3–4% per year. In the UK, NHL is approximately four times more common than HD, for which incident rates have remained relatively stable (Cancer Research Campaign 1998). The reasons for the increasing incidence of NHL remain unclear. The incidence of human immunodeficiency virus (HIV)-related lymphomas, improved diagnostic techniques and newer classification systems are all suggested as contributory factors. However, the increase is thought to be too great to be attributed to these factors alone (Sweetenham 1997).

Overall, both NHL and HD are commoner in men than women, except for the nodular sclerosing subtype of HD, which has a higher incidence in young females (Leukaemia Research Fund 1997).

HD is a potentially curable disease with standardised mortality rates being halved between 1988 and 1997 (Sweetenham 1998). Many subtypes of NHL are also curable, although there is still a significant mortality rate (Box 6.1).

Pathophysiology

Hodgkin's disease is characterised by the Reed–Sternberg cell, but the origin of this cell

---

Box 6.1   Risk factors

Hodgkin's disease	Non-Hodgkin's lymphoma
Risk factors remain unclear. Racial, genetic, social and infectious factors have all been implicated (Mack et al 1995, Meeiros & Greiner 1995, Gutensohn 1982)	Exposure to pesticides, hair-dye, and sunlight have all been implicated, but their impact as causative agents remains unproven (Zahm et al 1990, Adami et al 1995, Faustini et al 1996)
In the United States HD is commoner in Whites than in Blacks	Exposure to radiation, previous treatment with cytotoxic drugs and advancing age increase the risk of developing NHL
Those in higher social classes have increased risk of non-sclerosing HD (NSHD) and there is an increased incidence of other subtypes of HD associated with lower social class	Immunosuppressed individuals, such as those with HIV (Ziegler et al 1984), or recipients of organ transplants, especially renal and cardiac, have an increased incidence of lymphoma (Ultman & Jacobs 1985, Ioachim 1987)
The Epstein–Barr virus is strongly associated with HD (Jarrett et al 1996)	Infectious agents such as the Epstein–Barr virus (Klein 1991) and the human T-cell lymphoma virus-1 (HTLV-1) have also been associated with the development of NHL (Tajima 1990)
	Helicobacter pylori infection has been identified as a risk factor in gastric NHL (Wotherspoon et al 1991)
	Genetic susceptibility and chromosomal abnormalities, particularly of chromosomes 8, 14, 11 and 18, are commonly identified although their significance is unknown (Maloney 1995)

---

is uncertain, whereas non-Hodgkin's lymphomas originate from B or T lymphocytes (Mead 1998). Normal B and T lymphocytes are involved in cellular and humoral immunity. In lymphoma, cellular function may be abnormal, which may result in abnormal immunoglobulin secretion in B-cell lymphoma; whereas in T-cell lymphoma increased activation of lymphokines and macrophages may destroy normal blood cells, resulting in anaemia, neutropenia and thrombocytopenia (Rahr & Tucker 1990).

Lymphoma cells can infiltrate tissue, destroying normal structure, and lymphatic tissue, organs and the bone marrow may all be infiltrated. Lymph nodes are often the primary site of involvement, although lymphatic tissue outwith the nodes can also be affected. The most common presentation is a painless swelling of one group of lymph nodes. In HD the cervical nodes are most frequently affected first, although the mediastinal, axillary and inguinal nodes may also be the primary site. HD tends to follow a predictable course, with the disease progressing from one group of lymph nodes to adjacent groups, and is likely to be diagnosed at an early stage. Progression of NHL is less predictable and many patients have widespread or extranodal disease on diagnosis (Hughes-Jones & Wickramasinghe 1996) (Plates 4 and 5).

Clinical features

Painless, localised lymphadenopathy is frequently the only manifestation of HD. However, if the disease is more extensive, generalised lymphadenopathy and/or systemic symptoms such as general malaise, fever, night sweats, unexplained weight loss and pruritis may be present. Pain in affected lymph nodes with alcohol consumption has also been reported (Hoffbrand & Pettit 1993).

NHL may also present as painless, localised or generalised lymphadenopathy. Systemic symptoms are less likely to occur in NHL than in HD but extranodal involvement is more likely (Hughes-Jones & Wickramasinghe 1996). The gastrointestinal system is the commonest primary extranodal site, although primary disease is reported in most other organs (Sweetenham 1997). Gastrointestinal and central nervous system involvement are common in HIV-related lymphoma (Stanley et al 1991).

Clinical features depend on the extent and site of the disease. For example if mediastinal nodes are affected, respiratory symptoms such as cough or dyspnoea may be present and superior vena cava obstruction or pleural effusions may occur. Enlarged lymph nodes may cause pressure on other organs, resulting in pain or dysfunction. Obstruction of lymph drainage due to enlarged inguinal or axillary nodes may result in lymphoedema in upper or lower limbs. Anaemia or pancytopenia may be present if the bone marrow is involved. Hepatomegaly and splenomegaly may also be present if these organs are infiltrated.

Diagnosis

Lymph node biopsy is required for diagnosis and to determine the histology and classification of the lymphoma. Accurate histological classification and staging of the disease are important to ensure optimum treatment and management.

Classification

The presence of the giant Reed–Sternberg cell is diagnostic of HD and four subtypes of HD have been recognised since the 1960s:

■ nodular sclerosing
■ lymphoctye predominant
■ lymphoctye depleted
■ mixed cellularity.

(*Rye Classification of Hodgkin's disease*, Lukes et al 1966.)

The classification of NHL is more complicated. Difficulties have arisen in classifying NHLs because the immune system is, as yet, incompletely understood and classification schemes have continued to develop with increased knowledge. Several recognised systems have been used in recent years. The Kiel system devised by Lennert et al (1975) and updated by Stansfeld et al (1988) has been largely used in Europe and the Working Formula (Non-Hodgkin's Lymphoma Pathologic Classification Project 1982) in the USA (Box 6.2).

As different clinicians in different parts of the world have used different classification systems it is difficult to compare results of clinical trials, especially as subtypes of NHL appearing in one classification scheme do not always appear in the other. Furthermore, since these classifications were devised new disease subtypes have been recognised and in 1994 a new classification system the 'Revised European–American Classification of Lymphoid Neoplasms' (REAL) was proposed (Harris et al 1994). It is anticipated that this classification system will overcome the difficulties associated with other classification systems. The REAL classification includes Hodgkin's disease and consists of three categories:

■ B-cell
■ T-cell and putative natural killer cell neoplasms
■ Hodgkin's disease.

Box 6.2   Classifications of NHL

Updated Kiel system	Working formula
NHL is classified into categories, depending on whether it is thought to be of B or T cell origin. This system also categorises the aggressiveness of the tumour: high grade indicates a rapidly growing aggressive tumour and low grade indicates a slow growing, indolent tumour. The updated Kiel system therefore consists of four categories: low-grade B, high-grade B, low-grade T and high-grade T. Each of these categories contains a number of subtypes of NHL	NHL is classified into three categories, according to the aggressiveness of the tumour: high, intermediate and low grade. Again there are a number of disease subtypes in each category

---

Extranodal lymphomas are included within these categories. This classification system also recognises that not all presentations of lymphoma fit neatly into a category, and these are labelled unclassified cases. The REAL system no longer categorises lymphomas as high or low grade, as it is recognised that each individual subtype has a range of clinical aggressiveness and grading is thought to be an oversimplification of the clinical behaviour of a tumour (Harris et al 1994). However, Sweetenham (1997) states that many of the major subtypes of NHL can still be grouped into high, intermediate and low grade, depending on their clinical behaviour. This suggests that in practice, clinicians are likely to continue referring to grades of lymphoma.

The World Health Organization (WHO) is currently preparing a further classification of all haematological and lymphoid malignancies which is thought to be virtually identical to the REAL classification (Mason & Gatter 1998). Adoption of these newer classification systems worldwide is likely to reduce the difficulties and confusion associated with lymphoma classification. Classification of lymphomas is not, however, the only determinant of either prognosis or treatment.

Staging

Staging is undertaken to establish the extent of the disease and is a further determinant of prognosis and treatment. The Ann Arbor staging system was originally devised for HD based on the predictable progression of the disease (Carbone et al 1971) and, subsequently, modified slightly (Lister et al 1989). This staging system is also used in NHL but because of the unpredictable nature of NHL is less reliable as a prognostic indicator. The Ann Arbor staging system consists of four stages with stage I representing localised disease and stage IV representing advanced disease (Fig. 6.1).

- Stage I: one group of lymph nodes affected.
- Stage II: two or more groups of lymph nodes on the same side of the diaphragm affected.
- Stage III: one or more groups of lymph nodes on both sides of the diaphragm affected.
- Stage IV: extranodal disease present.

These four stages are also suffixed A or B. If an individual is asymptomatic, the suffix A is added. Whereas, systemic symptoms of night sweats, fever of over 38°C during the previous month, and a weight loss of >10% of body weight in the 6 months prior to diagnosis are indicated by the suffix B. The presence of B symptoms indicates more advanced disease.

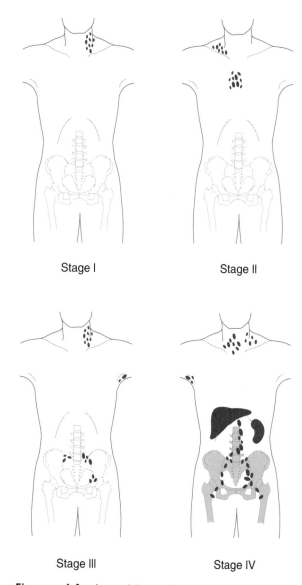

Stage I   Stage II

Stage III   Stage IV

Figure 6.1 Ann Arbor staging system (from Hoffbrand & Pettit 1993, reproduced with permission)

Additionally, localised extranodal involvement is indicated by the subscript E. Splenic involvement is frequently a precursor to widespread haematological spread and is classed as stage III$_s$ (Hoffbrand & Pettit 1993). A nodal mass of >10 cm in diameter, or widening of the mediastinum by more than one-third is classed as bulky disease and indicated by the subscript x. The presence of these subscripts indicates more advanced disease. The number of nodal areas affected may be

indicated by a numerical subscript: for example, stage II$_2$.

Staging is determined by both extensive clinical examination and a variety of investigations (Table 6.1). These investigations are mandatory, but further investigations may be undertaken if clinical indicators suggest involvement at a specific site (O'Reilly & Connors 1992).

Reflection point

Consider what support an individual undergoing staging investigations and their relatives/friends might require.

Prognostic indicators

It is now recognised that anatomical staging is no longer sufficient to determine prognosis and several prognostic indices have been developed. The presence or absence of adverse factors is a further determinant in treatment decisions. Approximately one-third of individuals with advanced HD fail to be cured with current treatment and it is estimated that a similar number of individuals are overtreated. Therefore, predicting the outcome of treatment allows identification of those who are unlikely to have a response to standard treatment and those who may benefit from reduced treatment (Hasenclever & Diehl 1998).

For individuals with early-stage HD, prognostic groups are favourable or unfavourable and are based on

- presence or absence of bulky mediastinal disease
- age <50 versus ≥50
- raised ESR <50 versus ≥50
- histological subtype (HD of mixed cellularity and lymphocyte depletion have a less favourable prognosis)
- extent and type of B symptoms
- number of disease sites

(Carde et al 1993).

For advanced HD a seven-factor prognostic scoring system has recently been identified (Hasenclever & Diehl 1998). This system predicts

Table 6.1 Staging investigations

Investigation	Findings
Full blood count	Normocytic, normochromic anaemia is common in both HD and NHL
	Eosinophilia may occur in some cases of HD
	Leucocytosis is present in approximately one-third of individuals with HD
	Reduced numbers of erythrocytes, leucocytes and platelets may occur in advanced disease if the bone marrow is involved
Erythrocyte sedimentation rate (ESR)	Frequently raised in HD especially if B symptoms present
Biochemical tests	Liver function may be abnormal if the liver is involved
	Raised serum lactate dehydrogenase levels indicate a poor prognosis
	Uric acid levels may be raised
Serum calcium levels	Hypercalcaemia may occur with bony involvement
Serum protein electrophoresis	Excess immunoglobulins may be secreted by some lymphomas
Chest X-ray	May show mediastinal involvement
Computerised tomography (CT) scan of chest, abdomen and pelvis	Provides information on presence and extent of organ involvement
Bone marrow aspiration and biopsy	Detects bone marrow involvement

5-year rates of freedom from disease and overall survival. Prognosis is determined by the number of adverse factors present at diagnosis. Adverse prognostic factors are identified as

- Hb $<10.5\,\text{g/L}$
- male
- stage IV disease
- age 45 or over
- white cell count $>15 \times 10^9/\text{L}$
- lymphocytopenia $<0.6 \times 10^9/\text{L}$ or $<8\%$ of total white cell count
- albumin $<4\,\text{g/L}$.

The presence of each factor reduces the 5-year failure-free survival by approximately 8%. For individuals with none of the adverse prognostic factors, 5-year failure-free survival was 84%.

In NHL five factors have been identified as predictors of outcome (Shipp et al 1993):

- age $\leqslant 60$ versus >60
- performance status 0 or 1 versus >2
- serum lactic dehydrogenase (LDH) levels $\leqslant 1$ times normal versus >1 times normal
- stage of disease – stage I or II versus stage III or IV
- number of extranodal sites involved $\leqslant 1$ versus >1.

Based on the number of prognostic indicators present at diagnosis, individuals are assigned to one of four risk groups:

■ low – score of 0 or 1
■ low intermediate – score of 2
■ high intermediate – score of 3
■ high – score of 4 or 5.

The low-risk group were found to have a 5-year overall survival of 73%, whereas in the high-risk group overall survival was 26%.

These indicators may be used as a basis for treatment decisions for individuals. For example those judged to be in the high-risk group may be considered for high-dose chemotherapy and BMT/PBSCT (bone marrow transplant/peripheral blood stem cell transplant) at an earlier stage. However, although these indicators are significantly more accurate predictors of prognosis than the Ann Arbor staging system, it is suggested that initial response to treatment remains the best indicator of survival (Johnson 1995).

TREATMENT

Hodgkin's disease

Both radiotherapy and chemotherapy are used in the treatment of HD and a high incidence of long-term disease-free survival has been achieved. At 5 years, survival rates are approximately 85% for stage I and II disease, 70% for stage IIIA and 50% for stages IIIB and IV (Hoffbrand & Pettit 1993). Both treatment modalities can be used either alone or in combination, depending on the stage of the disease.

Early-stage disease
Radiotherapy is used as a curative treatment for stage I and II disease except if bulky mediastinal disease is present. For several decades extended field radiotherapy techniques have been used to ensure treatment to all obviously diseased lymph nodes and adjacent, apparently normal lymph nodes at risk of containing subclinical disease. The 'mantle' technique includes all lymph node groups above the diaphragm and the 'inverted Y' technique

includes all lymph node groups below the diaphragm. (See Ch. 9 for further information on the mantle and inverted Y techniques.)

It is now recognised that these techniques (especially those involving the mediastinum) increase the risk of secondary malignancies, especially breast and lung cancer and other long-term effects such as pulmonary fibrosis and cardiac disease. Therefore, for individuals with stage II disease with mediastinal involvement, combined radiotherapy and chemotherapy is recommended (DeVita & Hubbard 1993). The inverted Y field was originally mainly used for treatment of stage III disease; however, chemotherapy is increasingly being used for stage III disease.

Optimum treatment for HD remains controversial. Recent research has focused on reducing the long-term toxicities of treatment, and clinical trials are ongoing. Results indicate that use of radiotherapy to include the involved area only and a short chemotherapy regimen produce similar long-term disease-free survival to extended field radiotherapy alone (Carde et al 1993, Horning et al 1997). However, these results need to be substantiated by longer-term studies.

Advanced disease
Combined radiotherapy and chemotherapy or chemotherapy alone may be used for stage III and IV disease. Combination chemotherapy is also used for stage I and II with bulky disease or B symptoms (Hoffbrand & Pettit 1993). The original, successful drug combination for HD was mechlorethamine, vincristine (Oncovin), procarbazine and prednisolone (MOPP). However, approximately one-fifth of patients either did not achieve complete remission with this regimen or relapsed shortly after completion of treatment (DeVita & Hubbard 1993). This was thought to be because of the development of drug resistance. Furthermore, successful treatment for HD unfortunately carried an increased risk of developing secondary leukaemias and myelodysplasia with a peak at 4 years (Hoffbrand & Pettit 1993). The alkylating agents have been identified as the greatest contributors to this, and different drug combinations have been investigated in an attempt to reduce the problems associated with drug resistance, the

risk of developing secondary malignancies and other long-term effects such as infertility.

Several drug combinations are commonly used as standard treatment for HD and there may be some variations between centres. A combination of doxorubicin (Adriamycin), bleomycin, vinblastine and dacarbazine (ABVD) has been found to be as effective and in some trials superior to MOPP in the treatment of HD (Canellos et al 1992). ABVD may be used alone or with MOPP in monthly alternate cycles. ABVD is less likely to cause infertility or induce secondary leukaemia than MOPP. Other centres use different combinations of drugs; for example, replacing mechlorethamine in the MOPP regime with chlorambucil (ChlVPP). A recent American study using the MOPP/ABV hybrid regimen has demonstrated a significantly increased 8-year overall survival compared to MOPP/ABVD, with a lower incidence of secondary leukaemia or myelodysplasia (Glick et al 1998). However, these results need to be substantiated by further studies.

Hodgkin's disease has a high 5-year failure-free survival rate. However, some individuals will relapse and the length of initial remission is related to the success of subsequent chemotherapy. Those who have an initial remission of over 1 year may well achieve a second lengthy remission with further chemotherapy, whereas those who relapse in under 1 year are unlikely to respond well to subsequent chemotherapy (Laport & Williams 1998). High-dose chemotherapy and autologous BMT/PBSCT offer a further chance of long-term remission for individuals who have relapsed. The optimum time for transplant and long-term toxicities associated with transplant in this group of individuals has yet to be determined.

Case study 6.1

Neil was diagnosed with stage IIIA Hodgkin's disease at the age of 23. He received combined treatment with chemotherapy and radiotherapy and 6 years later has recently married and remains disease free.

Non-Hodgkin's lymphoma
Low-grade lymphomas

Treatment of NHL is largely determined by histology and clinical aggressiveness. Generally, low-grade lymphomas (of which follicular lymphomas are the most common) are slow growing, indolent and currently incurable as most individuals are not diagnosed until the disease is at an advanced stage (Vose 1998). Individuals may be asymptomatic for several years and in asymptomatic individuals there currently appears to be no survival benefit from commencing curative chemotherapy at diagnosis. A period of watchful waiting commences where progression of the disease is monitored but treatment is not commenced until the patient becomes symptomatic.

Median overall survival for advanced disease is 8–10 years (Vose 1998). However, a minority of individuals will present with early-stage I or II disease and may be treated with involved field radiotherapy. This results in long-term disease-free survival in approximately 50% of people (Sweetenham 1997).

Interferon-α has also been investigated as a treatment in low-grade NHL. Interferon has been studied both alone and in combination with chemotherapy and although found to prolong remission in some individuals, to date, increased length of survival has not been demonstrated (Solal-Celigny et al 1993).

Individuals with symptomatic advanced low-grade disease are treated with either single-agent chemotherapy with chlorambucil or cyclophosphamide or combination chemotherapy regimens such as cyclophosphamide, doxorubicin, vincristine (Oncovin) and prednisolone (CHOP). Currently there appears to be no survival difference between these treatment options.

Individuals with low-grade lymphoma may benefit from high-dose chemotherapy and BMT/PBSCT; however, they may survive for lengthy periods of time without transplantation and the toxicities of this treatment and the potential for secondary malignancies need to be balanced against the slow progression of this form of lymphoma. Additionally, the optimum time for transplantation in low-grade

---

Box 6.3   Newer treatments

Hodgkin's disease	Non-Hodgkin's lymphoma
The use of immunotoxins mainly targeting CD30 antigen found on the Reed–Sternberg cell are being developed (Falini et al 1995)	The efficacy of the purine analogue drugs fludarabine and 2-chlordeoxyadenosine are currently being investigated in low-grade lymphomas
	Monoclonal antibodies are currently showing promise in clinical trials of treatment of B-cell NHL (Renner et al 1997, Scott 1998). Monoclonal antibodies bind with the antigen on the cell membrane, producing cell-mediated cytotoxicity and cell lysis. The advantage of monoclonal antibody treatment is that it is specific to the malignant cell and, unlike chemotherapy and radiotherapy, does not affect normal cells

---

lymphoma has yet to be determined (Horning 1997).

High-grade lymphomas

Aggressive tumours are rapidly fatal unless treated promptly. However, high-grade lymphomas are also extremely susceptible to chemotherapy and potentially curable. Most individuals have advanced disease at diagnosis, but a minority present with stage I disease for which treatment consists of a brief course of chemotherapy followed by involved field radiotherapy (Vose 1998).

Reflection point

Individuals with lymphoma face an uncertain future. Consider what help an individual may need to cope with this uncertainty.

For advanced disease, intensive combination chemotherapy is used with approximately 80% of individuals achieving a remission. However,

approximately 50% will relapse in the first 5 years (Johnson 1995). The CHOP drug regimen has been used for 30 years and, despite numerous clinical trials with newer chemotherapy regimens – including m-BACOD (methotrexate, bleomycin, doxorubicin (Adriamycin), cyclophosphamide, vincristine (Oncovin), dexamethasone); ProMACE-CytaBOM (prednisolone, doxorubicin (Adriamycin), cyclophosphamide, etoposide, cytarabine, bleomycin, vincristine (Oncovin), methotrexate); and MACOP-B (methotrexate, doxorubicin (Adriamycin), cyclophosphamide, vincristine (Oncovin), prednisolone, bleomycin) – none of these have so far shown improved survival rates.

Highly aggressive Burkitt's lymphomas and lymphoblastic lymphomas are treated with similar chemotherapy regimens to those for lymphoblastic leukaemia (see Ch. 4). If high-grade lymphomas recur or there is an incomplete response to initial chemotherapy, prognosis is generally poor although high-dose chemotherapy and autologous BMT may result in long-term remission (Philip et al 1995). However, many individuals with NHL are elderly and unsuitable for BMT/PBSCT procedures.

Palliative treatment

Radiotherapy is used as palliative treatment for both HD and NHL if organomegaly or lymphadenopathy are causing pain or dysfunction.

Surgery

Surgery has a small role in the treatment of NHL. Gastric lymphomas frequently present with acute abdominal pain and are frequently diagnosed at exploratory laparotomy and surgically excised.

Case study 6.2

Stuart, a 45-year-old man, was diagnosed with NHL 10 years ago. Following CHOP chemotherapy he experienced 6 disease-free years before his condition relapsed. A subsequent course of chemotherapy resulted in a further 4-year remission. At this time, Stuart experienced considerable difficulty swallowing and lost over a stone in weight. He was referred to the ear, nose and throat surgeons and, following a biopsy, Stuart was found to have a recurrence of NHL. He subsequently underwent high-dose chemotherapy and autologous BMT. Six months later he continues to do well.

Complications associated with HD and NHL

Tumour lysis syndrome

This syndrome is particularly likely with large bulky tumours. The high number of rapidly proliferating cells in high-grade lymphomas makes them particularly susceptible to chemotherapy. Rapid cell lysis may occur, resulting in a large circulating volume of the breakdown products of cell metabolism, which causes hyperuricaemia, hyperkalaemia, hyperphosphataemia and hypocalcaemia. The increased levels of these metabolites increases the demands on the kidneys for their excretion and may result in renal failure.

The cardiovascular and nervous systems may also be affected as a result of altered metabolite levels. Clinical manifestations of increased metabolite levels include nausea and vomiting, diarrhoea, lethargy and weakness, loin pain, haematuria, oliguria progressing to anuria and in severe cases renal failure, muscle cramps, paraesthesia, muscle twitching, carpopedal spasm, tetany, convulsions, hypotension, cardiac arrhythmias and cardiac arrest.

For those most at risk of tumour lysis syndrome, preventative measures should be implemented when chemotherapy is commenced. Renal failure is prevented by maintaining hydration with high-volume intravenous infusion. Uric acid is more soluble in an alkaline environment and sodium bicarbonate may be added to the fluid regimen to alkalinise urine, which helps to increase uric acid excretion. Urinary pH should be maintained at $\geqslant 7$ rather than the normal urinary pH of 5–6. Oral allopurinol is usually commenced 24 hours prior to the start of chemotherapy and decreases uric acid levels by altering purine metabolism. Diuretics may also be administered to aid in the dilution and excretion of urine.

Nursing management consists of close observation of the individual's condition. Accurate records of fluid balance should be maintained to ensure hydration and prevent fluid overload.

Superior vena cava obstruction

This may occur as a result of obstruction and pressure caused by the tumour and can be an oncological emergency. Clinical features include dyspnoea, cough, cyanosis with distension of the upper chest and neck veins and facial oedema. Raised intracranial pressure may result in dizziness, headache and visual disturbances.

Spinal cord compression

This is also an oncological emergency and occurs due to pressure on the spinal cord by the lymphoma. Nurses should be alert to warning signs of this condition. Complaints of pain, motor weakness, numbness or paraesthesia in the legs should be acted upon immediately. Prompt treatment with radiotherapy is required to prevent paralysis and irreversible damage.

Haemorrhage

Haemorrhage is a potential problem with gastrointestinal lymphomas (O'Reilly & Connors 1992).

SPECIFIC NURSING ISSUES

In common with individuals with other haematological malignancies, individuals with lymphoma are susceptible to a variety of side-effects associated with both the disease and its treatment and the related nursing issues are discussed in Section 3. Additionally, fatigue has been identified as a major problem for individuals with lymphoma (Persson et al 1995, 1997). Fatigue is now well recognised as problematic for individuals receiving chemotherapy and radiotherapy. Providing information about this side-effect is important as individuals can associate feelings of fatigue with worsening of their condition. Being forewarned can help the individual to develop coping strategies. Nurses also play an important role in assisting individuals to prioritise their activities and suggest interventions to reduce fatigue.

A number of psychological effects have been noted for individuals with lymphoma. Isolation, feelings of loss of control and living with uncertainty were particular issues for individuals with lymphoma and leukaemia in one retrospective Swedish study (Persson et al 1995). Raised levels of anxiety and depression have also been identified (Devlen et al 1987) and nurses need to be sensitive to individual needs and be ready to provide support (see Ch. 19).

Many lymphomas are potentially curable and individuals may experience prolonged disease-free survival. Younger individuals may want to start or add to their families and infertility may be a problem (see Ch. 18). Further problems may be experienced in relation to work, insurance and financial issues (see Ch. 20).

CONCLUSION

The lymphomas are a diverse group of diseases, many of which are potentially curable. For some individuals treatment will be successful and result in long-term disease-free survival. Others will experience a less-positive outcome. However, whatever the outcome of treatment, individuals with lymphoma and their relatives require both physical and psychological support to enable them to cope with the rigours of treatment, adjust to changed life circumstances and maintain quality of life.

DISCUSSION QUESTIONS

1. Many individuals with lymphoma are elderly. What issues might arise when an elderly person is receiving treatment for lymphoma?
2. What are the educational and informational needs of individuals with lymphoma?
3. What are the rehabilitation needs of individuals who are considered to be cured of their disease?

References

Adami J, Frisch M, Yuen J, Blimelius B, Melby M 1995 Evidence of an association between non-Hodgkin's lymphoma and skin cancer. British Medical Journal 310: 1491–1495

Cancer Research Campaign 1998 Factsheet 1.1 Incidence – UK. Cancer Research Campaign, London

Canellos G P, Anderson J R, Propert K J et al 1992 Chemotherapy of advanced Hodgkin's disease with MOPP, ABVD or MOPP alternating with ABVD. New England Journal of Medicine 327(21): 1478–1484

Carbone P P, Kaplan H S, Musshof K, Smithers D W, Tubiana M 1971 Report of the Committee on Hodgkin's disease Staging Classification. Cancer Research 31: 1860–1861

Carde P, Hagenbeek A, Hayat M et al 1993 Clinical staging versus laparotomy and combined modality MOPP versus ABVD in early stage Hodgkin's disease; the H6 Twin Randomized Trials from the European Organization for Research and Treatment of Cancer Lymphoma Cooperative Group. Journal of Clinical Oncology 11: 2258–2272

DeVita V T, Hubbard S M 1993 Hodgkin's disease. New England Journal of Medicine 328(8): 560–565

Devlen J, Maguire P, Phillips P, Crowther D, Chambers H 1987 Psychological problems associated with diagnosis and treatment of lymphomas. British Medical Journal 295: 953–957

Falini B, Pileri S, Pizzolo G et al 1995 CD30 (Ki-1) molecule: a new cytokine receptor of the tumour necrosis factor receptor superfamily as a tool for diagnosis and immunotherapy. Blood 85: 1–14

Faustini A, Settimi L, Pacifici R, Fano V, Zuccaro P, Forastiere F 1996 Immunological changes among farmers exposed to phenoxy herbicides: preliminary observations. Occupational and Environmental Medicine 53: 583–585

Glick J H, Young M L, Harrington D 1998 MOPP/ABV hybrid chemotherapy for advanced Hodgkin's disease significantly improves failure-free and overall survival: The 8 year results of the intergroup trial. Journal of Clinical Oncology 16: 19–26

Gutensohn N M 1982 Social class and age at diagnosis of Hodgkin's disease: new epidemiologic evidence for the 'two-disease hypothesis'. Cancer Treatment Reports 66: 689–695

Harris N L, Jaffe E S, Stein H et al 1994 A Revised European–American Classification of Lymphoid Neoplasms: A Proposal from the International Lymphoma Study Group. Blood 84(5): 1361–1392

Hasenclever D, Diehl V 1998 A prognostic score for advanced Hodgkin's disease. New England Journal of Medicine 339(21): 1506–1514

Hoffbrand A V, Pettit J E 1993 Essential haematology, 3rd edn. Blackwell Science, Oxford

Horning S J 1997 High-dose therapy and transplantation for low-grade lymphoma. Hematology/Oncology Clinics of North America 11(5): 919–935

Horning S J, Hoppe R T, Mason J et al 1997 Stanford-Kaiser Permanente G1 study for clinical stage I to IIA Hodgkin's disease: subtotal lymphoid irradiation versus vinblastine, methotrexate and bleomycin chemotherapy and regional irradiation. Journal of Clinical Oncology 15(5): 1736–1744

Hughes-Jones N C, Wickramasinghe S N (1996) Lecture notes on haematology, 6th edn. Blackwell Science, Oxford

Ioachim H L 1987 Neoplasms associated with immune deficiencies. Pathology Annual 22(part 2): 177–222

Jarrett R F, Armstrong A A, Alexander F A 1996 Epidemiology of EBV and Hodgkin's disease. Annals of Oncology 7(Suppl. 4): S5–S10

Johnson P W M 1995 The high grade non-Hodgkin's lymphomas. British Journal of Hospital Medicine 53(1/2): 14–19

Klein G 1991 Immunology of transforming viruses. Current Opinion in Immunology 3: 665–673

Laport G F, Williams S F 1998 The role of high-dose chemotherapy in patients with Hodgkin's disease and non-Hodgkin's lymphoma. Seminars in Oncology 25(4): 503–517

Lennert K, Mohri N, Stein H, Kaiserling E 1975 The histopathology of malignant lymphoma. British Journal of Haematology 31(Suppl.): 193–203

Leukaemia Research Fund 1997 The descriptive epidemiology of leukaemia and related conditions in parts of the United Kingdom 1984–1993. Leukaemia Research Fund, London

Lister T A, Crowther D, Sutcliffe S B et al 1989 Report of a committee convened to discuss the evaluation

and staging of patients with Hodgkin's disease: Cotswolds Meeting. Journal of Clinical Oncology 71(1): 1630–1636

Lukes R J, Craver L F, Hall T C et al 1966 Report on the nomenclature committee (on Hodgkin's disease). Cancer Research 26: 1311

Mack T M, Cozen W, Shibata D K et al 1995 Concordance for Hodgkin's disease in identical twins suggesting genetic susceptibility to the young-adult form of the disease. New England Journal of Medicine 332: 413–418

Maloney D G 1995 Non-Hodgkin's lymphoma. Current Opinion in Hematology 2: 255–261

Mason D, Gatter K 1998 The pocket guide to lymphoma classification. Blackwell Science, Oxford

Mead G M 1998 Malignant lymphomas and chronic lymphocytic leukaemia. In: Provan D, Henson A ABC of clinical haematology. BMJ Publishing Group, London, pp 47–50

Meeiros L J, Greiner T C 1995 Hodgkin's disease. Cancer 75: 357–369

O'Reilly S E, Connors J M 1992 Non-Hodgkin's lymphoma. I: characterisation and treatment. British Medical Journal 304: 1682–1686

Non-Hodgkin's Lymphoma Pathologic Classification Project 1982 National Cancer Institute sponsored study of classifications of non-Hodgkin's lymphomas: summary and description of a working formulation for clinical usage. Cancer 49: 2112–2135

Persson L, Hallberg I R, Ohlsson O 1995 Acute leukaemia and malignant Lymphoma – patients' experiences of disease, treatment and nursing care during the active treatment phase: an exploratory study. European Journal of Cancer Care 4: 133–142

Persson L, Hallberg I R, Ohlsson O 1997 Survivors of acute leukaemia and highly malignant lymphoma – retrospective views of daily life problems during treatment and when in remission. Journal of Advanced Nursing 25: 68–78

Philip T, Guglielmi C, Hagenbeek A et al 1995 Autologous bone marrow transplantation as compared to salvage treatment in relapses of chemotherapy – sensitive non-Hodgkin's lymphoma. New England Journal of Medicine 333: 1540–1545

Rahr V A, Tucker R 1990 Non-Hodgkin's lymphoma: understanding the disease. Cancer Nursing 13(1): 56–61

Renner C, Trumpter L, Pfreundschuh M 1997 Monoclonal antibodies in the treatment of non-Hodgkin's lymphoma: recent results and future prospects. Leukaemia 11(Suppl. 2): S55–S59

Scott S D 1998 Rituximab: a new therapeutic monoclonal antibody for non-Hodgkin's lymphoma. Cancer Practice 6(3): 195–197

Shipp M A, Harrington D P, Anderson J R et al 1993 The non-Hodgkin's lymphoma prognostic factors project: a predictive model for aggressive non-Hodgkin's lymphoma. New England Journal of Medicine 329(14): 987–994

Solal-Celigny P, Lepage E, Brousse N et al 1993 Recombinant Interferon Alfa-2b combined with a regimen containing doxorubicin in patients with advanced follicular lymphoma. New England Journal of Medicine 329: 608–1614

Stanley H, Fluetsch-Bloom M, Bunce-Clyma M 1991 HIV-related non-Hodgkin's lymphoma. Oncology Nursing Forum 18(5): 875–880

Stansfeld A, Diebold J, Kapanci Y et al 1988 Updated Kiel classification for lymphomas. Lancet 1: 292–293

Sweetenham J 1997 Cancer Research Campaign, Factsheet 10.1 Non-Hodgkins Lymphoma in Adults – UK. Cancer Research Campaign, London

Sweetenham J 1998 Cancer Research Campaign, Factsheet 27.1 Hodgkins Disease in Adults – UK. Cancer Research Campaign, London

Tajima K 1990 The 4th nation-wide study of adult T-cell leukaemia/ lymphoma (ATL) in Japan: estimates of risk of ATL and its geographical and clinical features. The T- and B-Cell Malignancy Study Group. International Journal of Cancer 45: 237–243

Ultman J E, Jacobs R H 1985 The non-Hodgkin's lymphomas. Ca: 35: 66–87

Vose J M 1998 Current approaches to the management of non-Hodgkin's lymphoma. Seminars in Oncology 25(4): 483–491

Wotherspoon A C, Ortiz-Hidalgo C, Falzon M R, Isaacson P G 1991 *Helicobacter pylori*-associated gastritis and primary B-cell gastric lymphoma. Lancet 338: 1175–1176

Zahm S H, Weisenburger D D, Babbit P A, Saal R C, Vaught J B, Blair A 1990 Use of hair colouring products and the risk of lymphoma, multiple myeloma and chronic lymphocytic leukaemia. American Journal of Public Health 82: 990–997

Ziegler J L, Beckstead J A, Volberding P A et al 1984 Non-Hodgkin's lymphoma in 90 homosexual men: relationship to generalized lymphadenopathy and acquired immunodeficiency syndrome. New England Journal of Medicine 311: 565–570

Further reading

Mason D, Gatter K 1998 The pocket guide to lymphoma classification. Blackwell Science, Oxford
A comprehensive guide to lymphoma classification.

Wallwork L, Richardson A 1994 Beyond cancer: changes, problems and needs expressed by adult lymphoma survivors attending an out-patients clinic. European Journal of Cancer Care 3: 122–132
One of the few British studies examining survivorship.

7 | **H**aematological malignancies and children

SAMANTHA HEATH

Key points
- Leukaemias and lymphomas are the commonest childhood cancers in the UK
- Treatment regimens can be intense and side-effects may be distressing to both the ill child and their family
- Understanding both the nature of treatment and its consequences is essential for both the child and their family
- Support of both the ill child and their family is an important component of care
- Long-term outlook is usually very good
- Survivors of childhood cancer may experience long-term physical, psychological and social sequelae.

INTRODUCTION

Childhood leukaemias and lymphomas constitute the highest incidence of all diagnoses of childhood cancers each year in Britain. However, in spite of being responsible for well over a third of all children's cancers, diagnosis of these diseases is still a rare occurrence (Cancer Research Campaign 1990). In context, this means that one general practitioner (GP) may see only one or two cases of childhood cancer throughout a career in medicine (Colliss 1996). Childhood leukaemias and lymphomas are treated quite differently to similar disease in adults although there remain many similarities in supportive care, and there are also significant differences in long-term survival. The implications of such successful treatment is perhaps most clearly seen in Meadows and Hobbie's (1986) suggestion that by the Year 2000, 1 in 1000 young adults will be cancer survivors. Therefore, the work of the children's cancer nurse is not only aimed at attempting to reduce and ameliorate the symptoms of the disease and its treatment but also at preparing families to live with the consequences of cancer throughout the rest of their lives.

Treatment for leukaemias and lymphomas in children often occurs over an extended period of time. The long-term outlook is generally very good, especially for those with acute lymphoblastic leukaemia (ALL) and Hodgkin's lymphoma. Such favourable outcomes have been made possible as a result of developments in multi-agent chemotherapy regimens, radiotherapy and bone marrow transplantation. Coupled with advances in supportive care – for example, prevention and treatment of infection, haematological support and the management of metabolic problems during therapy – the focus of care for children with such malignancies has significantly changed. Now, medical treatment and care is aimed at maintaining first remission, reducing side-effects of treatment, especially long-term problems, and avoiding death during therapy from opportunistic infection (Cancer Research Campaign 1990). Nursing care is initially focused on the physical and emotional support of the child and family during the treatment phase of the disease, both in hospital and at home. Increasingly this care is directed towards long-term survivorship, as previously outlined, but where this is not possible the role of the specialist children's oncology nurse in palliative care is key. Therefore, in this chapter the nature, causes and treatment of childhood leukaemias and lymphomas is considered but, in keeping with the particular concerns of children's cancer nurses, supportive care, family concerns and survivorship issues are also identified and discussed.

TYPES OF HAEMATOLOGICAL MALIGNANCIES IN CHILDREN

There are two broad groups of haematological malignancy in children: the leukaemias and the lymphomas.

The leukaemias

The acute leukaemias are by far the most common types found in children. Of the two major types, acute lymphoblastic leukaemia (ALL) and acute myeloblastic leukaemia (AML), ALL is most frequently encountered. Chronic leukaemia is rarely found in children, but can be divided into two groups, adult type and juvenile type (Pinkerton et al 1994).

The causes of leukaemia in children remain unclear (Reihm et al 1986). This is due to the rarity of the incidence of the disease and the subsequent inability to acquire the large volumes of data necessary from which to draw meaningful conclusions. However, currently available theories on causative factors include levels of paternal radiation exposure (Pinkerton et al 1994) and environmental factors – for example, living in close proximity to nuclear generating plants and electricity pylons (Gardener & Snee 1990). There is also some evidence to suggest that viral causes could be implicated (Greaves & Chan 1986). Chromosomal abnormalities have been positively identified and of particular note is the 14-fold increase in the incidence of ALL in children with Down's syndrome (Reihm et al 1986). The Philadelphia chromosome (translocation t9:22) is also present in some children

with ALL and AML. The United Kingdom Children's Cancer Study Group (UKCCSG) is conducting a major longitudinal study to investigate the possible causes of childhood cancers. When complete, this data may offer further valuable insights into the causes of this group of diseases among children.

Reflection point

The attempt to find causative factors and the most appropriate treatment methods for the child with a haematological malignancy is an ongoing concern within the speciality. As there are relatively few numbers of children presenting with this group of diseases it means that there is a potential for the same children and their families to be recruited into research studies time and again.

■ Consider the ethical implications for the child and family in these circumstances.
■ Think about the reasons why such families may feel compelled to be involved in research studies when approached.

Acute lymphoblastic leukaemia

Available statistical evidence indicates that the peak age of incidence among children is between 1 and 9 years, with 1 to 4 year olds most commonly affected (Cancer Research Campaign 1990). As a prognostic feature, the age of the child at diagnosis is significant (Ekert 1988). Children who are under 1 year or over 10 years appear to do less well than children aged between 2 and 9.

Presenting features of the disease are often pallor; tiredness; irritability; bruising; bone and/or joint pain; lymphadenopathy and enlargement of the liver and spleen (Pinkerton & Philip 1991). Since such symptoms are congruent with other disorders of childhood – for example, arthritis, osteomyelitis or mumps – careful diagnosis and classification is always undertaken. This involves peripheral blood screening to detect the presence of blast cells; bone marrow aspiration to determine cytochemistry and immunological markers; and lumbar puncture to identify blast cells in the cerebrospinal fluid at diagnosis. Additionally, ultrasound scans of the liver, spleen and kidneys and chest X-rays may be required if infiltration of these organs is suspected.

Case study 7.1

Ranjit, aged 6 years, had been well and very active at the end of his first year at school. During the summer holidays his mother noticed that he became progressively more lethargic and complained of pain in his knees. On an initial consultation with the family doctor Ranjit's mother was told to try and control his pain with generally available analgesia, and that an appointment would be made for him to see the paediatrician at the local hospital for further investigations. Three weeks later, there was no improvement in Ranjit's condition and, in addition, there were bruises on his legs which his mother could not explain. At a second consultation, this time with a locum general practitioner, Ranjit's mother was advised to wait for the appointment with the paediatrician which, she was assured, would be within the next two weeks. One week later, Ranjit began to have nosebleeds and his knees became too painful to walk for any length of time. Suspecting that something was seriously wrong with her son, Ranjit's mother took him to the local Accident and Emergency Department. The paediatrician examined Ranjit and a full blood count revealed abnormalities consistent with a diagnosis of leukaemia. Ranjit was referred to a regional cancer centre for further investigations.

The main form of treatment for ALL in children is chemotherapy (see Ch. 8), although for those children who present with significant central nervous system (CNS) disease at diagnosis, cranial or craniospinal irradiation may also feature (see Ch. 9). Each child diagnosed with ALL is entered into the current treatment trial and is randomised to receive a particular protocol, which in all cases can be divided into three distinct stages and lasts around 2 years.

During the first stage of treatment or 'induction' therapy, the aim is to achieve remission of disease within the bone marrow (Ekert 1988,

Pinkerton & Philip 1991). At present the drugs used include prednisolone, vincristine, daunorubicin and asparaginase. The major problems experienced at induction are associated with tumour lysis syndrome (particularly where there is a high white cell count at presentation), and the high risk of infection during the pancytopenic period following the first course of chemotherapy. Other problems include the more common side-effects anticipated with the use of cytotoxic agents (see Ch. 8).

The second stage is directed towards either prophylactic or actual treatment of CNS disease. This can be done in one of three ways: high-dose intravenous administration of methotrexate; intrathecal treatment of the CNS using methotrexate, or cranial/craniospinal irradiation. At present, the aim of treatment trials is to determine whether chemotherapy alone can achieve CNS disease ablation because of the long-term problems related to growth, endocrine function and intelligence associated with radiotherapy for children (Pinkerton & Philip 1991).

During the final or 'maintenance' stage of treatment the child receives oral chemotherapy (Pinkerton & Philip 1991). This stage of treatment is mostly carried out as an outpatient with regular monitoring of response. Risk factors at this stage of treatment include chronic myelosuppression and the attendant susceptibility of the child to infection, especially common childhood illnesses such as chicken pox and measles. For these reasons children in the maintenance stage of treatment are given septrin as a prophylactic antibiotic, and are advised to report all contacts with childhood infectious diseases to the regional cancer centre.

Reflection point

During the maintenance phase of treatment, the child and family still visit their regional centre regularly. Consider the way in which completion of this stage of the child's treatment may affect the family in the following months and years.

If initial treatment fails, relapse is usually found in the bone marrow, but may also be detected in the CNS or testes in boys. Depending upon the type of relapse, different types of retreatment can be offered. If the relapse is medullary (found within the bone marrow alone) then reinduction and bone marrow transplant (BMT) may be offered. However, there are significant risk factors associated with this procedure (see Ch. 10). In some cases peripheral stem cell harvest and transplant may be the treatment of choice. For those children who experience an extramedullary relapse (found outside the bone marrow – for example, the testes and CNS), chemotherapy and radiotherapy can be offered with a good success rate when relapse occurs after completion of initial treatment (Pinkerton et al 1994).

Acute myeloid leukaemia

Presenting features of acute myeloid leukaemia (AML) are less specific than those for ALL. However, the significant difference between the two is an increased incidence of a history of bleeding in AML. Diagnosis can be positively confirmed on peripheral blood and marrow aspirates. Prognostic indicators with AML are also less specific, but there is some evidence to suggest that the child with the promyelocytic hypergranular (M3) type of AML is more susceptible to disseminated intravascular coagulation at induction and the presence of the Philadelphia chromosome at diagnosis is less favourable (Ekert 1988, Pinkerton et al 1994). Involvement of the CNS is less likely in children with AML and in most cases where this is present, intrathecal methotrexate is usually effective (Pinkerton & Philip 1991).

Treatment for AML is extremely intense and susceptible to complication from either the disease or its treatment. Although remission from induction therapy is regularly achieved, maintenance of the first remission is more difficult; therefore, continuing, aggressive treatment is given. This takes the form of allogeneic BMT where there is a matched donor available, and for children for whom this type of transplant is not possible, high-dose chemotherapy and autologous bone marrow rescue is considered (Pinkerton et al 1994); (see Ch. 10).

Case study 7.2

Megan, aged 4 years, was diagnosed as having acute myeloid leukaemia 6 months ago and achieved remission quickly with chemotherapy. Megan was an only child and had no suitably matched donor available. Therefore, she received high-dose chemotherapy and autologous bone marrow rescue.

The bone marrow transplant specialist nurse prepared Megan and her family for this treatment during the weeks immediately preceding the planned time for the procedure. For Megan's parents, this preparation included an outline of the likely events during transplant; the precautions that would be necessary to protect Megan during her neutropenic phase; the ways in which her family could be supportive during the period of isolation; and the opportunity to ask questions about any aspects of the procedure, including a meeting with other families who had already experienced this type of treatment. Megan's preparation included the use of therapeutic play with the help of the ward play specialist, which gave her the opportunity to handle the equipment she was unfamiliar with and to see inside an isolation room. Megan was also invited to choose toys and games she would like to have in her room during the procedure.

Although the bone marrow rescue procedure was a difficult time for Megan and her family, the preparation was useful in reducing family anxieties. Megan, as expected, regressed to previous stages of behaviour, but her parents were able to understand this and responded positively, accepting that this was their daughter's way of coping with a very stressful event.

Chronic leukaemias

Chronic leukaemia is rare in children. When it is diagnosed it falls into two groups. The adult type is found in older children and is associated with the presence of the Philadelphia chromosome. There is a high white cell count at presentation, with significant enlargement of the spleen. By contrast the juvenile form of the disease, which is found in children under the age of 4 years, has no Philadelphia chromosome and the presenting white cell count is much lower.

Adult-type chronic leukaemia shows a good response to initial treatment. The white cell count is controlled using mild, often oral chemotherapy (Ekert 1988). However, where the presenting white cell count is very high, leucophoresis may be used to reduce the risk of cerebral infarction due to hyperviscosity of the blood. The chronic phase of the disease may last months if not years, but will eventually develop into the stage of 'blast crisis'. At present the best chance of cure lies in the success of early allogeneic BMT during the chronic phase of the disease.

The juvenile form of the disease is particularly resistant to treatment, and the best option at present is allogeneic BMT with intensive pre-conditioning (Pinkerton et al 1994).

The lymphomas

Lymphoma in children is divided into two groups, non-Hodgkin's lymphoma (NHL) and Hodgkin's lymphoma. The two types of disease have very different prognoses and treatment.

Non-Hodgkin's lymphoma

This type of lymphoma is closely related to ALL, but unlike leukaemia, lymphoma arises in the lymph nodes or thymus. Classification of the disease is complex, but the most commonly encountered subtypes of the disease are T-cell or B-cell lymphoma. Presentation of the disease is dependent upon the initial site. In T-cell lymphoma, this is commonly cervical lymphadenopathy, but in some cases where there is swelling of the thymus, there is the possibility that the child will present with superior vena caval or tracheal obstruction. In B-cell lymphoma there may be an abdominal mass and/or pain. Occasionally, where there is involvement of the ileum, intussusception may occur. In both types there may be CNS and bone marrow disease. Staging of the disease includes chest X-rays, CT scan, bone marrow aspirate and lumbar puncture.

Treatment for T-cell lymphoma is the same as for ALL and survival rates are equivalent, at around 60% at 5 years (Pinkerton et al 1994). In B-cell lymphoma, chemotherapy is pulsed over a period of 6–9 months. With early diagnosis,

survival rates can be as high as 95%, but where there is disseminated disease the outlook is poor.

Hodgkin's lymphoma

The cells of origin in this type of lymphoma are, as yet, unknown. However, there is some evidence to suggest that there may be a viral component (Pinkerton & Philip 1991). Presentation in children is by gradual enlargement of the lymph nodes of the neck. This lymphadenopathy is usually bilateral and some children may have identifiable mediastinal disease. In Hodgkin's disease there is the additional possibility of systemic symptoms, which include unexplained fevers, night sweats and weight loss.

Investigation and staging is by tissue biopsy, although in children this does not go to the extent of a laparotomy, and CT scans and chest X-rays are taken. Treatment for Hodgkin's lymphoma can be by use of either radiotherapy or chemotherapy. However, because of the unacceptable side-effects of radiotherapy use for children's treatment, chemotherapy is increasingly preferred and demonstrates the same extremely good outlook.

Fanconi's anaemia

Fanconi's anaemia or congenital aplastic anaemia is a thankfully rare condition among children. It usually occurs with multiple congenital abnormalities – for example, renal and cardiac anomalies; skeletal problems; shortness of stature; hyperpigmentation of the skin, and microcephaly – and is inherited via an autosomal recessive trait (Lankowsky 1989). Children with this disease generally present between 4 and 12 years with the effects of pancytopenia: for example, pallor, bruising and recurrent infections. Differential diagnosis of the condition is made by excluding other, similarly presenting conditions, such as acquired aplastic anaemia.

The mainstay of treatment for this group of children is found in supportive care by transfusion of packed cells, platelets and, occasionally, white cells. Combined steroid and androgen therapies can also be used. However, the best chances of survival with this condition are at present, allogeneic bone marrow transplantation. It is important to note that siblings of children with this disease have a higher incidence of acute myeloid leukaemia (Lankowsky 1989). (See Ch. 3 for further discussion of Fanconi's anaemia.)

CARE OF THE CHILD WITH LEUKAEMIA OR LYMPHOMA

The child with leukaemia or lymphoma will require a great deal of care and support from hospital staff. Usually, this is provided by one of the children's regional cancer centres distributed throughout the country. In many cases, however, this provision is complemented by a system of 'shared care' between the regional centres and the child's local hospital. The main reason for this is to reduce the amount of time spent travelling to the regional centre, particularly when this is a long or costly journey, and when the local hospital can duplicate equally effective support services. In most cases this support will be provided by a range of in-patient, outpatient and community liaison facilities.

Case study 7.3

Thomas is 9 years old and lives in a rural area in the Midlands. Following treatment for his acute lymphoblastic leukaemia, he needed to return for regular checks of his blood count. However, the journey to his nearest regional centre meant that he would miss a whole day at school for a relatively quick procedure.

To ensure that Thomas missed as little schooling as possible during the periods he did not need to be an inpatient at the regional centre, care was shared. This 'shared care' approach was set up by community liaison nurses who, through a planned teaching programme, helped nurses on Thomas' local children's ward to understand the nature and course of his treatment. Now, Thomas only returns to his regional centre for chemotherapy and aftercare, but returns to his local hospital for blood counts and blood product support when needed. So far, multidisciplinary communication has worked well and Thomas is benefiting educationally from reduced time loss at school.

The kind of support which needs to be provided for the child with leukaemia or lymphoma can be broadly divided into three areas:

- informational needs
- alleviation of physical side-effects of cancer treatment
- play and educational needs.

Informational needs of the child

Informational needs are clearly related to age of children during treatment and their level of cognitive development. It is possible to present quite complex information to children about their disease providing that this is done appropriately. There are various materials developed by individual centres that facilitate this process, as well as books which are widely available and written especially for the purpose.

In conjunction with developing their knowledge about the disease itself, children also require information about the types of procedures they will have to undergo. The results of Rodin's work in the early 1980s established that children whose informational needs are met prior to undergoing an invasive procedure are less likely to display signs of anxiety than those who have no preparation (Rodin 1983). In this respect, nurses have a key role in helping children to understand what will happen to them during their treatment. However, this role is greatly complemented by the work of the play specialist. The skill of a play specialist is essential in children's cancer care, since therapeutic play can help children to work through difficult emotional issues, allow experimentation and practice at problem-solving. There is also good evidence to suggest that through this kind of play misconceptions about treatment or disease can be rectified and subsequently reduce the stress experienced by the child (Kuykendall 1988).

Providing information for children can be a difficult task for the multidisciplinary team. However, it helps to remember that the child's stage of cognitive development and concept of illness can provide some indicators about useful techniques to use. For example, a child who is 5 years old will be at the pre-operational stage of development. The characteristics of thinking are that they are easily influenced by their visual perception and their thought patterns are often unreliable and illogical. Their concept of illness is often that disease is transmitted by magical means and that it can be a punishment for misbehaviour. In such cases, it is useful to use purposeful or 'therapeutic play' to help understanding of the reasons for their diagnosis and to use very visual props which can be handled by the child. Using teddies and dolls as a 'third person' through whom the child can 'talk' is also useful to reduce fear and anxiety.

Alleviation of physical side-effects

Alleviation of the physical side-effects of cancer treatment – for example, oral care, nausea and vomiting and haemorrhagic problems – are dealt with in Chapters 16, 15 and 14. However, there are some special aspects which need to be examined when considering children's care.

Venous access for children who are receiving particularly toxic therapy or intravenous drugs over an extended period must be carefully considered. Although the insertion of a central venous catheter requires a general anaesthetic, it is a preferred method of giving intravenous medication to children in these circumstances, and has benefits in terms of reducing the anxiety associated with repeated insertion of peripheral cannulae for both the child and family. In most cases, one catheter will last for the entire course of treatment (see Ch. 12 for the care of central venous catheters).

The maintenance of nutritional status is also important in the care of the child. Children receiving steroids as part of their treatment are likely to gain weight. However, children at other stages of treatment may actually lose weight and this is of great concern. Factors which contribute to weight loss in children are related to poor eating, where chemotherapy has affected the child's taste sensation, rendering food less appetising. Mucositis, nausea and vomiting are also problematic and must be addressed if they are not to make a detrimental

contribution to the child's nutritional status. Therefore, active and prophylactic treatment of these side-effects is of great importance.

Assessment of the child's nutritional problems begins with accurate measurement of weight and height and includes a dietary evaluation. Nutritional support is then aimed at maintaining the growth velocity of the child, rather than simply at weight maintenance (Hunter & Janes 1988). It is usual practice for recommendations to be made for changes in oral feeding in the first instance. This type of advice usually includes using calorie-dense foods and supplements in keeping with the child's preferences (Wellock 1992). Alternatively, where nutritional problems are severe, enteral and parenteral nutrition may be considered.

Play and educational needs

The long periods of regular hospitalisation and the necessity of outpatient visits can severely disrupt schooling. Therefore, when the child is well enough during treatment in hospital they are likely to attend the hospital school. Equally, the child who is not yet of school age also requires ongoing stimulation in the form of organised play sessions. The purpose of both these activities is to ensure that previously learned skills are not lost during admission and to ensure that all aspects of the child's development are promoted throughout the course of the illness.

Reflection point

The drugs used to treat leukaemia have many side-effects. The most obvious of these to the child are an initial weight gain following steroid therapy on some protocols and alopecia.

■ Consider the ways in which you could prepare a school-age child for such a marked change in their body image.

■ What resources do you have in your clinical area to help prepare children returning to school after initial chemotherapy treatment?

THE FAMILY

It is well recognised that the family is responsible for the greatest physical, psychological and social nurturing of children, and therefore the importance of family support cannot be underestimated. It is important to identify that the single biggest threat caused by diagnosis of childhood malignancy is the effect that this has on the entire family (Heath 1996a, Spinetta & Deasy-Spinetta 1981).

The dramatic improvements in the treatment for childhood leukaemia and lymphoma over the last 30 years has changed the way in which care by nursing, medical and allied health-care professionals is approached. The emphasis of care is not now that of an inevitably fatal disease but one which bears more resemblance to a chronic illness. While the professional view of childhood leukaemias and lymphomas may be that of a chronic illness, it is also important to recognise that the prevailing view of cancer within larger society may be far less positive. Associations are often made between cancer and pain, discomfort, mutilative treatment and uncertainty of outcome (McGee 1992). This has ensured that there has had to be a commensurate change in the way nursing staff respond to the needs of family members throughout the course of the disease.

Reflection point

Diagnosis of a haematological malignancy in a child has an enormous impact on the whole family.
- How are families assisted to cope with such a diagnosis?
- Reflect on your own helping skills and identify the areas you are good at. What aspects do you think need to be improved?

Parents

Binger et al (1969) asked 20 families whose children had died from leukaemia to describe their experience. They reported that diagnosis of cancer in their child was

> ...the hardest blow they had to bear throughout the course of the illness.
>
> *Binger et al 1969, p 414*

More recently, similar feelings have been reported by other researchers and it has been possible to identify feelings of guilt, anger, depression, helplessness and self-blame among parents of children with cancer (Lewandowski & Jones 1990, Overholser & Fritz 1990, Sales 1991).

In the initial period following diagnosis, these feelings are quite usual and, in general, will subside over a period of weeks when other coping responses and resources are mobilised (Culling 1988, Heath 1996b). At this stage of the disease, nurses have a significant role in facilitating parents to communicate the information about diagnosis to both the child with cancer and their well siblings, and encouraging them to be open and honest. As treatment begins, parents will often require factual information about the disease itself, treatment protocol and side-effects and regularly become extremely knowledgeable about their child's situation.

Support for parents is derived from many sources, including other family members and friends. The relationships developed between the family and health-care professionals are perhaps some of the most significant. Helping parents to cope with diagnosis and treatment can be facilitated by encouraging their involvement in the child's care while in hospital and ensuring that they are well informed at all stages. However, the importance of concurrently stressful events must not be overlooked (Heath 1996b). The kinds of life events that may add to the parent's difficulties include financial problems, occupational changes or the illness or death of another family member or friend (Kalnins et al 1980). In some cases health-care professionals can offer advice, support or referral to appropriate agencies to help in dealing with these events. Helping parents to restore the equilibrium and continue family functioning is essential. However difficult these problems are for parents to overcome, they must also ensure that the needs of their well children are met.

Siblings

The nature of sibling relationships are complex (Dominic 1993). Within the boundaries of these associations many life skills are acquired, social and emotional development is encouraged and the ability to comfort, protect and support is learned (Walker 1990, Dominic 1993). The diagnosis of malignancy in one sibling undoubtedly threatens these deep emotional bonds and has the potential to cause long-term psychological problems for the well child (Spinetta & Deasy-Spinetta 1981). Indeed, Spinetta & Deasy-Spinetta (1981) and Rollins (1990) identify that the greatest unhappiness within the family facing diagnosis of malignancy in a child is most apparent in the well children. This vulnerability of well siblings is largely attributable to the diversion of family resources to the needs of the sick child and changes in familiar family roles and expectations (Spinetta & Deasy-Spinetta 1981, Rollins 1990, Walker 1990). These changes can provoke many different emotions in the well sibling. Doyle (1987) has documented responses to this major family upheaval, which include anxiety, rejection, isolation, jealousy, guilt and resentment.

Anxiety in well siblings is often associated with fear for their own health (Cairns et al 1979, Walker 1990). This can be manifested by the mimicking of symptoms experienced by the sick child, or exacerbation of an underlying condition such as asthma or eczema (Dominic 1993). In many cases, this can be attributed to a lack of information about the sick child's condition. As Sepion (1988) rightly asserts, well siblings need the same information about the illness and, in many cases, need more reassurance than does the child with the disease. Well siblings need to know that the illness is not contagious and was not caused by them in any way.

Preoccupation with the sick child's needs, long periods of hospitalisation and over-indulgence have been cited as reasons for the basis of feelings of rejection in well siblings (Doyle 1987). In her seminal study, Iles (1979, p 373) found several informants who were able to articulate such feelings:

> Everyone asks how (child's name) feels, I feel left out.

> I can't invite friends over ... Mom's gone so much ... I never get to stay over at someone's house and I have only been to three parties.

Isolation felt by well siblings has been described as being both physical and emotional (Doyle 1987). Separation of the well child from the sick child and at least one parent to attend clinic appointments or treatment sessions is one of the most common reasons for physical isolation (Iles 1979). Emotional isolation is described when the well sibling lacks the emotional input from one or both parents as a result of the treatment or supportive care (Doyle 1987). The consequences here can manifest themselves in the form of fantasies about the causes and nature of the disease and imagination about likely outcomes.

Jealousy is not merely confined to the extra emotional attention given to the sick child, but can also extend to any new toys or presents. It is not unusual for attention-seeking behaviours to be exhibited by well siblings. Stealing and the use of abusive language towards parents has been reported in older children, while regression to old behaviours such as thumb-sucking and enuresis is most commonly found in children who are younger than the sick child (Doyle 1987).

Siblings often feel guilty that they are not suffering from the effects of the disease or its treatment (Dominic 1993). In some cases well children have been reported as believing that they are responsible for the onset of the disease because of a previous argument or fight with their sick sibling (Rollins 1990). It is not always the recency of these arguments that is relevant. Some incidents long forgotten by other members of the family have been noted as a trigger for sibling guilt.

Diversion of family resources and the lack of available funds for luxuries such as family holidays may cause feelings of resentment in the well sibling. This is often made worse by well-meaning relatives and friends who provide cards and presents for the sick child. The illness itself may also become a source of resentment. From the well child's perspective the appearance of the disease has transformed their normal life from one in which there were usual rules and boundaries to adhere to, to their current situation which has brought about change and inconsistency.

Help for well siblings must be provided on an age-appropriate and individual basis. In many cases this can take the form of provision of accurate information about the disease and treatment to reduce the incidence of misconceptions. Family and friends can be advised to treat the children in the same way as they have always done, with consistent rules and boundaries. Giving the well child responsibility for taking care of a treasured toy or pet at home can give an enormous sense of importance and belonging. Above all, recognition that the well child remains as much a part of the family as they have always done is essential.

Reflection point

Consider the types of support that could be offered to well siblings of children with leukaemia or lymphoma and the ways in which these measures could be implemented into your practice.

SURVIVORSHIP

Combination chemotherapy regimens and adjuvant radiotherapy have revolutionised treatment for childhood haematological malignancies and, in turn, have led to a greater number of children achieving 'cure'. As a consequence, the problems of survivorship have been highlighted. These problems are not only confined to the physical effects of treatment but must also include psychological and social sequelae.

Physical effects

Each treatment modality has its own late effects (Koocher & O'Malley 1981, Oakhill 1988, Weesner et al 1991). The exact nature of these physical effects depends entirely upon the child's age and the dosages of both chemotherapy and radiotherapy deemed necessary for treatment. There is convincing evidence to suggest that the late effects of cancer therapy

can manifest themselves months, if not years, after initial treatment (Fraser & Tucker 1988, Oakhill 1988).

Chemotherapy renders most body systems vulnerable to damage. The effects include impaired renal, cardiac, neurological and gonadal function (Fraser & Tucker 1988, Hydzik 1990). However, functional damage is not the only concern, since it is also possible that secondary malignancies may develop as a result of treatment for the first (Koocher & O'Malley 1981, Fraser & Tucker 1988, Oakhill 1988). Irradiation of sites containing endocrine glands can lead to later disruption in growth, delay in the onset of puberty, and a marked reduction in intelligence quotient in some survivors (Koocher & O'Malley 1981, Oakhill 1988).

Ongoing monitoring of the physical effects of treatment for childhood haematological malignancy takes place before each course of chemotherapy. This is often in the form of ultrasound scans, growth measurements, and kidney-functioning tests. Medical staff can reduce dosages of chemotherapy if there is concern that the effects of treatment are detrimental to the child's current and, therefore, future health.

Psychological effects

Koocher & O'Malley (1981) are key researchers in the field of psychological consequences of surviving childhood malignancies. Their findings illustrate several factors associated with positive long-term psychological outcomes, which include having a type of cancer for which treatment periods are relatively short and have few permanent side-effects; maintaining a long first remission; and developing the malignancy in infancy or early childhood. Survivors who appear to adjust less favourably are those who lack confidence in a positive outcome of their treatment or who have already suffered one relapse of their disease.

Psychological issues raised by the families of survivors involved in the study were often related to the long-term implications for their children, particularly in relation to physical effects of treatment, infertility problems, relapse and secondary malignancies (Koocher

& O'Malley 1981). Siblings reported feelings of resentment, jealousy and fears for their own health. Interestingly, Koocher & O'Malley (1981) note that well siblings of children with a malignancy found more difficulty in their adjustment to the disease than other siblings of children with a life-threatening illness.

Social effects

The most common social problem for survivors of childhood malignancies is cited as being employment discrimination. Koocher & O'Malley (1981) suggest that the reason for this may be attributable to the employer's fears of unreliability and absenteeism. Personal insurance is also difficult to obtain. Those respondents who eventually succeeded in acquiring this insurance communicated that these policies were subject to various clauses excluding cover relating to their cancer history (Koocher & O'Malley 1981).

Future care

The treatment for childhood haematological malignancies has the potential to affect all aspects of living and, as the number of survivors increases each year, nurses have a key role both in gathering data related to the physical consequences of survivorship and as part of a multidisciplinary team involved in comprehensive recognition of psychological and social problems experienced by survivors (Waterworth 1992). Health-care professionals need to consider how and where the most appropriate support can be offered to these children and families. This may be in the form of drop-in clinics and open door policies similar to those piloted in the United States. Alternatively, the pertinence of handing on this treatment to the adult oncology team also needs to be explored.

CONCLUSION

The nature of haematological malignancies in childhood means that the complex treatment protocols and supportive care are delivered over an extended period of time. As a result, the child and their family have ongoing and changing needs throughout the course of the illness and this requires that the children's cancer nurse undertakes a unique role in responding to these needs, and identifying and facilitating care. However, in order to carry out this role effectively, there are many skills that need to be developed, which has implications for day-to-day practice and ongoing professional development.

Understanding both the nature of treatment and its consequences, physically and psychologically, are essential; however, this means more than just having a simple appreciation of the facts. Such understanding needs to be used in practice in order to instigate thoughtful and appropriate nursing care. Using a partnership approach with the family can facilitate this, in conjunction with the effective use of a multidisciplinary team focused towards care activities. In addition, the children's cancer nurse also needs to be aware of the effects of diagnosis and treatment on all family members and to ensure that as far as possible the needs of individual members are met.

Such activities require that communication skills are foremost, especially in the way that support, information and advice are offered. Indeed, these skills are most clearly used in the development of relationships with the child and their family and in the coordination of care activities across the multidisciplinary team. As children's cancer nurses usually have the most contact with the child and family they are in an ideal position to do this, and to ensure that the mobilisation of appropriate resources is optimally facilitated throughout the cancer experience.

It is also important to identify that the ability to undertake such a role is developed over time, and that ongoing education makes a significant contribution to the nurse's personal development. This is most apparent in the way that helping and communication skills can be refined and the application of theoretical concepts to nursing practice can be used to develop a broader evidence base for personal practice.

The future for children's cancer nurses is likely to be one in which there is rapid change in the science of the discipline and the nature of nursing care offered. As more and more children survive first treatment for haematological malignancies, nurses will have to embrace and respond to new challenges, but they must also ensure that knowledge of good practice in children's nursing continues to be integrated into this specialist field.

DISCUSSION QUESTIONS

1. In the content of this chapter it has been assumed that the child will accept the treatment offered for their disease. Consider the implications for your sphere of practice when a 10 year old refuses treatment for a relapse of leukaemia on the grounds that previous treatment was unacceptable and that prognosis following a relapse is much poorer.

2. Specialist children's cancer nurses usually care for children with haematological malignancies and their families. What evidence is there to suggest that a specialist nurse may be the most appropriate person to undertake this kind of nursing?

References

Binger C M, Albin A R, Feuerstein R C, Kushner J H, Zoger S, Mikkelson C 1969 Childhood leukaemia: emotional impact on patient and family. New England Journal of Medicine 280(8): 414–418

Cairns N U, Clark G M, Smith S D, Lansky S B 1979 Adaptation of siblings to childhood malignancies. Journal of Pediatrics 95: 484–487

Cancer Research Campaign 1990 Childhood Cancer – UK Factsheet 15.1. Cancer Research Campaign, London

Colliss G 1996 Children having oncology treatment. In: McQuaid L, Huband S, Parker E (eds) Children's nursing. Churchill Livingstone, Edinburgh, Chapter 24

Culling J A 1988 The psychological problems of families of children with cancer. In: Oakhill A (ed) The supportive care of the child with cancer. Wright, London

Dominic K 1993 Left out in the cold. Paediatric Nursing 5(3): 28–29

Doyle B 1987 I wish you were dead. Nursing Times 83(45): 44–46

Ekert H 1988 Childhood cancer understanding and coping. Gordon & Breach, New York.

Fraser M C, Tucker M A 1988 Late effects of cancer therapy: chemotherapy related malignancies. Oncology Nursing Forum 15(1): 67–75

Gardener M J, Snee M P 1990 Results of a case control study of leukaemia and lymphoma among young people near Sellafield nuclear plant in West Cumbria. British Medical Journal 300: 423–429

Greaves M F, Chan L C 1986 Is spontaneous mutation the major cause of childhood acute lymphoblastic leukaemia? British Journal of Haematology 64: 1–13

Heath S 1996a Childhood cancer – A family crisis 1: the impact of diagnosis. British Journal of Nursing 5(12): 744–748

Heath S 1996b Childhood cancer – A family crisis 2: coping with diagnosis. British Journal of Nursing 5(13): 790–793

Hunter M, Janes E M H 1988 Nutrition in cancer care. In: Tiffany B, Webb P (eds) Oncology for nurses and health care professionals, 2nd edn, Vol. 2. Care and support. Harper and Row, London

Hydzik C A 1990 Late effects of chemotherapy: implications for patient management and rehabilitation. Nursing Clinics of North America 25: 423–445

Iles P 1979 Children with cancer: healthy siblings perceptions during the illness experience. Cancer Nursing 2: 371–377

Kalnins I V, Churchill M P, Terry G E 1980 Concurrent stresses in families with a leukaemic child. Journal Pediatric Psychology 5(1): 81–92

Koocher G P, O'Malley J E 1981 The Damocles syndrome. McGraw-Hill, New York

Kuykendall J 1988 Play therapy. In: Oakhill A (ed) The supportive care of the child with cancer. Wright, London

Lankowsky P 1989 Manual of pediatric hematology and oncology. Churchill Livingstone, New York

Lewandowski W, Jones S L 1990 The family with cancer: nursing interventions throughout the course of living with cancer. Cancer Nursing 11(6): 313–321

McGee R F 1992 Overview of psychosocial dimensions. In: Groenwald S L, Frogge M H, Goodman M, Henke Yarbro C (eds) Cancer nursing principles and practice, 2nd edn. Jones and Bartlett, Boston

Meadows A T, Hobbie W L 1986 The medical consequences of cure. Cancer 58(2 Suppl.): 524–528

Oakhill A 1988 The late effects of treatment. In: Oakhill A (ed) The supportive care of the child with cancer. Wright, London

Overholser J C, Fritz G K 1990 The impact of childhood cancer on the family. Journal of Psychosocial Oncology 8(4): 71–85

Pinkerton C R, Philip T 1991 Treatment strategies in paediatric cancer. Gardiner–Caldwell, Macclesfield

Pinkerton C R, Cushing P, Sepion B 1994 Childhood cancer management: a practical handbook. Chapman and Hall, London

Reihm H, Feikert H J, Lampert F 1986 Acute lymphoblastic leukaemia. In: Voute P A et al (eds) Cancer in children: clinical management, 2nd edn. Springer-Verlag, New York

Rodin J 1983 Will this hurt? Preparing children for hospital and medical procedures. Royal College of Nursing, London

Rollins J 1990 Childhood cancer: siblings draw and tell. Pediatric Nursing 16(1): 21–26

Sales E 1991 Psychosocial impact of the phase of cancer on the family: an updated review. Journal of Psychosocial Oncology 10(2): 1–26

Sepion B 1988 The impact of cancer on specific groups: children with cancer. In: Tiffany B,

Webb P (eds) Oncology for nurses and health care professionals, 2nd edn. Vol. 2, Care and support. Harper and Row, London

Spinetta J, Deasy-Spinetta P 1981 Living with childhood cancer. Mosby, St. Louis

Walker C L 1990 Stress and coping in siblings of childhood cancer patients. Nursing Research 37(4): 208–212

Waterworth S 1992 The long term effects of cancer on children and their families. British Journal of Nursing 1(8): 373–377

Weesner K A, Boedsoe M, Chauvenet A, Wofford M 1991 Exercise echocardiography in the detection of anthracycline cardiotoxicity. Cancer 68: 435–438

Wellock A 1992 Nutritional support. In: D'Angio D, Sinniah D, Meadows A, Evans A, Pritchard J (eds) Practical paediatric oncology. Hodder and Stoughton, London

Further reading

Darbyshire P 1994 Living with a sick child in hospital: the experiences of parents and nurses. Chapman and Hall, London
An enlightening account of hospitalisation and the relationships developed between children's nurses and their families. The book is based on Philip Darbyshire's research and offers a valuable account of family-centred care that is particularly useful to children's oncology nurses.

Faulkner A, Peace G, O'Keeffe C 1995 When a child has cancer. Chapman and Hall, London
Also based on a research study, this book offers invaluable insights into the feelings of families whose children are diagnosed with cancer. It is essential reading for anyone interested in children's cancer care.

SECTION TWO
Treatment

8 *Chemotherapy*

EVELYN THOMSON

Key points
- Cytotoxic drugs are the primary therapy for all forms of haematological malignancy
- An understanding of the cell cycle is necessary to understand the action of cytotoxic drugs
- Cytotoxic drugs are classified according to their mechanism of action
- An understanding of drug resistance is necessary to understand the underlying rationale of current treatment strategies
- Safe handling procedures are crucial as cytotoxic drugs are potentially hazardous to staff, patients and the environment
- Nursing strategies to minimise chemotherapy-associated toxicities are an essential element of patient care

INTRODUCTION

Cancer chemotherapeutic agents have had a profound influence on the treatment and survival of patients with cancer. Their purpose is to prevent cancer cells from multiplying, invading, metastasising, and ultimately killing the individual (Skeel 1987, DeVita 1989, Irani 1992). Current drug treatment is directed towards control of abnormal cell growth and reducing the number of actively dividing cells (Holmes 1990). Malignancies most susceptible to cancer chemotherapy are typically characterised by rapid growth and cell division; for example, acute leukaemia and lymphoma, which have a large growth fraction (Pitot 1981, Hoffbrand & Pettit 1993). The systemic nature of chemotherapy distinguishes it from radiotherapy or surgery, the therapeutic effects of which are confined to the local anatomical site to which they are applied. Cytotoxic chemotherapy is

therefore the primary therapy for all forms of haematological malignancy.

This chapter deals with the principles of chemotherapy and cytotoxic drug administration and focuses on the implications for nurses involved in the care of individuals receiving cytotoxic chemotherapy for haematological malignancies.

PRINCIPLES OF CHEMOTHERAPY

In order to appreciate the ways in which cancer chemotherapy affects cellular function and understand its beneficial and deleterious effects a basic knowledge of cell biology is essential.

The cell cycle

The cell cycle of cancer cells is qualitatively the same as that of normal cells (Fig. 8.1). The cell cycle is the sequence of events resulting in the replication of deoxyribonucleic acid (DNA) and equal division into daughter cells, known as *mitosis* (Fig. 8.2). It consists of five phases: G_1, G_2, S, M and G_0 (Maxwell & Maher 1992). Each cell begins its growth during a postmitotic period or phase (G_1), during which enzymes necessary for DNA production, other proteins, and ribonucleic acid (RNA) are produced. G_1 is followed by a period of DNA *synthesis* (S) in which essentially all DNA synthesis for a given cycle takes place. When DNA synthesis is complete, the cell enters a *premitotic period* (G_2), during which further protein and RNA synthesis occur. This gap is followed immediately by *mitosis* (M), at the end of which actual physical division occurs and two daughter cells are formed.

Figure 8.1 Cell cycle (from Maxwell & Maher 1992, reproduced with permission)

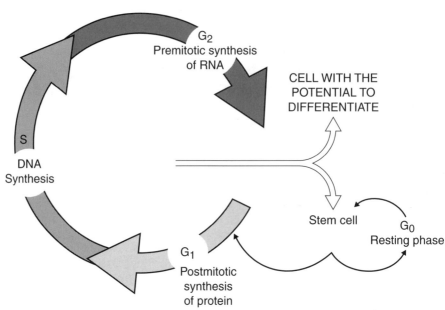

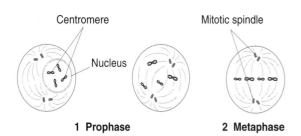

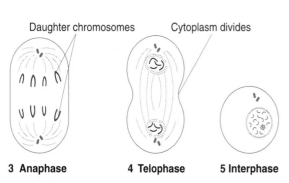

1 Prophase   **2 Metaphase**

3 Anaphase   **4 Telophase**   **5 Interphase**

Figure 8.2 Diagrammatic representation of the stages of mitosis (from Holmes S (1997) Cancer chemotherapy: a guide for practice, 2nd edn. Asset Books, Leatherhead, p 19, reproduced with permission)

Following cell division, the daughter cells may proceed in several ways (Fig. 8.3). They may enter G_1 prior to undergoing further cell division and continue to progress through the cell cycle. The second option is that the cell becomes a resting cell and does not undergo further cell division unless stimulated to do so. Such cells are said to be in G_0 (non-proliferating pool). This is an important concept, as cells in G_0 may not be susceptible to chemotherapeutic agents and thus form a reservoir of cells (clonogenic/stem cells) which retain the potential to divide and form more tumour cells. The third possibility is that the daughter cell becomes an end cell, incapable of further cell division, or capable of only a limited number of divisions (terminally differentiated pool). Cells enter programmed cell death (*apoptosis*) from either the differentiated or non-proliferating pools (G_0) (Tannock 1992).

The time required for completion of the cycle is called the *cell cycle time* and varies not only between tissues but also between malignant and normal cells. Variations in the cycle length usually occur in the G_1 phase, while the S, G_2 and M phases are relatively constant (Cline & Haskill 1980).

Tumour growth

Cancer cells are characterised by a growth process whereby their sensitivity to normal controlling factors has been completely or

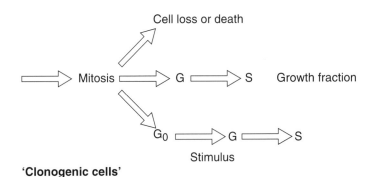

'Clonogenic cells'

Figure 8.3 Cell progression. Following cell division, the cell may progress in one of three ways: (a) it may die, be lost or have a limited number of cell divisions; (b) it may go into the cell cycle again; (c) it may go into G_0 and, following an appropriate stimulus, it may enter the cell cycle (from Calman et al 1980, reproduced with permission)

partially lost (Woolf 1986). Whereas proliferation in normal cells ceases once each cell comes into contact with adjacent cells (*contact inhibition*) proliferation of neoplastic cells appears autonomous and occurs regardless of the needs of the host (*i.e. loss of contact inhibition*) (Taussig 1979).

Tumour growth is dependent on several interrelated factors: the growth fraction, the clonogenic fraction (stem cells) and the end (non-clonogenic) cells (Fig. 8.4). The growth fraction represents cells which are actively dividing. With some tumours this fraction is very large (>70%), and the bulk of the tumour is composed of dividing cells, or very small (<10%) with only a small proportion of the tumour being composed of actively dividing cells (Calman et al 1980). Additionally, the growth fraction may vary during the growth of the tumour (Cline & Haskell 1980). The time taken for the mass to double in volume is known as the *doubling time*. This is extremely variable and may be as short as a few days in the leukaemias, to 100–200 days in some solid tumours (Irani 1992, Jenkins 1992).

During the early stages of tumour growth, doubling time is more rapid when the tumour is small than at later stages when the tumour is large (Hancock & Bradshaw 1981). This pattern of growth is called Gompertzian function, where exponential growth is matched by exponential retardation of growth (DeVita 1991) (Fig. 8.5).

The clonogenic fraction is composed of malignant cells which, though not in division at the time, are capable of dividing if given an appropriate stimulus (DeVita 1989). For example, if the growth fraction is reduced by effective therapy, clonogenic cells are recruited to maintain neoplastic growth. They may be considered as cells in an extended G_0 phase. The non-clonogenic fraction is composed of end cells; some may be viable but unable to divide while many are already dead (DeVita 1989). One of the principal aims of cancer chemotherapy is to increase the number of non-clonogenic cells, thus reducing the potential for further growth.

Cell kill hypothesis

As cancer cells grow from a few cells to a lethal cell burden, certain changes occur in the growth rate of the cell population that affect

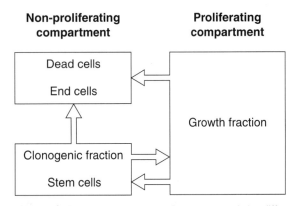

Figure 8.4 Tumour kinetics. Tumours contain different compartments of cells which are classified according to whether the compartment is proliferating (or growing). These compartments are interrelated as shown, (from Calman et al 1980, reproduced with permission)

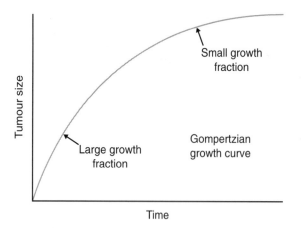

Figure 8.5 Tumour growth rate. Many tumours grow fast initially, and the growth fraction is large. However, as the size of the tumour increases, the growth rate and the growth fraction fall. This is described as Gompertzian growth kinetics (from Calman et al 1980, reproduced with permission)

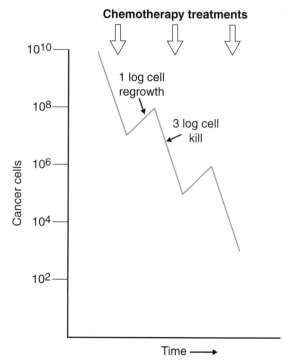

Figure 8.6 The effect of chemotherapy on cancer cell numbers. In an ideal system, chemotherapy kills a constant proportion of the remaining cancer cells with each dose. Between doses, cell regrowth occurs. When therapy is successful, cell killing is greater than cell growth (from Skeel R T 1987, reproduced with permission)

chemotherapy strategies. During initial development, tumour growth is slow; this is described as the *lag phase*. The lag phase is followed by a period of rapid growth called the *log phase* during which there is repeated doubling of the cell numbers (Skeel 1987). The basis of cell kill hypothesis is *log kill*. Because only a proportion of cells die with any given treatment, repeated doses of chemotherapy must be used to continue to reduce cell numbers. Each time the dose is repeated, the same *proportion* of cells, not the same absolute number, is killed. In the example shown in Fig. 8.6, 99.9% (3 logs) of the cancer cells are killed with each treatment, and there is a tenfold (1 log) growth between treatments for a net reduction of 2 logs with each treatment. Starting at 10^{10} cells it would take five treatments to reach less than 10^0, or one, cell (Cooper & Cooper 1991). Such a model, however, makes certain assumptions that are rarely strictly true in clinical practice (Skeel 1987):

1. All cells in the tumour population are equally sensitive to a drug.
2. Cell sensitivity is dependent on the location of the cells within the host and independent of local host factors, such as blood supply or surrounding fibrosis.

3. Cell sensitivity does not change during the course of therapy.

This hypothesis, together with the Gompertzian model of tumour growth, has directed the development of current chemotherapeutic regimens and strategies. For example, the use of combination chemotherapy regimens (Reich 1983), adjuvant therapy (Buzzoni et al 1991) and the prophylactic treatment of so-called sanctuary sites, where malignant cells are harboured beyond the reach of most cytotoxic drugs used in therapy (Hoffbrand & Pettit 1993). The latter is of particular importance for individuals being treated for acute lymphatic leukaemia, where leukaemic cells in the meninges are beyond the reach of most standard-dose chemotherapy regimens. Here the prophylactic use of intrathecal methotrexate is indicated during initial treatment and consolidation therapy, not only to reduce the risk of developing meningeal leukaemia but also to minimise the possible risk of subsequent systemic relapse (Henderson & Lister 1990).

Reflection point

Before proceeding pause and consider:

- the main similarities and differences between normal and malignant cells
- the rationale for using cytotoxic chemotherapy as first-line treatment in the management of haematological malignancies
- why the administration of intrathecal cytotoxic drugs, such as methotrexate, is indicated in the treatment of individuals with acute lymphatic leukaemia.

DRUGS USED IN CANCER CHEMOTHERAPY

Cytotoxic drugs can be described by their chemical structure, cell cycle activity and primary mode of action (Fisher et al 1993). Since the target of cytotoxic therapy is the malignant cell itself, the cell cycle has many

therapeutic implications and stages of the cell cycle are central to the action of antineoplastic agents. Drugs may be classified depending on their mechanism of action as follows:

- Cell cycle phase-specific – only toxic to cells in particular phases of the cell cycle
- Cell cycle non-phase specific – act on cells in any phase of the cell cycle.

It should be noted, however, that such a distinction is relative, as opposed to absolute, and that the concept of phase specificity may have marked therapeutic implications (Cline & Haskell 1980). Neoplastic cells may be in various stages of the cell cycle; therefore, if a phase-specific drug were used alone in treatment only some of these cells would be in the appropriate phase of the cell cycle (Priestman 1980). Hence the rationale for scheduling and combination chemotherapy.

Most chemotherapeutic drugs target DNA within the cell in some manner. This action may result in direct interference with DNA, inhibition of enzymes related to RNA or DNA synthesis, or both, and/or destruction of the cells' necessary proteins (Brown & Hogan 1993). There are, currently, four main groups of therapeutic agents: alkylating agents, antimetabolites, antitumour antibiotics and plant alkaloids (Table 8.1), plus a group of miscellaneous drugs which include a variety of agents with unique antineoplastic effects. While the primary

Table 8.1 Cytotoxic drugs – chemical groups

Alkylating agents	Antimetabolites	Vinca alkaloids	Antimitotic antibiotics	Miscellaneous
Busulphan	Cytarabine	Vinblastine	Actinomycin D	L-Asparaginase
Chlorambucil	Hydroxyurea	Vincristine	Bleomycin	Mitozantrone
Cyclophosphamide	Mercaptopurine	Vindesine	Daunorubicin	Procarbazine
Dacarbazine	Methotrexate		Doxorubicin	
Ifosfamide	Thioguanine		Epirubicin	
Melphalan			Mithramycin	
Mustine hydrochloride			Mitomycin	
Thiotepa				
Nitrosoureas				*Podophyllotoxins*
Carmustine				Etoposide
Lomustine				Teniposide

Table 8.2 Cytotoxic drugs – mode of action

Alkylating agents	Highly reactive compounds which cause cross-linking of DNA and impede RNA formation Generally cell cycle non-specific
Antimetabolites	Structural analogues of intracellular metabolites required during replication. Act by inhibiting pyrimidine or purine synthesis or incorporation into DNA Generally cell cycle phase-specific
Antitumour antibiotics	Derived from soil fungi. Act primarily by binding to the double-helical structure of the DNA molecule, inhibiting its synthesis and replication. Also disrupt RNA synthesis Generally cell cycle non-specific
Plant alkaloids	Derived from the periwinkle. Exert major antineoplastic effects during the metaphase of the mitotic process by binding to the microtubular proteins and causing mitotic arrest Generally regarded as cell cycle phase-specific

antineoplastic action may be similar for drugs within each class (Table 8.2), the pharmacokinetics, secondary mechanisms of action, spectrum of activity, and toxic effects may vary widely.

Another class of important compounds, active in lymphoid malignancies and modestly active in myeloid leukaemias, is the corticosteroids. The mechanisms by which corticosteroids are cytotoxic are unclear; in some systems, data clearly support the hypothesis that corticosteroids induce apoptosis, the process in which active synthetic processes associated with intracellular mechanisms lead to cell death (Trump & Smith 1994).

An understanding of the general classification of cytotoxic agents, their mode of action, methods of administration, common toxicities and side-effects, will help to ensure that appropriate care is planned for individuals (Krakoff 1977, Cline & Haskell 1980).

Therapeutic strategies

Although the first effective drugs for treating cancer were brought to trial in the 1940s, initial therapeutic results were disappointing. Impressive regressions of acute lymphocytic leukaemia (ALL) and adult lymphomas were obtained with single agents such as nitrogen mustard, antifolates, corticosteroids and vinca alkaloids, but responses were only partial and of short duration. When remissions were obtained, as in ALL, they lasted less than 9 months, and relapse was associated with resistance to the original drug (Kaufman & Chabner 1996). The introduction of cyclic combination chemotherapy for ALL of childhood in the late 1950s marked a turning point in the effective treatment of neoplastic disease. While cell kinetics, pharmacokinetics, mechanisms of action of cytotoxic drugs, host toxicity and clinical responses provided the basis for initial approaches to treatment regimens (Reich 1983, 1984), current understanding of mechanisms of resistance provide the rationale for today's treatment strategies (Chabner 1986).

Drug resistance

Drug resistance, either apparent with initial treatment or emerging at the time of relapse after an initial response, inevitably occurs in all but a few cancer types that are potentially curable with chemotherapy. Resistance to cytotoxic therapy is a combined characteristic of a specific drug, a specific tumour, and a specific host whereby the drug is ineffective in controlling the tumour without excessive toxicity. Such resistance may be temporary (*relative or biochemical*) or permanent (*phenotypic*) (Goldie 1983, Ozols & Cowan 1986, Knobf & Durivage 1993).

Factors associated with temporary drug resistance, include variations in drug bioavailability, metabolism or elimination, tumour present in sanctuary sites, limited drug diffusion, alteration in cell kinetics, host toxicity and blood supply to the tumour. These factors may be overcome but permanent drug resistance is genetically based and is now thought to be the major contributing factor in treatment failure (Calman et al 1980, DeVita 1983, Ozols & Cowan 1986). Furthermore, phenotypic drug resistance is either *intrinsic* or *acquired*. Intrinsic resistance describes the initial unresponsiveness of a tumour to a given drug without any prior drug exposure. Acquired resistance refers to the unresponsiveness that emerges after initially successful treatment.

These concepts of resistance help to explain treatment outcomes and Table 8.3 shows some possible resistant mechanisms that may contribute to treatment failure.

Mechanisms of resistance identified to date can be divided into three broad categories:

- those which prevent the drug reaching its target and effective cytotoxic levels
- those which increase the ability of the neoplastic cell to repair damage which has occurred
- those which permit the cell to tolerate an otherwise lethal amount of damage (Twentyman 1995).

A type of drug resistance receiving increasing attention is multidrug resistance (MDR). The main mechanism of MDR is believed to be the overexpression of P-glycoprotein, which has the ability to pump a chemically diverse range of drugs out of the cells by hydrolysing the energy-providing molecule ATP (Fig. 8.7) (Deuchars & Ling 1989, Dalton 1993). This not only reduces the efficacy of the primary cytotoxics, which belong to quite different chemical classes – for example, anthracyclines, vinca alkaloids and epipodophyllotoxins (e.g. etoposide) – but is also important in human haematological malignancies where increased levels of expression of P-glycoprotein are evident and, subsequently, at relapse when resistant cell clones often emerge (Hoffbrand & Pettit 1993).

Drugs aimed at inhibiting the action of P-glycoprotein, such as verapamil, tamoxifen and cyclosporin A, which are also pumped out by the protein, are currently being investigated in attempts to overcome MDR (Hoelzer & Seipelt 1991, Hoffbrand & Pettit 1993).

Combination chemotherapy

Combination chemotherapy utilises multiple agents, each with cytotoxic activity in the disease under consideration but with different mechanisms of action, allowing independent cell killing by each agent (Kaufman & Chabner 1996). Furthermore, cells resistant to one agent might still be sensitive to another drug in the regimen which increases the likelihood of a successful outcome. The goal of combination chemotherapy is maximum cell kill with tolerable toxicity (Knobf & Durivage 1993). Only drugs known to be partially effective when used alone should be selected for use in combination; drugs where possible should be selected on the basis that toxicity does not overlap with the toxicity of other drugs, used in their optimal dose and scheduled and given at consistent intervals determined by the shortest time period necessary for recovery of the most sensitive normal target tissue, which is usually the bone marrow (DeVita 1989). Combination chemotherapy is used as first-line treatment for the management of haematological malignancies.

Scheduling

The detailed scheduling of drugs in multidrug regimens was based initially on both practical and theoretical considerations. Traditionally, intermittent cycles of treatment were used to allow time for bone marrow, gastrointestinal tract and immune system recovery, with the expectation that recovery of the tumour cell population would be slower than that of injured normal tissues (Calman et al 1980). Such a strategy allowed retreatment with full therapeutic doses as frequently as possible in keeping with the cell kill hypothesis. Although, historically, most common anti-cancer regimens have used

Table 8.3 Mechanisms of drug resistance (from DeVita 1989, reproduced with permission)

General mechanisms	Drug	Result
Multidrug resistance	Vinca alkaloids Antitumour antibiotics Etoposide	Drug actively pumped out of the cell
Transport defect	Methotrexate Melphalan Nitrogen mustard Cytosine arabinoside	Low carrier-mediated uptake Low membrane binding
Poor activation	Cytosine arabinoside 5-Azacytidine 5-Fluorouracil 6-Thioguanine 6-Mercaptopurine Methotrexate Doxorubicin	Low deoxycytidine kinase Low uridine-cytidine kinase Low uridine kinase, orotic acid PRT, uridine phosphorylase Low hypoxanthine-guanine PRT Low polyglutamation Low P-450 enzymes
Drug inactivation	Cytosine arabinoside Alkylating agents 6-Thioguanine 6-Mercaptopurine	High cytadine deaminase High glutathione High alkaline phosphatase
Improved DNA repair	Alkylating agents Antitumour antibiotics Cisplatin	High efficiency repair of strand breaks, ligase
Gene amplification	Methotrexate PALA 2-Deoxycoformycin 5-Fluorouracil	Dihydrofolate reductase Aspartate transcarbamylase Adenosine deaminase Thymidylate synthetase
Alternate pathways	Methotrexate 5-Fluorouracil	Increased thymidine salvage Increased thymidine kinase
Altered pools of competing substrate	Cytosine arabinoside 5-Fluorouracil	High CTP and DCTP
Target alterations	Vincristine Methotrexate 5-Fluorouracil Hydroxyurea Steroids	Tubulin Dihydrofolate reductase Thymidylate synthetase Ribonucleotide reductase Receptor or receptor-DNA binding

Abbreviations:
CTP, cytidine triphosphate
DCTP, deoxycytidine triphosphate
PALA, N-phosphonacetyl-L-aspartic acid
PRT, phosphoribosyl transferase

intermittent bolus delivery of drugs, in recent years constant-infusion chemotherapy has been indicated to be advantageous with early clinical trials suggesting improved therapeutic ratios for several drugs, such as etoposide, cytosine arabinoside and doxorubicin (Bjornsson et al 1986). However, the only agents which have demonstrated superiority for constant infusion as opposed to bolus are anthracyclines, because of the decreased cardiotoxicity, and cytosine arabinoside in AML (Kauffman & Chabner 1996).

Figures 8.8 and 8.9 illustrate typical flow charts for the management of AML and ALL,

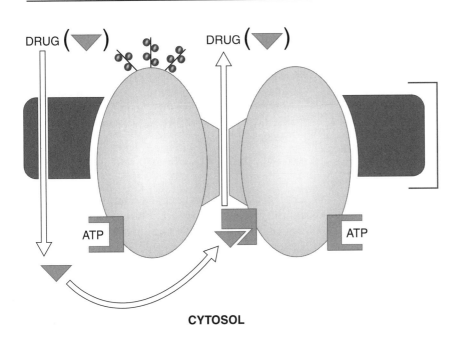

Figure 8.7 Schematic representation of P-glycoprotein, responsible for multidrug resistance (from Pastan & Gottesman 1988 reproduced with permission)

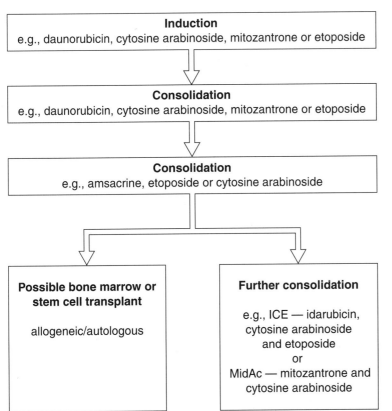

Figure 8.8 Typical treatment regimen for acute myeloid leukaemia

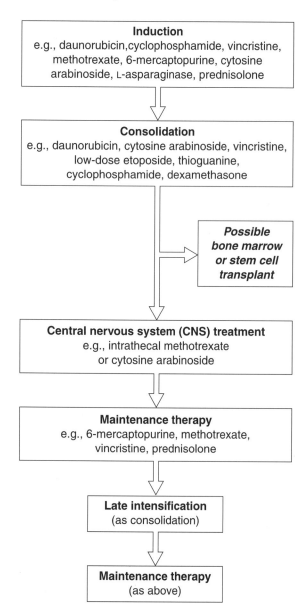

Figure 8.9 Typical treatment regimen for acute lymphatic leukaemia

respectively. In leukaemia, the aim of cytotoxic therapy is first to induce a remission (*induction therapy*). Thereafter, it is to prevent leukaemic recurrence related to undetectable, resistant disease (Hoffbrand & Pettit 1993, Seiter et al 1995) (*consolidation therapy*). This consists of one or two courses of further treatment with much higher doses of drugs than those used during induction therapy or with drugs, such as etoposide or cyclophosphamide, that are considered

to be non-cross resistant (Brown et al 1990). Additionally, in ALL some type of *intensification therapy*, consisting of further high-dose chemotherapy, followed by long-term (2 years) *maintenance therapy*, consisting of oral methotrexate and 6-mercaptopurine, has been found to reduce the risk of relapse (Cartwright & Staines 1992).

Dose

Dose intensification has received increasing emphasis in recent years as a strategy for overcoming resistance to chemotherapy. The importance of delivering maximum tolerated doses in potentially curable diseases has been repeatedly emphasised. Dose–response relationship is a fundamental principle of chemotherapy and is an important determinant of treatment outcome (DeVita 1991). Optimal dose intensity should be a composite of optimal drug dose and optimal duration of treatment (Hryniuk & Peter 1987, Harris & Mastroangelo 1991). To date, however, these are unknown for many current treatment regimens.

Outside the bone marrow transplant (BMT) setting, where marrow ablative doses of chemotherapy are used to increase tumour cell kill, dose intensification is frequently limited by haematological toxicity. It is here that the use

Case study 8.1

Peter, a 26-year-old married man with no family, has just been diagnosed with acute lymphatic leukaemia (ALL). Following initial investigations it is decided to enter him into the current United Kingdom ALL trial. It is planned that his induction therapy, consisting of combination chemotherapy daunorubicin, vincristine, L-asparaginase and oral prednisolone, will start within 24 hours.

Reflection point

What are the key nursing issues relevant at this stage, including specific informational/support needs, ethical issues and symptom management?

of haematopoietic growth factors has been proposed (Simon & Korn 1990). By alleviating bone marrow toxicity it is possible to achieve significant dose escalation (see Ch. 10).

CHEMOTHERAPY ADMINISTRATION

Handling cytotoxic drugs

In recent years an increasing number of articles have discussed the actual and potential hazards of cytotoxic chemotherapy (e.g. Cloak et al 1985, Frank-Stromborg et al 1986, Mayer 1991). Exposure to chemotherapy may occur during drug preparation, administration, disposal of equipment, or contact with human excreta through inhalation, absorption, direct skin contact or ingestion routes (Dewerk-Neal et al 1983, Miller 1987). The carcinogenic, teratogenic and mutagenic nature of cancer chemotherapeutic agents are well documented in animal models and at therapeutic levels in patients (Stellman & Zoloth 1986). Urinary mutagenicity has also been reported in nurses handling cytotoxic chemotherapy (Falck et al 1979) along with various anecdotal reports of acute symptoms being experienced (e.g. Falck et al 1979, Council on Scientific Affairs 1985, Selevan et al 1985). While conclusive evidence is not available to support the relationship between exposure and health risk, there is enough information to warrant prudent actions when handling cytotoxic agents.

National guidelines (e.g. Joint Council for Clinical Oncology 1994, Goodman 1998a) have been combined with local guidelines to provide a framework for practice development. These guidelines contain recommendations to prevent cytotoxic drug exposure to personnel and the environment. Box 8.1 summarises some of the general principles relating to the handling of cytotoxic drugs. Clearly, such guidelines are suggestions and form the basis for the development of local policies and procedures. However, compliance with guidelines has been found to be variable due to an unwillingness to change routines, variable access to disposal facilities and a lack of knowledge regarding the hazards of cytotoxic drugs (Mayer 1991). Little is known about current practice in relation to cytotoxic

---

Box 8.1   General principles of safe handling of cytotoxic drugs*

These principles aim to protect health-care professionals, patients and the environment from unnecessary exposure to potentially hazardous substances.

Only pharmacists with specialist knowledge and training should be involved in the preparation of cytotoxic drugs.

Proper aseptic techniques must be used in the preparation of chemotherapy to protect the patient and health-care professionals. The possibility of inadvertent ingestion or inhalation and direct skin contact or eye contact with drugs should be eliminated or avoided; for example, the use of laminar air flow cabinets or isolators.

Only nurses or medical staff with specialist knowledge and training should be involved in the administration of cytotoxic drugs.

All staff involved in the usage of cytotoxic drugs should be trained in the handling of cytotoxic drugs and be trained in the appropriate handling procedures relevant to their responsibilities. Anyone involved in the transportation of cytotoxic drugs should receive specific instructions related to hazardous waste and spillage precautions.

All equipment used in drug preparation and any unused drug(s) should be treated as hazardous waste and disposed of according to local policies and procedures.

*For further information on safe handling refer to Goodman I 1998a Clinical Practice Guidelines, The Administration of Cytotoxic Chemotherapy, Recommendations, Royal College of Nursing, London.

---

drug administration in either the UK or Europe. However, audit projects in the UK indicate that there is little consistency between different areas (Goodman 1998b, Grundy 1998). This has major implications for staff training and development.

    Reflection point

Compare your own local guidelines with current national guidelines and identify the issues which have implications for nursing practice.

Administration principles

The majority of cytotoxic drugs are administered intravenously, although they may also be administered orally, subcutaneously and, occasionally, intramuscularly or into specific body regions: for example, intra-arterially, intraperitoneally, intrapleurally, intraventricularly and intrathecally (Galassi et al 1996). The increase in the number of cytotoxic drugs now available, combined with the increasing sophistication of vascular access devices (see Ch. 12), the use of ambulatory infusion pumps and a move towards ambulatory and domiciliary chemotherapy provide unique challenges to healthcare professionals. Despite these changes, however, the basic principles of cytotoxic drug administration remain unchanged and are outlined in Table 8.4. However, it is frequently the education and support patients receive during treatment that determines the overall quality of care (Dennison 1993).

Management of extravasation

The most common mechanical complications of intravenous therapy administered via peripheral veins are thrombophlebitis and infiltration with extravasation of the infusate (Goodinson 1990). Extravasation refers to the leaking or infiltration of a drug into subcutaneous tissue. If the drug is a vesicant, it is capable of producing tissue necrosis or sloughing, whereas irritant drugs will cause inflammation and pain at the site of infiltration. Table 8.5 summarises known vesicant and irritant antineoplastic drugs (Skeel 1987, Yarbro 1992, Galassi et al 1996).

There is a lack of conclusive studies indicating the optimal management of drug extravasation. Guidelines for the management of extravasation have been proposed based on current level of knowledge and are outlined in Box 8.2 (Ford 1995). As the arguments on how best to treat extravasation remain equivocal it is essential to be aware of, and to adhere to, local policies and procedures. It is also imperative that an extravasation pack is available in the area where cytotoxics are being administered so treatment can be initiated promptly.

Antidotes specific to particular vesicants may be advocated: for example, sodium bicarbonate 8.4% (5 ml) + dexamethasone 4 mg (1 ml) or the use of hyaluronidase as a dispersant for extravasation of vinca alkaloids. Controversy surrounds the use of icepacks to an extravasation injury. While the rationale is to decrease the ability of the drug to disrupt cellular metabolism and reduce the destructive effects of enzymes released during the inflammatory response, it has been shown in animal studies to increase ulceration significantly when vinca alkaloids have been extravasated (Dorr & Fritz 1981). Conversely, the use of heat with vinca alkaloid extravasation increases vasodilation, facilitates fluid absorption and decreases local drug concentrations (Fingl & Woodbury 1975).

The management of doxorubicin extravasation is generally recognised as one of the most troublesome problems in the intravenous administration of chemotherapy. Tissue damage from extravasation of doxorubicin ranges from erythema, induration, and pain to excessive tissue breakdown requiring surgical debridement and spilt-thickness skin grafting. Contractures may be a long-term sequela of extravasation. Flushing around the extravasation site with normal saline to facilitate the removal of the remaining drug from the subcutaneous tissues has been advocated as a means of reducing extravasation injury (Gault 1993). However, early surgical intervention is recommended for serious extravasations, since doxorubicin can remain in the tissue for several months, causing continued damage (Coleman et al 1983). The first signs of extravasation may be subtle (McCaffrey Boyle & Engelking 1995). Individuals receiving cytotoxic drugs should be encouraged to report any burning, pain or other adverse sensation and continuous vigilance during administration is vital (Plate 9 illustrates damage caused by extravasation of a vesicant).

Considering the paucity of solid data on effective antidotes to extravasated drugs, prevention still must be considered the best way to avoid local tissue toxicity. While the incidence of vesicant drug extravasation among very experienced oncology nurses is low in cancer speciality settings (0.1%) in comparison

Table 8.4 Principles of intravenous cytotoxic drug administration (from Ford 1995, adapted with permission)

Action	Rationale
Selecting a site	
Most suitable: veins in the forearm	Ease of access. Sufficient tissue to protect nerves and tendons. Allows some flexibility and movement
Possible: veins on the dorsum of hand or wrist, anticubital fossa	Superficial veins easy to access and observe. Increased blood flow dilutes irritant drugs, reducing the likelihood of phlebitis. However, extravasation is difficult to detect
Avoid any limb with compromised circulation; e.g. lymphoedema or bruised areas	Detection of extravasation more difficult. Venous return less efficient/increased risk of infection
Avoid sites previously exposed to radiation	'Recall' phenomenon may occur.
Only one venepuncture per vein. If extravasation occurs, ideally select a site in the opposite limb. Avoid a distal point or the same vein	Potential for extravasation 'upstream'
Do not obscure injection site. Cannula should be lightly taped or covered with a transparent dressing	To detect extravasation at the earliest moment
Vesicants should be administered first if multiple drugs are being given	Integrity of vein is greatest following insertion and therefore extravasation is least likely
Chemotherapy infusions	
Inspect the cannula site for any signs of redness or swelling	To detect any condition which might render vein unsuitable for use
Check patency. Infuse 20–100 ml NaCl rapidly.	Tests vein integrity and flow and allows observation for extravasation
Check site frequently during administration	To detect any signs of extravasation
On completion of infusion flush with NaCl	To remove all drug from tubing and cannula
Administration of bolus chemotherapy	
Select site and assess patency	To test suitability and integrity of the vein
Assess 'flashback' by drawing blood back	To check correct insertion of the cannula
Flush between drugs with NaCl	To prevent interaction of the drugs
Administer over 3 min. Large volumes no greater than 5 ml/min	To allow drug dilution and minimise risk of extravasation
Observe continuously for extravasation	Many cytotoxics are vesicants and may cause serious tissue damage
Flush line prior to removal of cannula	To remove any residual drug from cannula

Table 8.5 Nonvesicant, vesicant and irritant drugs

Nonvesicant	Potential vesicant	Potential irritant
L-Asparaginase	Amsacrine	Carmustine
Bleomycin	Dacarbazine	Etoposide
Cyclophosphamide	Daunorubicin	Teniposide
Cytarabine	Doxorubicin	
Fludarabine	Epirubicin	
Ifosfamide	Esorubicin	
Methotrexate	Idarubicin	
Thiotepa	Mechlorethamine	
Topotecan	Mitomycin	
	Mitozantrone	
	Vinblastine	
	Vincristine	

to a somewhat higher incidence in general hospital settings (2–5%) (Rudolph & Larson 1987), there is no room for complacency. Currently, this has particular significance in the United Kingdom with the implementation of the recommendations of the Policy Framework for Cancer Services report (Department of Health 1995). Cancer networks consisting of cancer centres, cancer units and primary care services are being established and it is recommended that individuals will receive care as close to home as possible. This has particular implications for the development of cytotoxic drug administration and the associated requirements for education, training and support.

Allergic reactions

Some chemotherapeutic agents can potentially cause an allergic response. When administering a chemotherapeutic agent associated with a high incidence of allergic response, a test dose may be given: for example, L-asparaginase, where 10–20% of patients receiving it will experience a hypersensitivity reaction (Clavell et al 1986) with 10% of these patients progressing to life-threatening anaphylaxis (DeSpain 1992). For generalised allergic responses, such as anaphylaxis, intravenous adrenaline (1:10 000 solution) may be used. Usually 1–3 ml of adrenaline will be adminis-

---

Box 8.2   The management of extravasation

Treatment of extravasation may vary according to hospital policy

- Stop administration immediately and obtain expert advice.
- Mark extravasated area with a pen.
- Withdraw any solution by pulling back on syringe.
- Subcutaneous injection of 0.9% sodium chloride may be used to dilute the drug.
- Remove cannula.
- Apply warm compresses for vinca alkaloids or cold compresses for other vesicant agents.
- Prepare injection of hydrocortisone (100 mg) or dexamethasone (4 mg).
- Inject around entire area where extravasation is thought to have occurred, subcutaneously and intradermally, using 25 G needle.
- Apply hydrocortisone cream 1% to whole area.
- Cover site with icepack or equivalent for 24 hours.
- Continue to apply hydrocortisone cream 1% twice daily until redness disappears.
- Instruct patient to report any noticeable changes, e.g. blistering.
- Document, according to local policy.

For further information on the management of extravasation refer to Allwood M, Stanley A, Wright P 1997 The cytotoxics handbook, 3rd edn. Radcliffe Medical Press, Oxford.

---

tered slowly, with additional increments as needed to correct hypotension, bronchospasm and laryngospasm. Hydrocortisone may also be prescribed (Skeel 1987). Treatment of anaphylaxis requires prompt action; therefore a resuscitation kit containing the necessary drugs should be readily available in areas where chemotherapy is being administered.

Erythema multiforme, a reaction characterised by target lesions over the extremities and often involving the mucous membranes, has been infrequently associated with chemotherapeutic agents administered in high-dose combination therapy. Agents such as busulphan, VP16 (etoposide), procarbazine, hydroxyurea, bleomycin, methotrexate and cytosine arabinoside have been associated with such lesions which occasionally develop into generalised blistering (DeSpain 1992).

CHEMOTHERAPY: TOXICITY MANAGEMENT

Faced with the reality of a malignant disease, many patients will be prepared to accept a treatment of high toxicity for even a small chance of benefit (Slevin et al 1990). Treatment of haematological malignancies demands that treatment is intense, both in duration and in the number and range of side-effects and sequelae it causes. Consequently, there is a need for health-care professionals to be skilled in the administration of complex therapies and in monitoring and managing their toxic effects. Adequate assessment and documentation of side-effects, response to treatment and subsequent impact on quality of life are vital and provide the basis on which treatment decisions are made. To aid accurate and consistent assessment, toxicity-grading scales, such as the World Health Organization's (WHO) guidelines (1979) have been developed. Furthermore, nursing strategies to prevent the development of chemotherapy toxicities are essential for the care of patients (Travaglini & Nevidjon 1990).

Acute side-effects (those which occur immediately or a few days after chemotherapy administration) and chronic side-effects (occurring months to years after chemotherapy administration) are associated with most chemotherapeutic agents (Oldham & Smalley 1983). Drug toxicities will commonly determine the maximum amount of drug that can be administered safely. While cumulative and irreversible damage to certain vital organs, such as the heart, limits the total dose which can be administered (Goodman 1989), dose modification of chemotherapy agents because of toxicities, such as constipation, nausea, vomiting, or mucositis, may be preventable (Bertino & O'Keefe 1992).

Toxicities specific to individual, more commonly, used drugs are summarised in Table 8.6.

However, it is important to note that not only does the incidence and severity of toxicities relate to the drug dose, schedule and mode of action, but that they are also dependent on the underlying disease and interventions used to prevent or minimise toxicities, and may vary in severity according to the individual's condition and response to the drug therapy (Begg & Carbone 1983, Lydon 1986, Goodman 1989, Leslie 1992).

Systemic toxicities

Haematological toxicity

Haematological toxicities result from the drugs' ability to interfere with normal cell cycle function, by decreasing the absorption of necessary cellular nutrients, inhibiting the acquisition of required enzymes, or by other as yet unknown mechanisms (Griffin 1986, Caudell & Whedon 1991). The first blood cells to be affected are the neutrophils followed by a decrease in the circulating platelets; erythrocytes will be affected some weeks later (Hoffbrand & Pettit 1993). While bone marrow toxicity is generally temporary, recovering once treatment ceases, in some instances where the haematopoietic system is affected by primary or secondary malignant deposits recovery is less predictable. Blood component support may be required in some instances (see Ch. 11) until marrow recovery occurs. However, while anaemia is simpler to treat, if necessary, by transfusion, the treatment of neutropenia and thrombocytopenia is more problematic, particularly in patients undergoing bone marrow transplantation (Patterson 1992) (see Chs 10, 13 and 14).

Myelosuppression, a common side-effect of many agents, not only places the patient at increased risk for the development of opportunistic infections that are potentially lethal (see Ch. 13) but is the most common dose-limiting factor (Pastan et al 1986, Pederson-Bjergaard et al 1991). Chemotherapy may be withheld if the patient's white blood cell (WBC) count is between 1000 and 3000/mm^3 or if the actual neutrophil count (ANC) is <1500 cells/mm^3 (Hoffbrand & Pettit 1993). However, it is important to note that an ANC may be low

Table 8.6 Toxicities of commonly used cytotoxic drugs

Generic name	Side-effects		
	Immediate	Short-term	Long-term
Amsacrine	Venous pain, phlebitis if infused too fast	Mild/moderate nausea and vomiting. Stomatitis and oesophagitis	Bone marrow depression, cardiotoxicity
Asparaginase	Anaphylaxis and milder hypersensitivity reactions	Malaise, anorexia	Hepatotoxicity, CNS toxicity, pancreatic dysfunction
Busulphan			Bone marrow depression, irreversible pulmonary fibrosis
Cyclophosphamide	Hot flush. Dizziness. Strange taste	Nausea and vomiting at high doses	Bone marrow depression, haemorrhagic cystitis, alopecia, pulmonary toxicity, cardiotoxicity
Cytarabine		Nausea and vomiting at high doses. Flu-like syndrome	Bone marrow depression, hepatotoxicity (rare), hyperuricaemia, mucositis
Daunorubicin		Nausea and vomiting. Fever (often 2 h after therapy). Red urine	Bone marrow depression, alopecia, phlebitis, stomatitis, congestive cardiac failure, reactivation of radiation site
Etoposide	Severe hypotension if infused <30 min	Nausea and vomiting (very mild) greater with oral preparations	Alopecia, bone marrow depression, predominantly leucopenia
Melphalan	Hypersensitivity (very rare)	Nausea and vomiting (only in high single doses)	Bone marrow depression, alopecia with higher doses
Methotrexate		Gingivitis, stomatitis, mouth ulceration. CNS effects	Bone marrow depression, pulmonary toxicity, hepatotoxicity

while the total WBC may be within normal limits (4000–10 000/mm^3). Consequently, quantitating the ANC is essential.

As infection associated with myelosuppression is associated with significant morbidity and mortality (Pizzo 1989), much attention has been focused on the therapeutic administration of recombinant colony-stimulating factors to augment neutrophil counts (see Ch. 10). The aim of this therapy is to reduce morbidity and mortality from infections and allow full dosages of chemotherapeutic agents to be administered as scheduled, thus maximising therapeutic potential (Bronchud 1992).

Thrombocytopenia usually occurs 8–14 days after chemotherapy and in most cases concomitantly with neutropenia. Thrombocytopenia increases the risk of haemorrhagic complications (see Ch. 14). Consequently, chemotherapy may be withheld if the platelet count drops below 100 000/mm^3 (Mihich 1986).

Gastrointestinal toxicities

Gastrointestinal toxicity ranges from mild to severe and may be life threatening. Oral mucositis may be preceded by a sensation of dryness, followed by erythema and then by the formation of a white, patchy membrane, ulceration and necrosis. Enteric lesions may occur at any level, resulting in clinical symptoms of dysphagia, retrosternal burning, nausea and/or vomiting, watery diarrhoea and proctitis or constipation (Harris 1978, Holmes 1990, Grem 1996). Physical symptoms can result in significant distress that has a marked impact on the patient's quality of life (Ferrans 1990). Nurses have a significant role to play in minimising this distress, not only through practical interventions, such as regular mouth care (Daeffler 1980, Dudjak 1987) but in helping patients to cope with potential side-effects, thereby enhancing their quality of life.

Nausea and vomiting are the most commonly encountered, and often most distressing, side-effects of antineoplastic agents (Schulmeister 1991) (see Ch. 15) and may be accompanied by anorexia with subsequent alteration of nutritional status (see Ch. 17).

Diarrhoea may occur predominantly as a result of gastrointestinal mucosal irritation secondary to a direct toxic effect of the drugs on the bowel or infection. Diffuse mucosal changes can occur along the gastrointestinal tract; inflammation, oedema, subsequent degeneration, flattening or necrosis of intestinal crypt cells, and abnormalities of intestinal villous architecture appear (McDonald et al 1986). The absorptive surface area is reduced and mucosal irritability is common, leading to a rapid transit time and reduction in absorption

of nutrients (Wujcik 1992). The spectrum of toxicity varies according to agent, dose, schedule, route of administration and nadir (Hansen 1991, Camp-Sorrell 1993) and may be associated with abdominal distension, cramping and flatulence. In severe cases proctitis, mucosal ulceration and intestinal perforation may occur and without adequate management result in dehydration, nutritional malabsorption and circulatory collapse (Tchekmedyian et al 1992).

Although chemotherapeutic agents, such as methotrexate and doxorubicin, can cause diarrhoea it is important to remember that disruption of the integrity of the gut lining may permit access of enteric organisms into the bloodstream, with the potential for overwhelming sepsis, particularly if the granulocyte nadir coincides with diarrhoea (Grem 1996). Management of diarrhoea is varied and is dependent on the underlying cause. It may be controlled in some instances by dietary modifications, oral antibiotics if infection is confirmed (Figlin 1987), or may necessitate the use of various pharmacologic agents such as anticholinergic drugs (Camp-Sorrell 1993), loperamide (Levy 1991) and octreotide acetate (Mitchell & Schein 1992). Equally important are chemotherapeutic agents such as vincristine and vinblastine, which cause constipation – generally related to a direct effect on the nerve supply of the bowel, causing hypomotility. Constipation may occur within 3–7 days of drug administration and is often preventable through dietary management and the use of prophylactic stool softeners (Mitchell & Schein 1992).

Organ toxicity

Cardiotoxicity

The most common chemotherapeutic agents associated with cardiac toxicity are the anthracycline antibiotics doxorubicin and daunorubicin which damage myocyte cells. However, there are several other risk factors, summarised in Box 8.3 (Von Hoff et al 1982, Kaszyk 1986, Torti & Lum 1989), the most significant being the total cumulative dose of anthracycline. Guidelines have been established to minimise cardiac toxicity by limiting the total cumulative

---

Box 8.3   Risk factors that may potentiate cardiac toxicity

Specific agent
Total cumulative dose
Age
Administration schedule
Cardiac irradiation
Pre-existing heart disease

Box 8.4   Cytotoxic agents associated with neurotoxicity

Peripheral neuropathy
Vincristine
Vinblastine
Vindesine
Cytarabine
Procarbazine

Cranial nerve neuropathy
Vinblastine
Vincristine

Autonomic neuropathy
Vincristine

Subacute meningeal irritation
Intrathecal methotrexate

---

dose of doxorubicin to $550\,mg/m^2$ and daunorubicin to $600\,mg/m^2$ with a decrease to $450\,mg/m^2$ if mediastinal radiation has been administered (Camp-Sorrell 1991). While acute cardiotoxicity occurs in approximately 10% of patients receiving chemotherapy, and generally resolves quickly without serious complications, chronic effects involve non-reversible cardiomyopathy, which is generally poorly responsive to diuretics or digitalis and carries a 60% mortality rate (Torti & Lum 1989). In an attempt to reduce the risk of cardiotoxicity other anthracycline analogues, such as epirubicin, idarubicin, esorubicin and aclarubicin are being evaluated.

Nursing implications

- Nursing assessment is aimed at identifying individuals at risk of developing cardiomyopathy and observing for signs of congestive cardiac failure. Early signs include non-specific dry cough or tachycardia. As cardiomyopathy progresses, individual's may become dyspnoeic at rest, and physical examination may reveal peripheral oedema, distended neck veins and abdominal distension (Kaszyk 1986).
- Ensure a baseline electrocardiograph (ECG) is carried out prior to commencing any treatment.
- Record doses of cytotoxic drugs given accurately and be aware of total cumulative dose.
- Carry out cardiac monitoring; for example, when high-dose VP16 is administered.

If chronic cardiotoxicity develops:

- Focus on supportive care and rehabilitation within the constraints imposed by the condition.

- Focus on patient and family education; energy conservation; low sodium diet to minimise fluid retention; administer digitalis to improve cardiac function and monitor effects.
- Provide emotional support.

Neurotoxicity

Several cancer chemotherapeutic agents have been associated with neurotoxicities (Box 8.4) (Kaplan & Wiernik 1982, Weiss et al 1974, Goodman 1989). Neurotoxicity can occur as a direct or indirect result of damage to the central nervous system (CNS). Fortunately, for the majority of patients neurotoxicity is temporary; however, significant toxicity requires that the drug be withheld until symptoms resolve or may, in more severe cases, necessitate dose reduction or discontinuation of the drug (Macdonald & Axelrod 1992).

Nursing implications

- Carry out neurological assessments to observe for problems developing, such as:
  —peripheral neuropathy – paraesthesia, most commonly of the hands and feet, which may progress to muscle pain, weakness, gait disturbance and sensory impairment with continued drug dosing
  —cranial nerve neuropathy – recurrent laryngeal nerve $\rightarrow$ vocal cord paresis or paralysis

—oculomotor nerve → bilateral ptosis, diplopia

—trigeminal nerve → severe jaw pain after first dose

—autonomic neuropathy is very common, especially constipation and colicky abdominal pain. It may precede the onset of paraesthesiae or diminished deep tendon reflexes

—subacute meningeal irritation – stiff neck, headache, nausea and vomiting, and pyrexia – may begin 2–4 hours after drug administration and last for 12–72 hours (Kaplan & Wiernik 1984)

- Focus on rehabilitative care. Refer for occupational therapy assessment if motor function is affected.
- Implement and educate on safety measures required.
- Provide emotional support.

Pulmonary toxicity

Preventing pulmonary toxicities, which are usually progressive and irreversible if associated with chemotherapeutic agents, is the ideal as there is no specific method of treatment (Stover 1989). The drug most commonly associated with pulmonary toxicity is bleomycin, although other drugs have been implicated: for example, busulphan, methotrexate, cytosine arabinoside and cyclophosphamide (Hydzik 1990, Camp-Sorrell 1993), with combinations of these drugs leading to a higher morbidity (Ginsberg & Comis 1982). Patients present with a dry, hacking cough and exertional dyspnoea that can progress to resting dyspnoea, tachypnoea and cyanosis. Consequently, it is imperative that pulmonary toxicity is detected as early as possible.

Nursing implications

- Ensure that baseline X-ray has been carried out prior to commencing any treatment and is repeated prior to each treatment.
- Observe closely for any onset of symptoms previously outlined and report if present.
- Monitor oxygen saturation levels.
- If pulmonary toxicity is present, educate the patient to prioritise activities and support

them to implement effective breathing techniques and monitor in conjunction with the physiotherapist.
- Provide emotional support.

Hepatic toxicity

Hepatic toxicity is uncommon, but it can be a serious consequence of chemotherapy administration, ranging from transient elevation of liver enzymes to permanent cirrhosis (Camp-Sorrell 1993). While it is often difficult to attribute hepatic damage to specific agents due to the complexity of the disease itself and other treatment factors, drug dose may need to be reduced or treatment omitted (Perry 1992). Unless extensive fibrosis or necrosis has occurred, hepatotoxicity is reversible. (See Ch. 10 for discussion of veno-occlusive disease.)

Nursing implications

- Ensure regular monitoring of liver function tests.
- Observe closely for any signs of fluid shift: decreased blood pressure, increased pulse rate, low central venous pressure, decreased urine output, increased specific gravity of urine, low levels of serum albumin, weight gain or evidence of ascites.
- If hepatic impairment is evident, decrease protein intake in diet, monitor fluid balance closely, and administer intravenous albumin as prescribed.
- Provide emotional support, patient and family education.

Nephrotoxicity

Nephrotoxicity has been associated with a number of chemotherapeutic agents, such as cisplatin, high-dose methotrexate, mitomycin C, nitrosoureas, ifosfamide and cyclophosphamide for example, and is a dose-limiting side-effect (Weiss & Poster 1982, Camp-Sorrell 1993). While many of these agents are both metabolised and excreted by the kidneys, others are merely excreted as metabolites or as unchanged drugs. Primary treatment is aimed at prevention and often involves aggressive hydration, urinary alkalinisation, diuresis and monitoring biochemistry (Camp-Sorrell 1993). Renal insufficiency is a dynamic pathological process and exists on a continuum ranging from mild to severe (Ballard 1991). For patients who exhibit early signs of toxicity – for example, increased blood urea and creatinine and decreased renal clearance of creatinine – the dose may have to be reduced or the drug omitted from the treatment regimen. Therefore, observation for early signs of renal impairment, including decreased urinary output, fluid retention/oedema and weight gain, are essential.

Haemorrhagic cystitis

Within the BMT setting, haemorrhagic cystitis is a major toxicity associated with the administration of high-dose cyclophosphamide (120–200 mg/kg). The prophylactic administration of mesna (2-mercaptoethane sulphonate sodium) intravenously, at 40% of the cyclophosphamide dose, prior to and at 3, 6, and 9 hours following administration of cyclophosphamide, has been shown to reduce the incidence of haemorrhagic cystitis at a macroscopic level and allowed higher doses to be administered with minimal associated risk (Gordon-Smith 1992).

Haemorrhagic cystitis may occur as a direct effect of the deposition of acrolein, a by-product of cyclophosphamide or ifosfamide metabolism, on the urothelium (Stillwell & Benson 1988). While mild or transient haemorrhagic cystitis, associated with urinary frequency, urgency, dysuria and haematuria, may resolve spontaneously or with an increased fluid intake/output, moderate/severe haemorrhagic cystitis may necessitate bladder irrigation in addition to an increased fluid intake/output to clear developing clots. In more severe cases cystoscopy may be required to cauterise bleeding and in extreme cases cystectomy may be required (Camp-Sorrell 1993).

NURSING IMPLICATIONS

- Implement preventive measures, such as increasing fluid intake before and after treatment. Intravenous fluids may be prescribed and forced diuresis may be indicated, particularly when high-dose cyclophosphamide is being administered.
- Monitor fluid balance accurately.
- Test urine for haematuria, proteinuria and creatinine clearance.

- Administer mesna, which offers protection of the bladder mucosa, alongside cyclophosphamide or ifosfamide administration.
- Report any symptoms which become manifest.
- Provide emotional support, patient and family education.

Hyperuricaemic neuropathy

This condition may occur as a separate entity, or if accompanied by the rapid release of intracellular ions is called tumour lysis syndrome (TLS), which is considered a metabolic emergency. It involves a sudden increase in uric acid in the plasma, which may lead to a deposition of urate crystals in the kidney and subsequent renal damage. This is particularly relevant in some leukaemias and lymphomas with a large tumour volume, where rapid destruction of neoplastic cells following chemotherapy is accompanied by increased catabolism of cellular nucleic acids (Skipper et al 1993) (see Ch. 6).

Gonadal toxicity

Chemotherapeutic agents, singly or in combination, have a profound effect on male and female gonadal function in terms of both germ cell production and endocrine function and may alter sexual function directly or indirectly (Ostroff & Lesko 1991). For a full discussion of fertility issues refer to Chapter 18. However, provision of accurate information and sensitive discussion on such issues as sexual performance, fertility, childbearing abilities and risk of osteoporosis can make a significant difference to the individual's ability to deal with sexual concerns and the late effects of therapy.

Second malignancy

The development of a second malignancy is the most serious long-term effect of chemotherapy. Alkylating agents and nitrosoureas are the agents implicated in chemotherapy-related malignancies (Coleman & Tucker 1989). Prognosis is poor and treatment for second malignancies is often unsuccessful. Currently, however, the risk of second malignancy is small and treatment for the primary malignancy usually outweighs that risk (Sugarman et al 1985).

Case study 8.2

Peter, having undergone his induction and consolidation treatment, is now receiving maintenance chemotherapy while awaiting allogeneic bone marrow transplantation from his sister. He is also beginning to look to the future and family life.

During the course of his treatment he developed peripheral neuropathy in both his hands and feet which meant that some of his treatment required to be omitted and, on one occasion, experienced headache, neck stiffness and nausea following a lumbar puncture.

Reflection point

Consider why Peter experienced the symptoms outlined and the other side-effects he may have experienced during the course of his treatment. What are the implications for Peter in the future?

CONCLUSION

Cytotoxic chemotherapy will, for the foreseeable future, continue to be the mainstay of treatment for haematological malignancies (Summerhayes 1995). Nurses have major responsibilities in caring for patients receiving cytotoxic agents as part of their treatment regimen. It is important that nurses know treatment goals, drug classifications with modes of action, principles of tumour growth and cell kill and current treatment protocols. Chemotherapeutic agents should be administered only by nurses who have a thorough understanding and knowledge of such issues and who are educated, trained and skilled in the various procedures. Furthermore, patient and family education on the many aspects of chemotherapy (e.g. procedure, potential side-effects and toxicities, and follow-up care) requires competent nursing assessment and intervention based on each individual's needs. The field of cancer chemotherapy is constantly changing and nurses must strive to keep abreast of new developments in order that they provide optimal care to both the patient and their family.

DISCUSSION QUESTIONS

Choose one chemotherapy regimen commonly used in your area. Relating this directly to a case with which you are familiar, explore and discuss the following:

1. What drugs were used? In what phase of the cell cycle do these drugs act and how are they classified?
2. What are the nursing implications of systemic and organic toxicities which may accompany the administration of cytotoxic drugs?
3. What are the informational and educational needs of individuals undergoing treatment and their families?

References

Ballard B 1991 Renal and hepatic complications. In: Whedon M B (ed) Bone marrow transplantation: principles, practice and nursing insights. Jones and Bartlett, Boston

Begg C B, Carbone P P 1983 Clinical trials and drug toxicity in the elderly: the experience of the Eastern Co-operative Oncology Group. Cancer 52(11): 1986–1992

Bertino J R, O'Keefe P 1992 Barriers and strategies for effective chemotherapy. Seminars in Oncology 8(2): 77–82

Bjornsson T D, Huang A T, Roth P, Jacob D S, Christenson R 1986 Effects of high dose chemotherapy on the absorption of digoxin in two different formulations. Clinical Pharmacology and Therapeutics 39(21): 25–28

Bronchud M 1992 The importance of dose in cancer chemotherapy. Gardiner-Caldwell, Macclesfield

Brown J K, Hogan C M 1993 Chemotherapy. In: Groenwald S L, Frogge M H, Goodman M, Yarbro C H (eds) Cancer nursing principles and practice, 3rd edn. Jones and Bartlett, Boston

Brown R A, Nerzig R H, Wolff S N 1990 High dose etoposide and cyclophosphamide without bone marrow transplantation for resistant haematologic malignancy. Blood 76(3): 473–479

Buzzoni R, Bonadonna G, Valagussa P, Zambetti M 1991 Adjuvant chemotherapy with doxorubicin plus cyclophosphamide, methotrexate and fluorouracil in the treatment of resectable breast cancer with more than three positive axillary nodes. Journal of Clinical Oncology 9(12): 2134–2140

Calman K C, Smyth J F, Tattersall M N H 1980 Basic principles of cancer chemotherapy. Macmillan, London

Camp-Sorrell D 1991 Controlling adverse effects of chemotherapy. Nursing 91(4): 34–42

Camp-Sorrell D 1993 Chemotherapy: toxicity management. In: Groenwald S L, Frogge M H, Goodman M, Yarbro C H (eds) Cancer nursing: principles and practice, 3rd edn. Jones and Bartlett, Boston

Cartwright R A, Staines A 1992 Acute leukaemias. Clinical Haematology 5(1): 1–26

Caudell K A, Whedon M B 1991 Haemopoietic complications. In: Whedon M B (ed) Bone marrow transplantation: principles, practice and nursing insights. Jones and Bartlett, Boston

Chabner B A 1986 The oncologic end game. Journal of Clinical Oncology 4(5): 626–638

Clavell L A, Gelber R A, Cohen H J et al 1986 Four agent induction and intensive asparaginase therapy for treatment of childhood acute lymphocytic leukaemia. New England Journal of Medicine 315(11): 657–663

Cline M, Haskell C 1980 Cancer chemotherapy. W B Saunders, Philadelphia

Cloak M, Connor T, Stevens K et al 1985 Occupational exposure of nursing personnel to antineoplastic agents. Oncology Nursing Forum 12(5): 33–39

Coleman C N Tucker A 1989 Secondary cancer. In: DeVita V T (ed) Cancer principles and practice of oncology. J B Lippincott, Philadelphia

Coleman J J, Walker A P, Didolkar M S 1983 Treatment of adriamycin induced skin ulcers: a prospective controlled study. Journal of Surgical Oncology 22(2): 129–135

Cooper M R, Cooper M R 1991 Principles of medical oncology. In: Holleb A I, Fink D, Murphy G (eds) Clinical oncology. American Cancer Society, Atlanta

Council on Scientific Affairs 1985 Guidelines for Handling Parenteral Antineoplastics. Journal of the American Medical Association 253(11): 1590–1592

Daeffler R 1980 Oral hygiene measures for patients with cancer. Cancer Nursing 3(5): 347–356

Dalton WS 1993 Drug resistance modulation in the laboratory and the clinic. Seminars in Oncology 20(1): 64–69

Dennison S 1993 An exploration into the verbal communication that occurs between the nurse and the patient whilst the nurse is delivering intravenous chemotherapy. Unpublished MSc Thesis, University of Surrey

Department of Health 1995 A policy framework for commissioning cancer services: Report on the Advisory Group on Cancer Department of Health, London

DeSpain J D 1992 Dermatologic toxicity. In: Perry M C (ed) The chemotherapy source book. Williams and Wilkins, Baltimore

Deuchars K L, Ling V 1989 P-glycoprotein and multidrug resistance in cancer chemotherapy. Seminars in Oncology 16(2): 156–165

DeVita V T 1983 The James Ewing Lecture. The relationship between tumour mass and resistance to chemotherapy: implications for surgical adjuvant treatment of cancer. Cancer 51(7): 1209–1220

DeVita V T 1989 Principles of chemotherapy. In: DeVita V T, Hellman S, Rosenberg S A (eds) Cancer: principles and practice of oncology, 3rd edn. J B Lippincott, Philadelphia

DeVita V T 1991 The influence of information on drug resistance on protocol design. Annals of Oncology 2(2): 93–106

Dewerk-Neal A, Wadden R A, Chiou W L 1983 Exposure of hospital workers to airborne antineoplastic agents. American Journal of Hospital Pharmacists 40(4): 597–601

Dorr R T, Fritz W L 1981 Cancer chemotherapy. Elsevier, Amsterdam

Dudjak L A 1987 Mouth care for mucositis due to radiation therapy. Cancer Nursing 10(3): 131–140

Falck K, Grohn P, Sorsa M, Vainio H, Heinonen E, Holsti L 1979 Mutagenicity in urine of nurses handling cytotoxic drugs. Lancet 1(8128): 1250–1251

Ferrans C E 1990 Quality of life: conceptual issues. Seminars in Oncology Nursing 6(4): 248–254

Figlin R A 1987 Biotherapy with interferon in solid tumours. Oncology Nursing Forum 14(6 Suppl.): 23–31

Fingl E, Woodbury D M 1975 General principles. In: Goodman L, Gilman A (eds) Pharmacologic basis of therapeutics, 5th edn. Macmillan, New York

Fisher R J, Gaynor E R, Dahlberg S et al 1993 Comparison of a standard regimen (CHOP) with three intensive chemotherapy regimens for advanced non-Hodgkin's lymphoma. New England Journal of Medicine 328(14): 1002–1006

Ford M 1995 Cytotoxic drug therapy: guidelines for safe practice. Airedale National Health Service Trust Policy Document

Frank-Stromborg M, Krafka B, Gale D, Porter N 1986 Carcinogenesis: are some risks acceptable? American Journal of Nursing 86(7): 814–817

Galassi A, Hubbard S M, Alexander H R, Steinhaus E 1996 Chemotherapy administration: practical guidelines. In: Chabner B A, Longo D L (eds) Cancer chemotherapy and biotherapy: principles and practice. Lippincott-Raven, Philadelphia

Gault D T 1993 Extravasation injuries. British Journal of Plastic Surgery 46(2): 91–96

Ginsberg S J, Comis R L 1982 The pulmonary toxicity of antineoplastic agents. Seminars in Oncology 9(1): 34–51

Goldie J H 1983 Relevance of drug resistance in cancer treatment strategy. In: Muggia F M (ed) Cancer chemotherapy. Martinus Nijhoff, New York

Goodinson S M 1990 The risks of IV therapy. Professional Nurse 5(5): 235–238

Goodman I 1998a Clinical practice guidelines: the administration of cytotoxic chemotherapy, recommendations. Royal College of Nursing, London

Goodman I 1998b Development of national, evidence-based clinical guidelines for the administration of cytotoxic chemotherapy. European Journal of Oncology Nursing 2(1): 43–50

Goodman M 1989 Managing the side effects of chemotherapy. Seminars in Oncology Nursing 5(Suppl. 1): 29–59

Gordon-Smith E 1992 Bone marrow transplantation for acquired aplastic anaemia. In: Treleaven J, Barrett J (eds) Bone marrow transplantation in practice. Churchill Livingstone, London

Grem J L 1996 5-Fluoropyrimidines. In: Chabner B A, Longo D L (eds) Cancer chemotherapy and biotherapy, 2nd edn. Lippincott-Raven, Philadelphia

Griffin J P 1986 Physiology of the haemopoietic system. In: Griffin J P (ed) Haematology and immunology: concepts for nursing. Appleton-Century-Crofts, Norwalk, CT

Grundy M 1998 Chemotherapy administration by nurses: an audit of practice and educational preparation. National Board for Nursing, Midwifery and Health Visiting for Scotland, Edinburgh

Hancock B W, Bradshaw J D 1981 Lecture notes on clinical oncology. Blackwell, Oxford

Hansen R M 1991 5-Fluorouracil by protracted venous infusion: a review of recent clinical studies. Cancer Investigation 9(6): 637–642

Harris D T, Mastroangelo M J 1991 Therapy and application of early systemic therapy. Seminars in Oncology 18(6): 493–503

Harris J 1978 Nausea, vomiting and cancer treatment. Ca: A Cancer Journal for Clinicians 28(4): 194–201

Henderson E S, Lister T A 1990 Leukaemia, 5th edn. W B Saunders, Philadelphia

Hoelzer D, Seipelt G 1991 Myeloid malignancies. Gardiner-Caldwell, Macclesfield

Hoffbrand A V, Pettit J E 1993 Essential haematology, 3rd edn. Blackwell, London

Holmes S 1990 Cancer chemotherapy. Austin Cornish, London

Holmes S 1997 Cancer chemotherapy: a guide for practice, 2nd edn. Asset Books, Leatherhead

Hryniuk W M, Peter J L 1987 Implications of dose intensity for cancer clinical trials. Seminars in Oncology 14(Suppl. 4): 1–44

Hydzik C A 1990 Late effects of chemotherapy: implications for patient management and rehabilitation. Nursing Clinics of North America 25(2): 423–446

Irani M A 1992 Improving chemotherapy patient outcomes. Highlights on Antineoplastic Drugs 10(1): 5–8

Jenkins J 1992 Biology of cancer: current issues and future prospects. Seminars in Oncology Nursing 8(1): 63–69

Joint Council for Clinical Oncology 1994 Quality control in cancer chemotherapy: managerial and procedural aspects. Royal College of Physicians, London

Kaplan R S, Wiernik P H 1982 Neurotoxicity of antineoplastic drugs. Seminars in Oncology 9(1): 103–130

Kaplan R S, Wiernik P H 1984 Neurotoxicity of antitumour agents. In: Perry M C, Yarbro J W (eds) Toxicity of chemotherapy. Grune and Stratton, Orlando

Kaszyk L K 1986 Cardiac toxicity associated with cancer therapy. Oncology Nursing Forum 13(4): 81–88

Kaufman D, Chabner B A 1996 Clinical strategies for cancer treatment: the role of drugs. In: Chabner B A, Longo D L (eds) Cancer chemotherapy and biotherapy, 2nd edn. J B Lippincott, Philadelphia

Knobf M T, Durivage H J 1993 chemotherapy: principles of therapy. In: Groenwald S L, Frogge M H, Goodman M, Yarbro C H (eds) Cancer nursing: principles and practice, 3rd edn. Jones and Bartlett, Boston

Krakoff I 1977 Cancer chemotherapeutic agents. Ca: A Cancer Journal for Clinicians 27(3): 130–143

Leslie W T 1992 Chemotherapy in older cancer patients. Oncology 6(Suppl. 2): 74–80

Levy M H 1991 Constipation and diarrhoea in cancer patients. Cancer Bulletin 43(2): 412–422

Lydon J L 1986 Nephrotoxicity of cancer treatment. Oncology Nursing Forum 13(2): 68–77

McCaffrey Boyle D, Engelking C 1995 Vesicant extravasation: myths and realities. Oncology Nursing Forum 22(1): 57–67

McDonald G B, Shulman H M, Sullivan K M, Spencer G D 1986 Intestinal and hepatic complications of human bone marrow transplantation. Gastroenterology 90(3): 460–477, 770–784

Macdonald J S, Axelrod R 1992 Adjuvant therapy of colon and rectal cancer. In: Ahlgren J D, Macdonald J S (eds) Gastrointestinal oncology. J B Lippincott, Philadelphia

Maxwell M B, Maher K E 1992 Chemotherapy-induced myelosuppression. Seminars in Oncology Nursing 8(2): 113–123

Mayer D K 1991 Hazards of chemotherapy. Cancer Supplement 70(4): 988–992

Mihich E 1986 Future perspectives for biological response modifiers: a viewpoint. Seminars in Oncology 13(2): 234–254

Miller S 1987 Issues in cytotoxic drug handling safety. Seminars in Oncology Nursing 3(2): 133–141

Mitchell E P, Schein P S 1992 Gastrointestinal toxicity of chemotherapeutic agents. In: Perry M C (ed) The chemotherapy source book. Williams and Wilkins, Baltimore

Oldham R K, Smalley R V 1983 Immunotherapy: the old and the new. Journal of Biological Response Modifiers 2(1): 1–37

Ostroff J S, Lesko L M 1991 Psychosexual adjustment and fertility issues. In: Whedon M B (ed) Bone marrow transplantation: principles, practice and nursing insights. Jones and Bartlett, Boston

Ozols R F, Cowan K 1986 New aspects of clinical drug resistance: the role of gene amplification and reversal of resistance in drug refractory cancer. In: DeVita V T, Hellman S, Rosenberg S A (eds) Important advances in oncology. J B Lippincott, Philadelphia

Pastan I H, Gottesman M M 1988 Molecular biology of multidrug resistance in human cells. In: Devita V T, Hellman S, Rosenberg S A (eds) Important advances in oncology. J B Lippincott, Philadelphia, p 9

Pastan I, Willingham M C, Fitzgerald D J 1986 Immunotoxins. Cell 47(5): 641–648

Patterson K 1992 Blood and blood product transfusion during bone marrow transplantation. In

Treleaven J, Barrett J (eds) Bone marrow transplantation in practice. Churchill Livingstone, London

Pederson-Bjergaard J, Daugaard G, Hansen S W, Philip P, Larsen S O, Rorth M 1991 Increased risk of myelodysplasia and leukaemia after etoposide, cisplatin and bleomycin for germ cell tumours. Lancet 338(8763): 359–363

Perry M C 1992 Hepatotoxicity of chemotherapeutic agents. In Perry M C (ed) The chemotherapy source book. Williams and Wilkins, Baltimore

Pitot H C 1981 Fundamentals of oncology, 2nd edn. Marcel Dekker, New York

Pizzo P A 1989 Combating infections in neutropenic patients. Hospital Practice 24(7): 93–100, 103–104, 107–110

Priestman T J 1980 Cancer chemotherapy: an introduction. Farmitalia Carlo Erba, Barnet, Hertfordshire

Reich S D 1983 Rationale for anticancer drug dosing schedules. Cancer Nursing 6(6): 465–467

Reich S D 1984 The clinical application of drug dosing schedules in cancer therapy – Part II. Cancer Nursing 7(1): 59–61

Rudolph R, Larson D L 1987 Etiology and treatment of chemotherapeutic agent extravasation injuries: a review. Journal of Clinical Oncology 5(7): 1116–1126

Schulmeister L 1991 Establishing a cancer patient education system for ambulatory patients. Seminars in Oncology Nursing 7(2): 118–124

Seiter K, Miller W H, Feldman E J, Ahmed T, Arlin Z 1995 Pilot study of *all*-trans-retinoic acid as post remission therapy in patients with acute promyelocytic leukaemia. Leukaemia 9(1): 15–18

Simon R, Korn E L 1990 Evolving concepts in the systemic adjuvant treatment of breast cancer. Cancer Research 52(8): 2127–2137

Skeel R T 1987 The biologic and pharmacologic basis of cancer chemotherapy. In: Skeel R T (ed) Handbook of cancer chemotherapy, 2nd edn. Little, Brown and Company, Boston

Skipper A, Szeluga D J, Groenwald S L 1993 Nutritional disturbances. In: Groenwald S L, Frogge M H, Goodman M, Yarbro C H (eds) Cancer nursing: principles and practice, 3rd edn. Jones and Bartlett, Boston

Slevin M L, Stubbs L, Plant H J et al 1990 Attitudes to chemotherapy: comparing views of patients with cancer with those of doctors, nurses and general public. British Medical Journal 300(6737): 1458–1460

Stellman J, Zoloth S 1986 Cancer chemotherapeutic agents as occupational hazards: a literature review. Cancer Investigation 4(2): 127–135

Stillwell T J, Benson R C Jr 1988 Cyclophosphamide induced haemorrhagic cystitis: a review of 100 patients. Cancer 61(3): 451–457

Stover D E 1989 Pulmonary toxicity. In: DeVita V T (ed) Cancer principles and practice of oncology. J B Lippincott, Philadelphia

Sugarman B J, Aggarwal B B, Hass P E, Figari I S, Palladino M A Jr, Shepard H M 1985 Recombinant tumour necrosis factor-alpha: effects of proliferation of normal and transformed cells in vitro. Science 230(4728): 943–945

Summerhayes M 1995 Developments in the chemotherapeutic treatment of cancer. The Hospital Pharmacist 2(1): 113–116

Tannock I F 1992 Cell proliferation. In: Tannock I F, Hill R P (eds) The basic science of oncology, 2nd edn. McGraw-Hill, New York

Taussig M J 1979 Processes in pathology. Blackwell, Oxford

Tchekmedyian N H, Hickman M N, Siau J et al 1992 Megestrol acetate in cancer anorexia and weight loss. Cancer 69(5): 1268–1274

Torti F M, Lum B L 1989 Cardiac toxicity. In: DeVita V T (ed) Cancer principles and practice of oncology. J B Lippincott, Philadelphia

Travaglini J, Nevidjon B 1990 Complications related to cancer therapy. Clinical Advances in Oncology 2(3): 1–13

Trump D L, Smith D C 1994 Systemic therapies. In: Love R R (ed) Manual of clinical oncology, 6th edn. Springer-Verlag, London

Twentyman P R 1995 Multidrug resistance. Current Medical

Literature: Leukaemia and Lymphoma 3(4): 99–103

Von Hoff D D, Rozencweig M, Piccard M 1982 The cardiotoxicity of anticancer agents. Seminars in Oncology 9(1): 23–33

Weiss R B, Poster D S 1982 The renal toxicity of cancer chemotherapeutic agents. Cancer Treatment Review 9(1): 37–56

Weiss R B, Walker M D, Wienik P H 1974 Neurotoxicity of commonly used antineoplastic agents. New England Journal of Medicine 291(2): 75–81

WHO 1979 World Health Organisation handbook for reporting results of cancer treatment. World Health Organisation Offset Publication No. 48, World Health Organization, Geneva

Woolf N 1986 Cell, tissue and disease: the basis of pathology, 2nd edn. Baillière Tindall, London

Wujcik D 1992 Current research in side effects of high dose chemotherapy. Seminars in Oncology Nursing 8(2): 102–112

Yarbro C H 1992 Nursing implications in the administration of cancer chemotherapy. In: Perry M C (ed) The chemotherapy source book. Williams and Wilkins, Baltimore

Further reading

Fisher D S, Knobf M T 1993 The cancer chemotherapy handbook, 4th edn. Mosby-Yearbook, St. Louis
A compact and useful source book for chemotherapeutic treatment regimens and toxicity management.

**Galassi A, Hubbard S M, Alexander H R, Steinhaus E 1996 Chemotherapy administration: practical guidelines.
In: Chabner B A, Longo D L (eds) Cancer chemotherapy and bio-therapy: principles and practice. Lippincott-Raven, Philadelphia**

A text which offers an in-depth exploration of chemotherapy-related issues predominantly from a medical and scientific perspective.

Holmes S 1997 Cancer chemotherapy: a guide for

practice, 2nd edn. Asset Books, Leatherhead, UK
A comprehensive book which examines the use of cytotoxic chemotherapy as a treatment for cancer, side-effects and nursing management.

Joint Council for Clinical Oncology 1994 Quality control in cancer chemotherapy: managerial and procedural aspects. Royal College of Physicians, London
A short text which outlines key managerial and procedural aspects of delivering a quality controlled cancer chemotherapy service.

Knobf T, Durivage H J 1993 Chemotherapy: principles of therapy. In: Groenwald S L, Frogge M H, Goodman M, Yarbro C H (eds) Cancer nursing: principles and practice. 3rd edn. Jones and Bartlett, Boston
A comprehensive American cancer nursing text which explores in detail the principles of chemotherapy, administration issues and toxicity management.

Summerhayes M 1995 Developments in the chemotherapeutic treatment of cancer. The Hospital Pharmacist 2(1): 113–116

An article which offers an overview of drug developments in cancer treatment and management.

Yarbro C H 1992 Nursing implications in the administration of cancer chemotherapy. In: Perry M C (ed) The chemotherapy source book. Williams and Wilkins, Baltimore
A text which provides theoretical as well as 'hands on' information to assist the oncology nurse in providing comprehensive cancer nursing care to patients.

9 $\mathbf{R}$*adiotherapy*

DIANE SPREADBOROUGH AND JOANNE READ

Key points
- Radiotherapy can be used alone or in conjunction with chemotherapy in the treatment of haemato-oncological disorders
- Radiotherapy is used as both a curative and palliative treatment
- Radiotherapy affects all cells within the treatment field
- Side-effects of radiotherapy are the result of radiation on normal cells within the treatment field
- All potential side-effects of radiotherapy may occur following TBI

INTRODUCTION

Radiotherapy is a treatment modality which uses ionising radiation to kill cancer cells and has a variety of uses in haemato-oncology. A major role is total body irradiation (TBI) given as part of the conditioning regimen prior to bone marrow transplant (BMT). Radiotherapy is also used:

- as a curative treatment for lymphoma either alone or in combination with chemotherapy
- to prevent and treat disease recurrence in sanctuary sites in acute lymphoblastic leukaemia
- palliatively as a means of pain and symptom control for lymphoma and myeloma.

This chapter aims to facilitate a greater understanding of the use of radiotherapy within haemato-oncology. Basic concepts of radiotherapy will be discussed along with an overview of the effects of radiation on the cell.

The chapter focuses mainly on TBI and examines its purpose, dosages and positioning techniques; acute and long term side-effects and subsequent nursing management. Other uses of radiotherapy in haemato-oncology are discussed in the final part of this chapter.

PRINCIPLES OF RADIOTHERAPY

Radiotherapy is the use of ionising radiation which causes damage and destruction to normal and malignant cells, within the treatment field (Copp 1989). To fully comprehend this statement a clear understanding of atomic structure, ionising radiation and the overall effect of radiation on living cells is required. It is essential to appreciate the effects of radiotherapy so that nursing management can be planned and implemented to a high standard for each individual.

Atomic structure

An atom (Fig. 9.1) is the basic unit of an element from which all living matter is formed. It consists of protons (+ve charged particles), electrons (−ve charged particles) and neutrons (neutral particles).

Within an atom protons and neutrons are bound together by a strong nuclear force to form the nucleus, which is the centre of the atom. Orbiting the nucleus are the electrons. A stable atom has equal numbers of protons and electrons; positive and negative charges are therefore the same and the atom has electrical neutrality. Some atoms may, however, have differing numbers of protons and electrons

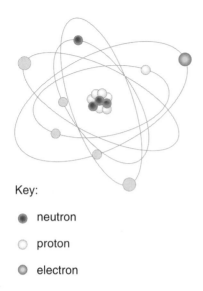

Key:

● neutron

○ proton

● electron

Figure 9.1 Three-dimensional representation of an atom

and are termed unstable. Unstable atoms are known as ions and undergo a process of breakdown in an attempt to achieve a more stable state. During this process of breakdown or decay, radiation is emitted in the form of alpha (α), beta (β) or gamma (γ) rays (Holmes 1996).

Radiation used therapeutically in cancer treatment is capable of disrupting the electrical neutrality of atoms within the tissues that it passes through, causing loss or gain of an electron: hence the term ionising radiation. Ions formed as a result of radiation are capable of causing further damage to cell structure.

Ionising radiation

Ionising radiation can be categorised as electromagnetic and particulate radiation. Electro-magnetic radiation, which consists of high-energy X-rays and γ rays, is the focus of this chapter. Electromagnetic radiation is delivered by machine in the form of external beam radiation (teletherapy); all radiotherapy in haemato-oncology for both palliative and curative treatment is delivered in the form of external beam therapy, with a calculated therapeutic dose of ionising radiation being delivered to a particular body area.

Radiation used to be measured in units called rads (radiation absorbed dose) but, since 1985, radiation dose has been measured in grays (Gy): 1 Gy = 100 rad. Doses smaller than a gray are measured in centigrays and 1 cGy = 1 rad.

Biological effects of radiation

A clear understanding of the cell cycle is essential in order to appreciate the concepts of radiotherapy and this is discussed in Chapter 8. Radiation has both a direct and an indirect effect on the cell. Radiation directly damages DNA and as all biochemical processes within the cell are controlled by DNA, cells are most sensitive to radiation-induced damage during the specific phases of the cell cycle when these processes may be disrupted: specifically, during G_2 and M phases of the cell cycle when protein synthesis, chromosomal changes and cell replication occur. DNA may be damaged by radiation in the following ways:

■ one of the four nitrogenous bases (thymine, adenine, cytosine or guanine) may be damaged or lost
■ the hydrogen bond between the two chains of the DNA molecule may be broken
■ one or both chains of the DNA molecule may be broken
■ after breakage, cross-linking of the chains of the DNA molecule may occur.

This damage results in mutations and, consequently, impaired cellular function or cell death (Hilderley 1993).

Radiation affects cells indirectly by transferring some of its energy to the cell as it passes through. Cellular products called free radicals are formed when radiation combines with intracellular water. Free radicals are highly reactive and may combine with both oxygen and other free radicals, resulting in a variety of chemical reactions and causing early cell death, inhibition of mitosis or cellular mutations (Holmes 1996).

Cells with a short cell cycle time appear to be most sensitive to radiation as there are more cells in active replication. These cells exhibit signs of damage more rapidly than those with a longer cell cycle time or resting cells (Holmes 1991). Other factors which impact on sensitivity to radiation include the degree of cell differentiation and oxygenation of the cell. Poorly differentiated and immature cells are more radiosensitive than well-differentiated cells. Well-oxygenated cells are also more radiosensitive.

Radiation has the same effect on both malignant and normal cells within the treatment field; however, normal cells have greater reparative powers than cancer cells and can repair partial but not total damage. The dose of radiotherapy administered therefore needs to be high enough to fatally damage malignant cells while allowing normal cells to recover. Dividing the radiation dose into fractions given over a number of days or weeks allows normal cells to recover from radiation damage. However, in some instances radiotherapy cannot be used as a curative treatment as the dose of radiation required to cause fatal damage to malignant cells would also irreparably damage normal cells.

The side-effects and the level of cellular radiation damage are dependent upon:

- duration of treatment
- dosage
- area size
- type of radiation
- radiosensitivity of tissues involved.

However, at this time, the molecular basis of radiation damage repair is incompletely understood. Cell death may occur within a few hours of radiation exposure, be delayed until mitosis or cells may continue to function while degenerating slowly. In many cells radiation-induced death is not instantaneous because cells continue to function and even undergo several divisions before biological death occurs (Perez et al 1998). Cell necrosis, which is degenerative, is the most usual type of cell damage, consequently, the full impact of radiation on cancer cells does not become apparent until 4–6 weeks after treatment.

TOTAL BODY IRRADIATION

Total body irradiation is the exposure of the whole body to a high dose of ionising radiation, in the form of external beam treatment. Many individuals with haematological malignancies are conditioned for BMT with a regimen that includes the use of TBI and chemotherapy. TBI is often used in conjunction with chemotherapy in the conditioning regimen because of its ability to penetrate the central nervous system and other sites that chemotherapy is unable to reach; no cell is resistant to TBI (Driefke & De Mayer 1992).

TBI has three essential functions:

1. Sufficient immunosuppression to allow engraftment of foreign donor marrow for allogeneic transplants
2. Eradication or reduction of systemic disease
3. Provision of sufficient marrow space for donor marrow (Silverman & Goldburg 1996).

Duration and doses of TBI

In the early days of BMT, TBI was given as a single fraction, the usual dose being 8–10 Gy (Lawton 1994). However, too low a dose of radiation led to regeneration of tumour cells and too high a dose caused irreversible long-term damage to normal cells. Therefore TBI is now given in fractionated doses over several days to overcome these problems.

Many studies have sought to establish an effective treatment plan that will meet the essential functions of TBI and yet reduce toxicities (Thomas et al 1982, Deeg 1983, Dinsmore et al 1983, Kim et al 1990, Gale et al 1991). Overall, they show that multiple fractions of TBI allow the main objectives of TBI to be achieved with the advantages of

- a decrease in leukaemic relapse
- increased survival rates due to the decrease in fatal complications, such as interstitial pneumonitis and veno-occlusive disease (VOD).

However, within differing medical protocols, dosages still remain variable and range from 1000 cGy to 1400 cGy.

Treatment techniques

Generally, the selection of a treatment technique should include the following considerations:

- the beam energy
- the treatment distance
- the beam direction and patient position (i.e. anterior, posterior, lateral fields or a combination)
- the dose rate (Bentel et al 1989).

These considerations vary from centre to centre depending upon factors such as the equipment available, the size of the treatment room and the established protocols used with regard to shielding. Lead shielding is sometimes used to reduce the toxicity to organs such as the eyes and lungs, but since leukaemia can reoccur anywhere in the body, the benefits of shielding are controversial.

Figure 9.2 shows an example of TBI given at a centre in Manchester. This regimen is used so that the whole body is exposed to the radiation beam.

SIDE-EFFECTS AND NURSING MANAGEMENT

TBI affects the whole body whereas radiotherapy used therapeutically for other purposes only affects the area within the treatment field. All potential side-effects of radiotherapy may therefore occur following TBI and knowledge of side-effects and nursing management related to specific body sites can be elicited from the following information.

TBI is given in combination with immuno-suppressive drugs. Consequently it is difficult to distinguish between chemotherapy-induced or TBI-induced toxicities. Some of these effects are also discussed in Chapters 8 and 10.

Radiation side-effects can occur, days, weeks or months following treatment and can be acute and long term. Side-effects are specific to the body part in the treatment field and related to the total dose of radiation given. Acute (or immediate) effects of radiation on tissues can

be seen within the first 6 months (Hilderley 1993). Holmes (1996) further subdivides acute side-effects, distinguishing between acute and sub-acute effects: acute side-effects occur during or immediately after treatment and sub-acute side-effects occur in the weeks or months after treatment. Long-term side-effects occur between 1 and 5 years after treatment.

Acute effects of TBI

Acute reactions occur when tissues with a high mitotic rate are exposed to radiation. The main effects are

1. bone marrow depression
2. effects on the gastrointestinal tract, including oral complications, nausea and vomiting and bowel changes
3. effects on the bladder
4. alopecia
5. effects on the skin
6. veno-occlusive disease.

Bone marrow depression

Bone marrow depression is the ultimate aim of TBI. However, it can also be life threatening, as the cells produced by the bone marrow are particularly radiosensitive, causing thrombocytopenia, anaemia and leucopenia. These complications are exacerbated by adjuvant cytotoxic agents. Bone marrow depression also occurs when smaller areas of the body containing a large percentage of bone marrow are treated with radiation. Each person having TBI will have a full blood count taken daily to monitor their blood counts. Actions to be taken if the blood count is low are discussed in the following sub-sections.

Thrombocytopenia

Thrombocytopenia can be manifested by superficial bleeding: for example, purpura, bruising, nose bleeds, bleeding per vagina. Individuals need to be informed of these potential effects prior to transplantation and preventative advice given in order to promote early detection, reduce the risk of bleeding and give reassurance. A full body check should be conducted each day and findings documented

Dosage   Total dose 1200 cGy given twice a day for 3 days

Figure 9.2 Example of TBI regimen

Shielding   No lead shielding

Positioning

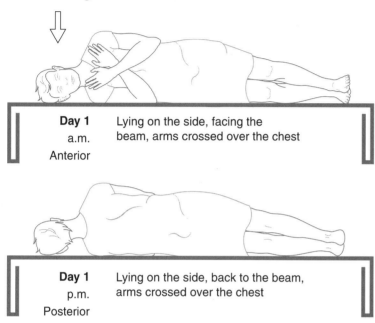

Day 1   Lying on the side, facing the
a.m.   beam, arms crossed over the chest
Anterior

Day 1   Lying on the side, back to the beam,
p.m.   arms crossed over the chest
Posterior

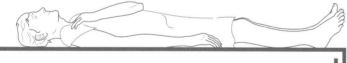

Day 2   Lying on the back with the right
a.m.   side to the beam, left arm across
Right lateral   the chest, right arm down the side

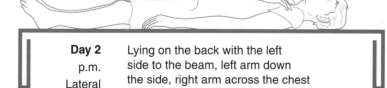

Day 2   Lying on the back with the left
p.m.   side to the beam, left arm down
Lateral   the side, right arm across the chest

Day 3   Repeat Day 1

accordingly. (See Chs 11 and 14 for further discussion of thrombocytopenia and its treatment.)

Leucopenia

Leucopenia can result in infection, indicated by pyrexia and fever, low blood pressure and tachycardia. Again, it is imperative that individuals are aware of this risk before commencement of treatment. Prevention of infection is discussed in greater detail in Chapter 13.

Anaemia

Anaemia is usually seen approximately 2 weeks after administration of radiotherapy but may occur sooner due to the additional effects of cytotoxic agents. Indicators of anaemia include pallor, lethargy, shortness of breath and reduction in haemoglobin levels. It is corrected by administration of a blood transfusion. Information may be helpful in alleviating anxieties and the individual should be encouraged to rest. It is important to maintain a haemoglobin level greater than 10 g/L as hypoxic cells are less radiosensitive (Perez et al 1998).

Gastrointestinal tract

When tissues are exposed to radiation, an inflammatory response is produced causing oedema. Cells slough off mucosal surfaces, leading to ulceration and resulting in mucositis, nausea, vomiting and diarrhoea (Holmes 1991).

Oral complications

Generally, mucosal changes begin 2 days before and peak 8 days after completion of TBI and cytotoxic agents (Zerbe et al 1992). Radiation damages the epithelial cells of the oral mucosa, causing cracked lips, an ulcerated mouth and mucositis. Loss of oral epithelium can exacerbate oral infections and potentiate bleeding. As the mucosa becomes denuded and atrophies it may become covered with a patchy white membrane known as radio-epithelite. This resembles oral candida and is a result of extravasation of plasma from damaged capillaries and dead cells. Removal of radio-epithelite may result in bleeding (Holmes 1996).

Significant xerostomia may follow TBI due to reduced saliva production as a result of irradiation of the parotid glands. Radiation changes the consistency of saliva, which becomes thick, viscous and clings to teeth and mucosal surfaces. Individuals may find that the consistency of saliva makes it difficult to swallow or spit out and the reduced amount of saliva makes swallowing and chewing difficult. The normal pH of saliva is also reduced and the more acidic environment along with loss of the normal antibacterial and lubricating functions of saliva predispose to dental caries as bacteria and food debris cling to the teeth.

Radiation also causes taste changes, oesophagitis and a sore, hoarse throat due to the effects on the pharyngeal and laryngeal mucosa. Overall, these symptoms can be distressing and lead to a poor dietary intake, problems with communication and extreme discomfort and pain.

NURSING MANAGEMENT Dental assessment is required prior to treatment to reduce the possibility of complications. The importance of attending for regular dental appointments to detect future problems such as dental caries should also be emphasised (Kusler & Rambur 1992).

Daily assessment and documentation of the oral cavity is imperative to detect problems and evaluate the care given.

Mouthwashes should be encouraged to promote oral hygiene, as should the use of a soft toothbrush to prevent trauma. Aqueous creams should be applied to prevent and treat cracked lips (for further discussion on mouthwashes see Ch. 16).

Frequent drinks, sugar-free chewing gum, sucking boiled sweets or ice and the use of artificial saliva sprays have all been suggested as means of reducing oral dryness.

Oral antibacterial and antifungal medication may be indicated after swabs have been taken for culture and sensitivity.

Food consumption should be monitored and, if necessary, dietary supplements, soft diet and high-protein foods should be encouraged to maintain an adequate nutritional intake (see Ch. 17). Parenteral feeding may be required if daily weight is reducing.

Advice should be given on avoiding hot spicy food, alcohol and smoking which can exacerbate the dryness and soreness of the mouth and delay the healing process.

Pain control is essential. Local analgesics such as Difflam mouthwashes may be helpful and if tolerated, mist paracetamol is sometimes effective but care should be taken to ensure that a pyrexia is not masked. However, frequently pain is so severe as to require intravenous diamorphine infusion.

Oral care is discussed in further detail in Chapter 16.

Nausea and vomiting

Vomiting, which may be severe, can occur in the first 48 hours post-irradiation becoming less frequent after the second or third day (Deeg 1983). There are various explanations for this, ranging from anticipatory vomiting due to external stimuli to stimulation of the vomiting centre based in the medulla by toxic waste produced by radiation-induced cell destruction. Nausea and vomiting can be a difficult symptom to control depending upon the circumstances (see Ch. 15).

NURSING MANAGEMENT An effective antiemetic regimen is essential with constant review and assessment; the use of sedatives can sometimes be beneficial.

Fluid intake and output should be monitored for signs of dehydration and intravenous fluids administered as needed.

Dietary intake should be monitored and dietary advice offered to maintain an adequate nutritional intake. Liaising with the dietician is essential.

Mouthwashes should be encouraged, to reduce oral acidity post-vomiting and to maintain comfort and dental protection.

Diversional and/or complementary therapies, such as relaxation tapes and acupressure bands, may be helpful.

For further information on nursing management refer to Chapter 15.

Bowel changes

The epithelial lining of the bowel has a rapid cell turnover with a cell life-span of approximately 2 days (Holmes 1991). Radiation to this area causes mucosal damage, leading to abdominal gripes, flatulence, diarrhoea, tenesmus and anal ulceration. However, it should be remembered that these symptoms may not be due to radiation alone and factors such as graft versus host disease (GVHD), chemotherapy, intravenous antibiotics and parenteral nutrition may also contribute.

NURSING MANAGEMENT Bulk-forming laxatives are usually effective in controlling the above symptoms and preventing further exacerbation. However, individuals are unlikely to be able to tolerate this particular medication due to an accumulation of other side-effects.

Antidiarrhoeal medication, analgesics and antispasmodics help to promote comfort.

Weekly faecal specimens for culture and sensitivity should be taken to eliminate the possibility of infections such as *Clostridium difficile*.

Frequency, consistency and colour of faeces should be monitored as should the presence of blood or mucus, which are indications of radiation-induced bowel changes.

Fluid intake and output should be monitored to assess hydration.

Good personal hygiene and regular use of a bidet to prevent excoriation of the perianal region is important.

Effects on the bladder

The epithelium of the bladder mucosa consists of highly proliferating radiosensitive cells. Radiation can cause inflammation and oedema of the mucosa, producing symptoms of cystitis and dysuria.

NURSING MANAGEMENT A fluid intake of 2–3 litres daily should be encouraged to keep urine osmolarity low and reduce the risk of urinary tract infection. Fluid intake and output should be carefully monitored to ensure adequate intake and detect frequency of micturition.

Weekly urine specimens should be obtained to exclude the presence of infection.

Mist potassium citrate may help to alleviate symptoms of cystitis but use is dependent on serum potassium levels.

Alopecia

This is generally a reversible side-effect which occurs approximately 2 weeks after commencement of radiation and administration of some cytotoxic agents. Hair re-growth is usually seen 3–6 months after completion of treatment.

Alopecia is likely to have occurred before admission for BMT as a result of previous treatments and appropriate measures have usually already been initiated. However, it is important that the patient is aware that TBI also causes alopecia and ongoing psychological support is offered.

Skin

Skin cells have a high mitotic rate, making them highly sensitive to radiation. Skin reactions are frequently seen within the treatment field despite the skin-sparing effect of many modern treatment machines. The extent of the reaction depends upon the dose of radiation given, the total treatment time and the area being irradiated. Areas where skin surfaces meet, such as the groin and axilla, are particularly likely to be affected. Cytotoxic drugs also exacerbate skin reactions. Skin reactions can range from mild erythema to dry and moist desquamation that requires intensive nursing care. Erythema is not unlike a sunburn reaction and is characterised by reddening of the skin. Itching and peeling of skin are features of dry desquamation and in moist desquamation the epidermis is destroyed and serous fluid oozes from the affected area. Individuals receiving TBI tend to develop mild erythema in the first few days following treatment. More severe skin reactions are usually due to a combination of chemotherapy and TBI in the preconditioning regimen.

NURSING MANAGEMENT Advice on skin care needs to be given prior to treatment to reduce further trauma and irritation to the epithelium:

- non-perfumed toiletries should be used
- individuals should be advised to wear loose cotton clothing
- gentle washing and drying of the skin should be encouraged – patting skin dry rather than rubbing is preferable
- for men, an electric razor should be used.

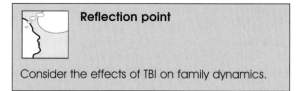

Reflection point

Consider the effects of TBI on family dynamics.

Daily monitoring and recording of any skin changes should be undertaken.

Steroid-based creams, such as hydrocortisone 1%, can alleviate skin irritation and promote comfort in individuals with mild erythema.

Individuals should avoid exposure to direct sunlight and advice should be given on use of high-factor sun-creams and clothing.

Veno-occlusive disease

VOD affects approximately 10–20% of individuals undergoing TBI/BMT and in a third, the disease is life threatening or lethal (Deeg 1983). It can develop rapidly within days to weeks. VOD is a disease of the liver diagnosed by both biopsy and clinical presentation and characterised by ascites, raised serum bilirubin levels, sudden weight gain, hepatomegaly and jaundice (Deeg 1983, Silverman & Goldburg 1996).

VOD appears to be a poorly understood condition thought to depend upon factors such as prevailing liver disease and the severity of the conditioning regimen used. TBI is therefore considered to be only a contributing factor and research in this area is ongoing.

Currently, medical and nursing management consists of the administration of continuous intravenous heparin infusions prior to BMT, followed by weekly liver function tests and daily weight and body checks.

Fatigue

Fatigue is a well-documented side-effect of radiotherapy. However, fatigue is also a side-effect of chemotherapy and a result of anaemia. For those undergoing TBI/BMT or suffering from other haematological malignancies, fatigue may be exacerbated by these other contributing factors. The impact of fatigue should not be underestimated. If individuals are unaware of the likelihood of its occurrence they may feel that their disease is not responding to treatment. Fatigue may also continue for a lengthy period of time once treatment is completed. In one study individuals were still experiencing fatigue 3 months after radiotherapy had been completed (King et al 1985). Fatigue may not be relieved by sleep and individuals should be advised that they are likely to experience this side-effect. Nursing interventions are aimed at helping the individual to conserve energy and prioritise their activities.

Long-term effects of TBI

General long-term effects occur from 3 months after administration of the conditioning regime and affect the individuals quality of life to varying degrees depending upon their severity and duration. Long-term effects are attributed not only to TBI but also to cytotoxic agents and GVHD (see Chs 8 and 10). However, a study by Vowels & Ford (1994), investigating people who survived longer than 2 years post-transplant, noted late side-effects in 100% of individuals given TBI compared with only 16.5% of people receiving chemotherapy alone, which suggests that TBI does contribute to long-term complications.

Long-term effects caused specifically by TBI include

- interstitial pneumonitis
- cataracts
- infertility
- psychological effects
- secondary cancers.

Interstitial pneumonitis

The lungs are particularly sensitive to ionising radiation. Interstitial pneumonitis is one of the major causes of morbidity and mortality after BMT (Latini et al 1992). TBI is a causative factor but links have also been made to cytomegalovirus, GVHD, cytotoxic agents and pre-existing lung disease (Deeg 1983, Silverman & Goldburg 1996).

Interstitial pneumonitis is characterised by dyspnoea, coughing, wheezing, facial oedema and poor lung function. It can occur from approximately 3 months to 2 years post-transplant. Some treatment centres use shielding over the lung area in an attempt to minimise this side-effect, but studies have found that the benefits of shielding are inconclusive (Labar et al 1992, Latini et al 1992).

Medical and nursing management initially involves educating the individual to be aware of any chest abnormalities after completion of treatment. On diagnosis of interstitial pneumonitis, appropriate intervention includes antibiotics, steroid therapy and referral to a chest physician.

Cataracts

Cataract formation occurs within 1½–3 years post-treatment, the main symptom being deteriorating vision. Cataracts have been seen in 80% of individuals given single-dose TBI compared with 18% of those given fractionated TBI (Deeg 1984). They can often be corrected surgically.

Infertility

Future reproduction may not be the first priority when confronted with the diagnosis of cancer

---

Case study 9.1

Jeff, a 42 year old, was diagnosed with acute myeloid leukaemia and following three courses of conventional chemotherapy was admitted to the bone marrow transplant unit prior to receiving peripheral stem cell transplant. His pre-transplant conditioning regime included TBI, consisting of 200 cGy twice a day for the 3 days immediately before transplant. The following 16 days were spent in isolation.

The main side-effects Jeff experienced included nausea and vomiting, diarrhoea, pancytopenia, a sore mouth and cystitis. These side-effects could have been due to either chemotherapy or TBI or a combination of both. One side-effect experienced specifically from TBI was skin erythema.

Three days after transplant Jeff complained of itchiness on his lower abdomen and back and observation of the areas showed a reddening of the skin. Jeff was informed that his symptoms were due to the radiation and symptoms would subside. Hydrocortisone cream 1% was applied sparingly to the areas of erythema and daily full body checks ensured no other areas were affected. The use of non-perfumed toiletries and gently patting skin dry after showering were advised. The erythema resolved after a further 7 days.

and impending treatment, but the long-term impact of infertility can have great psychological implications. Individuals need to be informed of the effect of treatment on fertility before treatment commences and it is essential that the topic is discussed honestly and openly.

The dose of radiation given in TBI causes infertility in both men and women. In men, damage to the germ cell epithelium of the testes leads to impaired sperm production and in women, permanent cessation of ovulation and menstruation results (Sanders et al 1983, Yarbro & Perry 1985).

Other effects on sexuality such as impotence, decreased libido, decreased vaginal lubrication, dyspareunia and psychological implications due to changes in body image and self-esteem may also occur. (See Ch. 18 for further discussion of fertility.)

Psychological effects

Individuals receiving radiation treatment may have underlying misconceptions of the treatment, such as fear of severe burns and becoming radioactive and potentially harming family and visitors. For those receiving TBI, a further consideration is leaving a controlled, sterile environment to attend the Radiotherapy Department when the importance of prevention of infection and isolation has been emphasised. During radiotherapy treatment the individual is left alone and expected to remain still once positioned, which may lead to feelings of claustrophobia. Other areas of concern may include changes in body image, sexuality, separation from family, isolation and fears and uncertainty about the future.

In order to deliver holistic nursing care psychological issues need to be addressed, information given to alleviate any fears or misconceptions and support offered as appropriate. It is important to recognise the need for further psychological assessment (see Ch. 19).

Secondary cancers

The risks of developing secondary malignancies post-radiation have been examined in several studies (Deeg 1983, Kaldor 1990, Chessells 1992). Findings are generally unclear and inconclusive, although radiotherapy does appear to increase the risk of secondary cancers. Further ongoing research is needed within this area.

Reflection point

Examine the information available to individuals undergoing BMT in your area. Do you feel enough emphasis is given to total body irradiation?

OTHER USES OF RADIOTHERAPY IN HAEMATO-ONCOLOGY

Lymphomas

Radiotherapy can be used as a curative treatment either alone or in combination with chemotherapy and surgery for the treatment of lymphomas. Generally the type of treatment given depends upon staging, presence of B symptoms and disease characteristics (see Ch. 6). Common techniques include the mantle technique and the inverted Y field. The mantle technique encompasses the major lymph nodes above the diaphragm with the upper margin being below the eyes (Fig. 9.3). This ensures effective delivery of radiation to tumour sites.

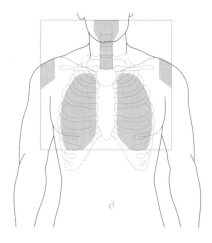

Key:
▨ Lead shielding

Figure 9.3 The mantle technique

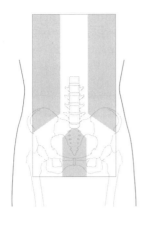

Key:
▨ Lead shielding

Figure 9.4 Inverted Y technique

Lead lung shields are individually positioned to protect the lungs from radiation damage.

For disease below the diaphragm, the inverted Y field is used to cover the para-aortic nodes and the pelvic nodes, while protecting the kidneys (Fig. 9.4). Radiotherapy may also be used to treat specific areas of bulky disease after completion of chemotherapy.

Acute lymphoblastic leukaemia

Previously all individuals with acute lymphoblastic leukaemia (ALL) received cranial irradiation to prevent disease recurrence in the central nervous system (CNS). However, clinical trials have indicated that administration of intrathecal and high-dose systemic chemotherapy early in the disease is effective CNS prophylaxis (Cortes et al 1995). Cranial irradiation is therefore not always used and may be reserved for patients with a high white cell count or at high risk of CNS relapse.

For those individuals who do receive cranial irradiation, side-effects include nausea and vomiting, drowsiness, somnolence syndrome, increased fatigue and cerebral oedema. Antiemetics are required to control nausea and vomiting and cerebral oedema may be treated with dexamethasone. It is important that patients and their relatives are advised about

the occurrence of these symptoms as they may fear that their symptoms are due to disease progression.

Testicular relapse occurs in approximately 10% of males with ALL within 1 year of completing treatment (Whittaker & Judge 1990). Gonadal irradiation is usually the treatment of choice. Side-effects include infertility and delayed puberty if administered to younger boys (see Chs 4 and 7).

Palliative radiotherapy

Radiotherapy is also used as a palliative treatment in haemato-oncology, mainly for lymphomas and myelomas. Palliative radiotherapy tends to be given in lower doses, as single or reduced multiple fractions. Consequently, benefits of radiation can be appreciated and side-effects minimised as the overall aim is improving quality of life.

Palliative radiotherapy is useful for symptom control and specific complications such as superior vena cava obstruction and spinal cord compression. It has a well-recognised role in the management of pain, particularly in myeloma, and may also be used to reduce the threat of pathological fractures (Rowell & Tobias 1991) (see Ch. 5).

CONCLUSION

It can be seen that radiotherapy plays a major role in the management of haematological malignancies both curatively and palliatively. It is hoped that this chapter has enabled the reader to appreciate the short- and long-term effects that radiation can impose on an individual's overall quality of life. In achieving this, nursing care can then be planned and implemented to identify and minimise radiation reactions.

As treatment of haematological malignancies continues to advance and life expectancy increases it is apparent that ongoing research is required to fully comprehend the implications of radiotherapy and develop appropriate nursing interventions to alleviate the distress they may cause.

DISCUSSION QUESTIONS

1. The majority of research on radiotherapy is medically orientated. What, in your opinion, are the priority areas for nursing research in relation to the short- and long-term effects of radiation?
2. How can common misconceptions such as radiation sickness, skin burns, genetic

mutations and radioactivity be allayed prior to radiotherapy treatment?

3. How much information should be given to patients about the long-term side-effects of TBI?
4. What support groups/systems are required for individuals pre- and post-radiotherapy treatment?

References

Bentel G, Nelson C, Thomas N K 1989 Total body irradiation. In: Treatment planning in radiation oncology. Pergamon Press, Oxford, pp 304–305

Chessells J M 1992 Treatment of childhood acute lymphoblastic leukaemia: present issues and future prospects. Blood Reviews 6(4): 193–203

Copp K 1989 Nursing patients having radiotherapy. In: Tiffany R (ed) Oncology for nurses and health care professionals, Vol 3, Cancer nursing. Harper & Row, London, Ch. 2

Cortes J, O'Brien S M, Pierce S, Keating M J, Freireich E J, Kantatjian H M 1995 The value of high-dose systemic chemotherapy and intrathecal therapy for central nervous system prophylaxis in different risk groups of adult acute lymphoblastic leukaemia. Blood 86: 2091–2097

Deeg H G 1983 Acute and delayed toxicities of total body irradiation. Int Radiat Oncol Biol Phys 9: 1933–1939

Deeg H G 1984 Cataracts after total body irradiation and marrow transplantation – a sparing effect of dose fractionation. Int Radiat Oncol Biol Phys 10: 957–964

Dinsmore R, Kirkpatrick D, Flomenburg N 1983 Allogeneic bone marrow transplantation for

patients with acute lymphoblastic leukaemia. Blood 62: 381–388

Driefke L, De Meyer E 1992 Information guide for patients receiving total body irradiation before bone marrow transplantation. Cancer Nursing 15(3): 206–210

Gale R P, Butturinia A, Bortin M M 1991 What does total body irradiation do in bone marrow transplants for leukaemia. Int J Radiat Oncol Biol Phys 20: 631–634

Hilderley H 1993 Radiotherapy. In: Groenwald S L, Frogge M H, Goodman M, Yarbro C H (eds) Cancer nursing, principles and practice, 3rd edn. Jones and Bartlett, Boston, Ch. 13, pp 235–269

Holmes S 1991 Radiotherapy. The Lisa Sainsbury Foundation Series. Austen Cornish, London

Holmes S 1996 Radiotherapy: a guide for practice. Asset Books, Leatherhead, UK.

Kaldor P A 1990 Second cancer following chemotherapy and radiotherapy: an epidemiology perspective. Acta Oncologica 29(5): 647–655

Kim T H, McGlane P B, Ramsay N 1990 Comparison of two total body irradiation regimens in allogeneic bone marrow transplantation for acute non-lymphoblastic leukaemia in first remission. Int Radiat Oncol Biol Phys 19: 889–897

King K, Nail L, Kreamer K, Strohl R, Johnson J 1985 Patients' descriptions of the experience of having cancer. Oncology Nursing Forum 12(4): 55–61

Kusler D, Rambur B 1992 Treatment for radiation induced xerostomia. Cancer Nursing 15(3): 191–195

Labar B, Bogdanic V, Nemet D et al 1972 Total body irradiation with or without lung shielding for allogeneic bone marrow transplantation. Bone Marrow Transplantation 9: 343–347

Latini P, Aristei C, Aversa F et al 1992 Interstitial pneumonitis after hyperfractionated total body irradiation in H.L.A. matched T-depleted bone marrow transplantation. Int J Radiat Oncol Biol Phys 23: 401–405

Lawton C A 1994 Radiation therapy for bone marrow transplants. In: Cox J D Moss' Radiation oncology, 7th edn. Mosby, London, Ch. 35

Perez C A, Brady L W, Rotiroti J L 1998 Overview. In: Perez C A, Brady L W (eds) Principles and practice of radiation oncology, 3rd edn. Lippincott Raven, Philadelphia, Ch. 1, pp 1–78

Rowell N P, Tobias J S 1991 The role of radiotherapy in the management of multiple myeloma. Blood Rev 15: 84–89

Sanders J E, Buckner D C, Leonard J M 1983 Late effects of gonadal function of cyclophosphamide total body irradiation and marrow transplantation. Transplantation 36: 252–255

Silverman C L, Goldburg S L 1996 Total irradiation in bone marrow transplantation and advanced lymphomas: a comprehensive overview. In: Tobias J S, Thomas P R M (eds) Current radiation oncology, Vol 2. Arnold, London, Ch. 14

Thomas E D, Clift R A, Hersman H 1982 Marrow transplantation for acute non-lymphoblastic leukaemia and first remission using fractionated or single dose irradiation. Int J Radiat Oncol Biol Phys 8: 817–821

Vowels M R, Ford D 1994 Allogeneic and autologous bone marrow transplantation for acute non-lymphoblastic leukaemia. Journal of Paediatric and Child Health 30(4): 319–323

Whittaker J A, Judge M 1990 Acute leukaemias. In: Ludlam C A (ed) Clinical haematology.

Churchill Livingstone, Edinburgh, pp 121–148

Yarbro C H, Perry F 1985 The effect of cancer therapy on gonadal function. Seminars in Oncology Nursing 1(1): 3–8

Zerbe M B, Parkerson S G, Lynch-Ortlieb N, Spitzer T 1992 Relationships between oral mucositis and treatment variable in bone marrow patients. Cancer Nursing 15(3): 196–205

Further reading

Buschel P C 1993 Bone marrow transplantation. In: Groenwald S L, Frogge M H, Goodman M, Yarbro C H (eds) Cancer nursing, principles and practice, 3rd edn. Jones and Bartlett, Boston, Ch. 18
An extensive chapter in a comprehensive book covering all aspects of cancer nursing.

Hoffbrand A V, Pettit J E 1993 Essential haematology, 3rd edn. Blackwell, London
A detailed textbook on haematology.

Holmes S 1996 Radiotherapy: a guide for practice. Asset Books, Leatherhead, UK
A comprehensive book which covers all aspects of radiotherapy.

Snape D, Robinson A 1996 Radiotherapy. In: Tschudin V (ed) Nursing the patient with cancer, 2nd edn. Prentice Hall, Hertfordshire, Ch. 4
A basic introduction to principles of radiotherapy and nursing care.

10 *Blood and marrow transplantation*

HELEN OUTHWAITE

Key points

- Blood and marrow transplantation (BMT) is used to treat a wide variety of haematological and non-haematological disorders
- BMT is designed to cure (or induce long-term remission of) the underlying disease
- BMT involves administration of myeloablative doses of chemotherapy with or without irradiation
- BMT involves transfer of stem cells to establish haematopoiesis
- Autologous BMT allows dose intensification with rescue from the effects of pancytopenia
- Allogeneic BMT aims to replace the haematopoietic system with donor cells
- BMT is associated with significant complications, morbidity and mortality.

INTRODUCTION

The care of people undergoing bone marrow transplantation is an area that many nurses find exciting and fulfilling as it encompasses so many different, and sometimes conflicting, nursing skills. Other nurses would argue that a bone marrow transplant unit is a frightening and depressing place in which to work. The role of transplantation within the field of malignant haematology has become increasingly recognised and is now an established procedure. Recent advances have increased the role of transplants and encouraged investigation into their use for other malignancies.

Inevitably more nurses are now coming into contact with people having this form of treatment. Confusion surrounds the terminology of transplantation – even the word 'transplant' conjures up inaccurate images and does not sufficiently describe the different treatment and procedures of the process. Recent guidelines, produced in Europe and the USA, indicate the resources needed in transplant units to look after this special group of patients so that adequate numbers of dedicated staff are trained to deal with the specific problems they may encounter. These guidelines have been coordinated by the European Group for Blood and Marrow Transplantation (EBMT 1998) and the International Society for Haemopoietic and Graft Engineering (ISHAGE 1997). This chapter provides an overview of the process of transplantation, the different types of transplant and the complications that can arise as a result of treatment.

Rationale for transplantation

People may have their bone marrow replaced if the bone marrow is

- not functioning correctly (e.g. in aplastic anaemia)
- diseased (e.g. in leukaemia)
- suppressed (e.g. after high-dose chemotherapy and/or radiotherapy).

Blood and marrow transplantation is concerned with the transfer of the stem cells required to establish haematopoiesis. Pluripotent stem (or progenitor) cells are the undifferentiated cells in the bone marrow from which all other blood cell lines arise (see Ch. 1). When progenitor cells are infused into someone whose bone marrow has been destroyed by high-dose therapy, they can replace the previously existing bone marrow and restore normal marrow function. BMT is no longer considered an experimental treatment and results have improved enormously in recent years with reduced transplant-related mortality and a reduced risk of relapse from the original disease (Gratwohl 1998).

Patient selection

Originally, bone marrow transplantation was indicated for people for whom all other treatment modalities had failed, and therefore had a very poor prognosis. As transplantation has become safer, so people with an overall better chance of survival, but for whom conventional therapy offers a poor prognosis, have been offered the treatment, and it is now felt that in some diseases patients treated with high-dose therapy earlier in the course of their disease are likely to do better. Randomised trials are being undertaken to determine who should be transplanted and when the transplant should take place in various different diseases. It is generally recommended that people should be in remission at the time of transplant, or have minimal, or responding disease, with good organ function and performance status. Transplantation includes aggressive therapy with the aim of inducing a long-term disease-free survival and individuals need to be as fit as possible to withstand treatment. Most centres therefore have guidelines to exclude people for whom transplantation may not offer significant benefit. Such guidelines might include criteria such as

- age (for allografts, over 50 years; for autografts, over 70 years)
- relapse – or blast crisis of chronic myeloid leukaemia (CML)
- life expectancy – severely limited by other disease
- symptomatic cardiac disease
- neurological disease – not controlled by conventional therapy

- uncontrolled infection
- psychologically unable to withstand treatment.

Table 10.1 indicates the diseases for which transplants are carried out and the type of transplant generally recommended for a particular disease.

TYPES OF TRANSPLANT

Transplant can be either syngeneic, allogeneic or autologous.

Syngeneic transplants

Transplants between identical twins are termed syngeneic. The bone marrow in each twin is genetically identical. This type of transplant is inevitably rare.

Allogeneic transplants

Allogeneic transplantation involves cells being transferred from one person to another, therefore a donor is always involved. Choosing a donor depends upon a human leucocyte antigen (HLA) match between the recipient and donor. Donors are usually HLA-compatible siblings but may be an HLA-mismatched family member (mismatched transplants) or an unrelated HLA-matched donor (volunteer unrelated donor (VUD) transplants). Allogeneic transplantation is more complex and risky than autologous transplantation with the complexity increasing in mismatched and VUD transplants.

In allogeneic BMT the donor's immune system is part of the transplant. The immuno deficiency that ensues following transplant predisposes the recipient to severe complications. A matched donor decreases the risks of complications such as graft versus host disease (GVHD) and graft rejection and therefore tissue typing is of prime importance.

Tissue typing

Tissue typing is the process of matching donor and recipient tissue. Each potential donor gives a blood sample which is tested for the major

Table 10.1 Indications for and types of transplant

Indications for transplant	Type of transplant
Leukaemias	
Acute myeloid leukaemia	Allogeneic/autologous
Acute lymphoblastic leukaemia	Allogeneic/autologous
Chronic myeloid leukaemia	Allogeneic
Chronic lymphocytic leukaemia	Allogeneic/autologous
Myelodysplastic syndrome	Allogeneic
Multiple myeloma	Allogeneic/autologous
Lymphomas	
Hodgkin's disease	Mainly autologous
Non-Hodgkin's lymphoma	Mainly autologous
Burkitt's lymphoma	Mainly autologous
Solid tumours	
Ewing's sarcoma	Autologous
Teratoma	Autologous
Neuroblastoma	Autologous
Carcinoma of the breast	Autologous
Malignant melanoma	Autologous
Non-malignant disorders	
Bone marrow failure syndromes	Allogeneic
Aplastic anaemia, Fanconi's anaemia	
Immunodeficiency states	
Severe combined immunodeficiency	Allogeneic
disease, Wiskott–Aldrich syndrome	
Haematological disorders	
Thalassaemia, sickle cell disease	Allogeneic

histocompatibility complex (MHC). MHC is determined by identifying HLAs. These antigens are genetically inherited proteins found on the surface of all human cells. The unique combination of antigens on the cell determines the tissue type. The group of genes that codes for the HLA antigen is called the HLA complex and is found on chromosome 6. Four specific HLA loci are identified and compared. If a donor and recipient are identical at all four loci, they are considered matched.

Donor registries

For allograft transplants the donor of choice is a matched sibling. However, with small family sizes in Europe only 30% of people needing a transplant will have a matched sibling donor. In cases where there is no family donor it may

be appropriate to search for a volunteer donor from one of the donor panels. There are two donor registries in the UK – the Anthony Nolan Bone Marrow Trust in London (established in 1979, this was the first panel and was named after Anthony Nolan, who died before finding a donor; it was founded in his memory by his mother) and the British Bone Marrow and Platelet Donor Panel, based in Bristol. The extremely large number of possible HLA tissue types means that finding an unrelated donor can be difficult. Currently the chance of obtaining a match from the bone marrow registry (all the panels are computer linked to facilitate searching) depends on the frequency of the person's HLA profile in the donor population (Campbell 1997). It is particularly difficult to find donors for people from ethnic minorities and mixed racial backgrounds as the majority of volunteer donors are of Caucasian background. The donor panels have undertaken large-scale advertising to increase awareness of this problem and attempt to establish a more varied donor pool.

Autologous transplants

Autologous transplantation uses the patient's own cells, which can then be used to shorten the period of pancytopenia following high-dose therapy, thus allowing safe dose escalation. The cells are taken (usually when the disease is in remission), preserved and then returned following high-dose therapy. Autologous transplantation is very different from allogeneic transplantation and is considered much simpler, with fewer and less devastating side-effects. Due to the decreased risks it is possible for older people to have autografts relatively safely. The main concern with autografts is relapse of the original disease – especially in haematological malignancies. Various methods to attempt to ensure that the replaced cells do not contain malignant cells are under investigation. These are now described.

Negative selection (or purging)

This method is a way of removing contaminated and unwanted cells from the graft before returning the cells. Techniques include the use of immunomagnetic approaches, monoclonal antibodies and chemotherapy, but more trials are needed to see if purging improves relapse rates.

Positive selection

This method involves retaining only those cells which have specific receptors identifying them as needed for reconstitution of marrow function. The CD34+ receptor is currently used for selection and cells not carrying this antigen are discarded. The major advantages of this approach are

- the reduction of unwanted cells
- less infusional toxicity
- less storage space required for frozen cells
- further handling and processing is possible.

However, the benefits of this procedure have not yet been established.

Sources of stem cells

Stem cells may be obtained from bone marrow, peripheral blood or the umbilical cord. At any given time 90% of haematopoietic progenitor cells will be found in the bone marrow. Traditionally this source of stem cells was used in transplantation – hence the term bone marrow transplant. In the late 1980s it became possible and was considered more advantageous to collect the stem cells from the peripheral blood. As the understanding and practicality of using peripheral blood stem cells has increased this source of stem cells has superseded the use of bone marrow in most transplant centres. Initially, peripheral blood stem cell transplants (PBSCT) were restricted to autologous use, but are now also commonly used in the allogeneic setting.

No mechanism is currently available to identify and measure the pluripotent stem cell. The pluripotent stem cell is responsible for maintaining marrow function throughout the life of an individual while more differentiated stem cells progress and evolve into differentiated blood cells (see Ch. 1). It is therefore important that transplanted cells include pluripotent cells to sustain a functioning marrow and to ensure haematopoietic reconstitution.

COLLECTION OF MARROW AND STEM CELLS

Harvesting bone marrow

The technique of harvesting bone marrow is the same for both donors and patients. Various investigations may be carried out before collecting marrow and these are outlined below:

- full blood count
- biochemistry
- virology – cytomegalovirus (CMV), herpes simplex virus (HSV), varicella zoster virus (VZV), hepatitis screen, human immunodeficiency virus (HIV)
- blood group and save (autologous blood donations may be made by donors)
- chest X-ray
- electrocardiogram (ECG).

Bone marrow harvest requires a general anaesthetic, and following admission the usual preoperative checks are carried out to ensure safety. In theatre, marrow is harvested by repeated bone marrow aspirations from the posterior iliac crests using bone marrow biopsy needles. If a sufficient number of cells cannot be gathered from this site the anterior iliac crests and sternum may also be used. Usually 800–1000 ml of bone marrow is removed to acquire 100–300 million cells per kilogram of the recipient's body weight. The marrow may be processed on a cell separator to remove any bone chips and the red cells. The cells may then be cryopreserved in liquid nitrogen until needed or given immediately to the patient. People usually remain in hospital overnight following the procedure. Simple analgesia may be required for back pain, but a bone marrow harvest is usually well tolerated. The aspiration of the cells does not significantly alter the peripheral blood count and the marrow is quickly regenerated. Occasionally, top-up blood transfusions are required; however, donors are not thought to suffer any permanent loss from providing their bone marrow.

Mobilising and collecting cells from peripheral blood

An increase in the number of circulating stem cells during the recovery phase from chemotherapy was demonstrated by Richman et al (1976). Cells could be successfully collected but repeated apheresis procedures were required. The breakthrough in the collection and use of blood stem cells was heralded by the development and application of haematopoietic growth factors. These growth factors, such as granulocyte–colony-stimulating factor (G-CSF) and granulocyte, monocyte–colony-stimulating factor (GM-CSF), have allowed the numbers of progenitor cells in the blood to be deliberately expanded. The ability to collect these cells using a blood cell separator is a far less invasive procedure than the traditional method of bone marrow harvesting. The advantages of using peripheral blood stem cells instead of marrow stem cells are outlined in Box 10.1.

Stem cells may be collected from the peripheral blood:

■ with no attempt to increase their number (steady state)
■ during recovery following chemotherapy (although not donors)
■ after the administration of haematopoietic growth factors
■ after both chemotherapy and haematopoietic growth factors.

Box 10.1 Advantages of using peripheral blood stem cells

● Less-invasive procedure, which does not require a general anaesthetic
● More rapid engraftment therefore less blood product and antibiotic therapy required
● Available for individuals with tumour involving their bone marrow
● Available for patients with fibrotic marrow following pelvic radiotherapy
● Possibly reduces tumour contamination
● Cheaper?

Box 10.2 Investigations required prior to peripheral blood stem cell collection

Full blood count, including haematocrit
Blood group and save – irradiated, leucocyte-depleted blood
Vital signs and temperature
Compliance to G-CSF administration
Venous access
Virology – CMV, HIV, hepatitis screen

If cells are collected in the steady state, multiple aphereses are required to collect an adequate number of stem cells. It is possible to expand the number of cells available for collection by stimulating (or mobilising) them following chemotherapy and growth factor administration. Potential side-effects associated with the administration of haematopoietic growth factors include fever, chills, bone pain and reactions at the subcutaneous injection site. Investigations required prior to stem cell collection are shown in Box 10.2.

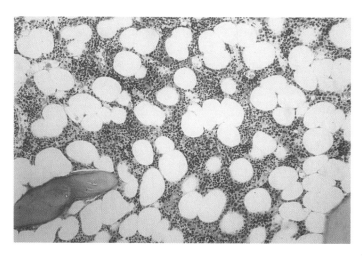

Plate 1 Normal bone marrow showing normal mixed haematopoiesis (courtesy of Dr David Swirsky, with permission of Dr Inderjeet Dokal, Hammersmith Hospital, London)

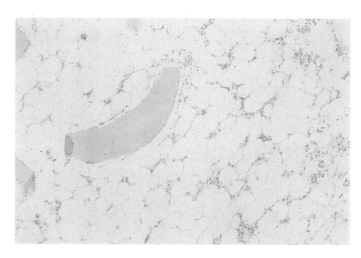

Plate 2 Aplastic bone marrow showing gross hypocellularity with replacement by fat cells (courtesy of Dr David Swirsky, with permission of Dr Inderjeet Dokal, Hammersmith Hospital, London)

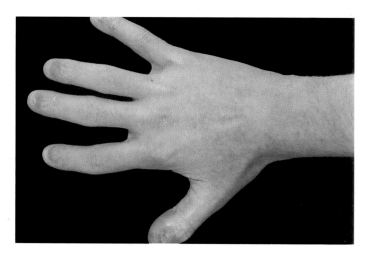

Plate 3 Nail dystrophy in dyskeratosis congenita (courtesy of Dr David Swirsky, with permission of Dr Inderjeet Dokal, Hammersmith Hospital, London)

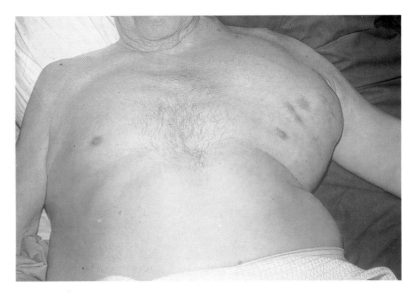

Plate 4 Gross axillary lymphadenopathy in lymphoma (courtesy of Dr Dominic Culligan, Aberdeen Royal Infirmary)

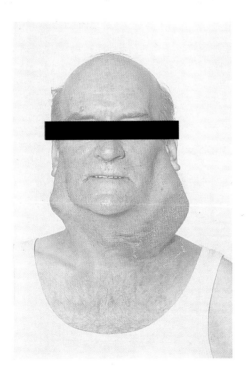

Plate 5 Gross cervical lymphadenopathy in lymphoma (courtesy of Dr Dominic Culligan, Aberdeen Royal Infirmary)

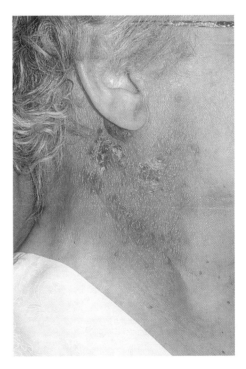

Plate 6 Neutropenic sepsis: cellulitis of the neck in acute leukaemia (courtesy of Dr Dominic Culligan, Aberdeen Royal Infirmary)

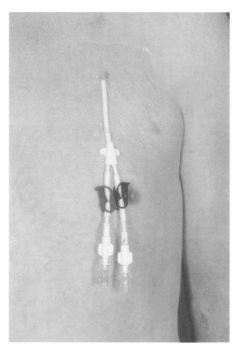

Plate 7 Hickman-type catheter (courtesy of Dr Rachel Green and Mr Douglas Watson, Glasgow Royal Infirmary)

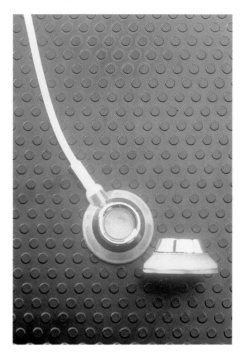

Plate 8 Subcutaneous port (courtesy of Bard Ltd)

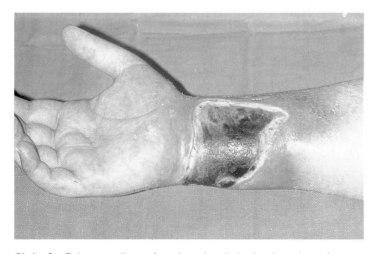

Plate 9 Extravasation of vesicant cytotoxic drug (courtesy of
Dr Andrew Hutcheon, Aberdeen Royal Infirmary)

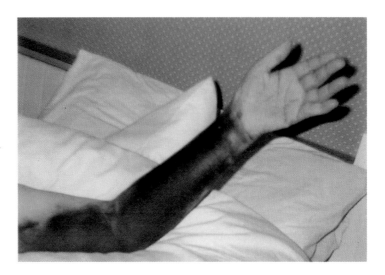

Plate 10 Bruising in thrombocytopenia

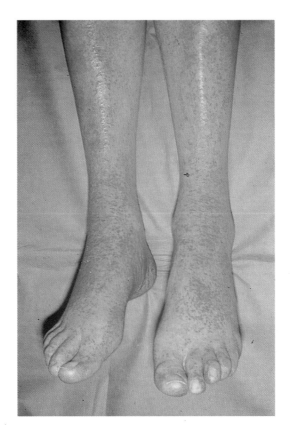

Plate 11 Thrombocytopenic purpura (courtesy of Grampian University Hospitals NHS Trust)

Mobilisation of stem cells in the autologous setting

Mobilisation is the movement of the progenitor cells from the bone marrow into the peripheral blood ready for collection. It was originally noted that the number of circulating progenitor cells increased as blood counts recovered from chemotherapy. Growth factors were also noted to increase progenitors in the blood. However, combined use of chemotherapy and growth factors shows increased efficacy compared to the use of only one agent (Sheridan et al 1992).

Many transplant units operate a mobilisation programme in which people are given cyclophosphamide chemotherapy followed by the administration of growth factors over a set period of time followed by cell collections. The dosages and timing of the chemotherapy and growth factors differ between centres. Most centres give mobilisation treatment on an outpatient basis, and therefore it is essential that patients understand the procedure and are able to comply with it. Growth factors are given on a daily basis as small subcutaneous injections. Where possible, patients are advised and taught how to give this injection themselves. Blood counts are monitored closely during the mobilisation process, and once the white cell count starts to rise cell collections are begun. Many centres recommend starting cell collections when the white blood cell count is greater than 3×10^9/L. Using a standard mobilisation regimen such as $1.5 \, g/m^2$ of cyclophosphamide followed by $10 \, \mu g/kg$ of G-CSF, average white blood cell recovery time is 9–10 days, although it is not always easy to predict this exactly. This can cause operational difficulties if the apheresis unit is based in a day-care setting, operating office hours.

Mobilisation of stem cells in the allogeneic setting

Mobilisation of donor stem cells for allograft patients is achieved by growth factors alone. Chemotherapy cannot be given to donors because of the obvious toxic effects. The first report of peripheral blood stem cells being used for allografting was by Kessinger et al (1989). They reported successful engraftment,

but nine collections were required to obtain sufficient cells without any mobilisation. By giving donors growth factors, cells may be collected more conveniently and efficiently. Donors are given between 5 and $15 \, \mu g/kg/day$ of growth factor (G-CSF) subcutaneously and their cells are collected after approximately 4–5 days. The long-term effects of administering growth factors to a healthy donor are as yet unknown. This must be explained to all potential donors and they must be told that the procedure is still being researched. Informed consent should be obtained before administration of growth factor is commenced.

Conversely, the advantages of using peripheral blood stem cells for the recipient are well known and are outlined in Table 10.2.

Apheresis

Since the mid-1980s peripheral blood stem cells have been collected from the blood using blood cell separators in a process called apheresis. A number of companies manufacture apheresis machines, among the most common of which are Cobe, Baxter, Haemonetics and Fresenius.

There are various problems associated with obtaining cells via apheresis, particularly with venous access. A 16-gauge needle is required in order to maintain adequate flow rates of at least 30 ml/min blood flow. In people with poor venous access, this may prove difficult, and central venous line insertion may be required. Standard Hickman-type catheters are not rigid enough to allow collections, although they may be used for the return flow. Apheresis skin

Table 10.2 Advantages of PBSC allografts

For the donor	For the recipient
No general anaesthetic required	Accelerated engraftment
No hospitalisation required	Less blood component support required
No blood transfusions required	Possibly less GVHD
No post-procedure pain	

tunnelled catheters are now available and have helped to combat this problem.

Apheresis is a safe, if rather time-consuming, procedure with patients experiencing minimal problems either during or after the procedure. The patient is attached to the machine via intravenous lines and the disposable circuit acts as a closed system. Approximately 10 litres of blood are processed per apheresis procedure, depending on the individual's body mass. Blood is anticoagulated in the machine, usually using citrate solutions such as acid citrate dextrose (ACD); this may induce a transient hypocalcaemia, often manifested by tingling of the lips, which can be easily treated with calcium supplements. Each apheresis session lasts approximately 3–4 hours. The total number of collections required depends upon the target cell count, which may vary between centres but a CD34+ cell dose of 2×10^6/kg is generally recommended.

Box 10.3 Advantages and disadvantages of umbilical cord blood cells	
Advantages of cord blood	**Disadvantages of cord blood**
Ease of procurement with no risk to mother or donor	Not yet demonstrated to successfully transplant adults as insufficient numbers
Less immunoreactivity, therefore less rejection and GVHD	
Minimal risk of graft infection (particularly cytomegalovirus)	Less graft versus leukaemia effect
Off-the-shelf supply	

Reflection point

If insufficient cells are collected, the mobilisation procedure may need to be repeated. If mobilisation attempts fail, a bone marrow harvest may be considered as an alternative source of stem cells. Consider what information an individual may require prior to commencing the apheresis procedure.

Stem cells from umbilical cords

The most recently identified source of stem cells is the umbilical cord. During development the fetus produces large quantities of CD34+ cells in the liver and bone marrow and these cells seem to be more active than normal, with a capacity for rapid increase. The advantages and disadvantages of using cord blood cells are outlined in Box 10.3.

The first cord blood transplant was carried out in Paris in 1988 by Dr Elaine Gluckman, who successfully treated a child with Fanconi's anaemia by transplanting his sibling's cord cells (Gluckman et al 1997). Currently, researchers

are investigating how to optimise the cell collections from cord blood by ex-vivo expansion to allow their use in the adult setting. Cord blood banks are being established with women making voluntary donations of umbilical cords – evidence from Switzerland shows that pregnant women of all backgrounds are happy to donate cords after delivery (Surbeck 1998). In the USA, some cord banks are allowing parents to pay to have cords stored in case their child might require them at a later date. There are currently four cord blood banks in the UK – in Belfast, Bristol, London and Newcastle.

Freezing and storage

Cryopreservation techniques for marrow and peripheral blood stem cells are the same, although the quantities involved are very different. During a bone marrow harvest approximately 1 litre of marrow is collected compared to 100–150 ml of cells per apheresis procedure. Cells are preserved with a cryoprotectant – dimethyl sulphoxide (DMSO) – which is added to the cells prior to freezing. The cells are frozen gradually at 1–2°C/min to at least −40°C, and stored below −120°C in mechanical freezers or liquid nitrogen tanks. Cells may be stored for many years prior to their use.

ADMISSION FOR TRANSPLANT

Before admission for intensive treatment people undergo a thorough medical evaluation which includes a wide variety of baseline investigations. This is a means of testing the function of vital organs prior to the onslaught of highly toxic therapy and may alert the team to any extra risks so that treatment can be modified accordingly. Investigations might include:

- chest X-ray
- echocardiogram for cardiac ejection fraction and ECG
- pulmonary function tests
- creatinine clearance
- nose, throat and Hickman-line swabs for methicillin-resistant *Staphylococcus aureus* (MRSA) and culture
- complete blood profile – full blood count, biochemistry and liver function tests, clotting screen, virology
- test dose for total body irradiation – if required
- placement of central venous catheter.

Before admission people are usually given the opportunity to visit the ward, meet some of the staff and discuss their care in order to alleviate some of their anxieties. Some centres also carry out pre-transplant psychosocial assessments to consider whether extra psychological support will be required. Family and carers are also encouraged to visit prior to admission to discuss any concerns they may have. Most people need repeated explanations concerning the timetable of events and expected complications. Many units have written information booklets with full explanations of all procedures. A general information booklet about transplants is also available from the British Association of Cancer United Patients (BACUP) and the Leukaemia Research Fund (LRF).

Conditioning treatments

Following admission conditioning treatments, which are preparatory regimens for transplantation, are commenced. The aim of conditioning treatments is three-fold:

- To create space within the bone marrow cavity. Apperley et al (1998) explain that this is a controversial idea which originates from the thought that stem cells occupy defined niches in the bone marrow.
- To cause immunosuppression to prevent rejection (important in allografting).
- To eradicate residual disease.

The type of myeloablative therapy regimen varies, depending on the disease, the disease state and the transplant centre. Conditioning regimens consist of high-dose chemotherapy either alone or in combination with other high-dose cytotoxic drugs or total body irradiation (TBI). The benefits of each conditioning regimen has to be balanced against associated toxicities. Treatment-related mortality is closely associated with more toxic regimens.

In the transplant setting, chemotherapy is administered in supralethal doses, resulting in side-effects that are generally more severe than those experienced with conventional chemotherapy. Drugs commonly used include cyclophosphamide, melphalan, etoposide, cytarabine and busulphan.

Total body irradiation was originally given as a single dose at a low-dose rate, but is now more commonly fractionated with the hope of improving toxicities (see Ch. 9). The aim of TBI is to deliver the maximum tolerated dose in an even distribution across the body. Doses between 0.02 and 0.50 Gy/min are given. The radiotherapist usually sees the patient prior to TBI to give a full explanation, including the immediate and late side-effects: some of these are the same as those for chemotherapy, others are unique to TBI treatment. As the patient receives chemotherapy and radiotherapy in combination, toxicities are expected to be more severe. Common acute effects and late effects are outlined in Box 10.4.

THE TRANSPLANT

The day the patient receives their transplant is called Day 0. Stem cells are infused through a

Box 10.4 Common acute and late effects of BMT	
Common acute side-effects	**Late side-effects**
Nausea and vomiting	Chronic GVHD
Diarrhoea	Infections
Mucositis and	Cataracts
parotitis	Secondary
Dry mouth or	malignancies
excessive salivation	Gonadal
Skin rash	dysfunction
Alopecia	Endocrine
Somnolence	dysfunction
Pancytopenia	Immunodeficiency
Electrolyte imbalance	Pulmonary
	complications

blood administration set via the central venous catheter.

Allografts: Patients receiving cells from a donor may have a fresh product to be infused. This is more likely with bone marrow cells than peripheral blood stem cells. It is possible for allergic reactions to occur in allograft infusions and an antihistamine and steroid injection are often given as prophylaxis.

Autografts: Patients receiving their own cells will obviously always have a frozen product. Frozen cells are taken to the patient in a liquid nitrogen container, thawed in a water bath, and given to the patient. When frozen cells are infused, there is often a sweet smelling unpleasant odour in the patient's breath and perspiration. This is due to the preservative used when freezing the cells and may be present in the atmosphere around the patient for approximately 24 hours. Some patients also experience a strange taste sensation at the time of cell infusion. Other potential problems following the infusion of preserved cells include:

- nausea and vomiting
- diarrhoea
- haematuria (possibly resulting from the lysis of red cells after thawing)
- dyspnoea
- abdominal cramps.

Stem cells migrate to the bone marrow space by a poorly understood mechanism.

The transplant day is often a nerve-racking occasion for the patient – who knows the dire effects of not having a functioning bone marrow – but it is not as exciting as some people seem to expect. Most people feel a great sense of anticlimax at the simplicity of the procedure, mingled with a sense of relief that the mechanism is now in place for recovery to begin.

 Reflection point

While infusing cells is a relatively simple procedure it is important to ensure staff have sufficient skills and knowledge to deal with any potential complications that may occur. Consider what skills and knowledge are required to deal with any potential complications.

THE RECOVERY

The road to recovery is not always an easy one. The degree and severity of complications and side-effects depend upon the type of transplant, age and fitness of the individual and the nature of the conditioning regime.

The care of people in the recovery phase concerns:

- preventing complications
- detecting complications quickly
- managing complications promptly.

Skilled nursing care is important in each of these areas and requires a theoretical knowledge base of potential complications and their management. Some complications are typical to all cancer therapies and are dealt with in depth in other chapters of this book, while some are unique to, or specially concern, the post-transplant patient.

Complications of post-transplant
Infection

Post-transplant, with profound neutropenia, people are particularly at risk from infection (see Ch. 13). Susceptibility to infection is increased by depressed T- and B-cell function, use of immunosuppressive drugs as well as the risks of indwelling central venous catheters. Within the transplant field, special attention has been paid to ways of minimising infection risk through prophylactic antibacterial, antiviral and antifungal drugs and by protective isolation. Poe et al (1994) conducted a nationwide study in the USA and discovered little standardisation of infection-prevention methods, with some centres following more stringent guidelines than others – this is probably also true of transplant units in the UK. The benefits of strict protective isolation (sometimes using laminar air flow or high-efficiency particulate air (hepa) filters) are now being questioned. Russell et al (1992) carried out a study in which no isolation procedures were used and concluded that transplantation may safely occur without protective isolation, or indeed confining patients in hospital, without any added risk. However, concern remains that isolation is necessary to prevent aspergillus infection in the immediate post-transplant period.

For the patient, protective isolation can be an extremely lonely and frightening experience. Being kept in a small room with minimal visitors and decreased human contact can seem like a prison sentence (see Ch. 19). There are also issues of staffing as more nurses are required to care for patients in side rooms, especially if patients are unwell and cannot easily be monitored without a nurse actually being in the room.

The use of peripheral blood stem cells and the availability of haematopoietic growth factors have radically reduced the length of the post-transplant neutropenic period. However, the prompt treatment of infections with empirical broad-spectrum antibiotics remains essential for people with neutropenic fevers.

Haemorrhage

Anaemia and thrombocytopenia occur as a result of the bone marrow suppression following high-dose therapy. Thrombocytopenia in the transplant patient is potentially life threatening and may be transient or prolonged. Bleeding complications are often avoided by the administration of prophylactic platelets. BMT units usually have a limit to which the haemoglobin and platelet count may fall following which transfusions must be instigated. Commonly, patients have blood transfusions to maintain their haemoglobin above 10 g/L and the platelet count above 10×10^9/L. The frequency and amount of platelet transfusions may need to be increased in patients who have increased platelet consumption due to infection or haemorrhage. Bleeding can occur from any site and may be internal or external. Close monitoring of daily blood counts and thorough assessment of the clinical situation is imperative in the prevention of catastrophic bleeding (see Ch. 14 for further discussion of haemorrhagic problems).

Gastrointestinal toxicity
Mucositis
The incidence of mucositis among BMT patients is extremely high. Particularly severe mucositis is associated with regimens containing busulphan, etoposide, thiotepa and TBI. Often the pain associated with mucositis can only be controlled using opiates, and parenteral nutritional support may be required. Mucositis develops early following BMT, commonly occurring shortly after infusion of cells, and starts to resolve as the neutrophil count recovers. Good oral hygiene is essential throughout the transplant process – it does not prevent mucositis but may reduce the incidence of superimposed infections (see Ch. 16). Mucositis is often described by BMT patients as their most distressing symptom.

Diarrhoea
Many patients will develop diarrhoea post-high-dose therapy. Damage to the mucosa results in an increase of fluid secreted by the intestine. Diarrhoea usually resolves with time but is an extremely distressing and unpleasant experience which may be helped by the use of antidiarrhoeal agents such as loperamide.

Interstitial pneumonia
This condition is characterised by diffuse pulmonary disease, fever, hypoxia and respiratory distress. It is a particularly nasty complication and many people die as a result of it.

Treatment is supportive and often includes the use of steroids. Any pneumonia that is not bacterial can be called interstitial. There are many possible causes including:

- idiopathic – probably due to lung damage caused by TBI, chemotherapy or disease
- cytomegalovirus – the incidence is reduced by the administration of CMV-negative products to people who are not seropositive and the prophylactic use of acyclovir and immunoglobulin
- *Pneumocystis carinii.*

Interstitial pneumonia can be extremely distressing for patients and their families due to the often rather sudden onset of acute life-threatening symptoms. With rapidly progressing pulmonary infiltration ventilatory support is often required, with the patient moving to the intensive care unit.

In allografts

Graft versus host disease

GVHD is a disorder in which immunocompetent donor lymphoid cells react to a foreign immunosuppressed host (the recipient). T lymphocytes in the donor stem cells recognise the host tissue as being foreign and attack it. GVHD can occur in acute (less than 100 days after transplant) or chronic (more than 100 days after transplant) forms. Chronic GVHD need not be preceded by the acute phase, although it is more likely to occur in people who have had the acute form.

GVHD affects:

- skin: ranging from a mild maculopapular rash on the body surface to generalised erythroderma with peeling that resembles a third-degree burn
- liver: elevated serum bilirubin, jaundice and increased girth
- gastrointestinal tract: abdominal cramps, severe diarrhoea – classically, green coloured.

Symptoms are graded according to their severity and the number of organs involved. Grade 1 is mild GVHD and needs no treatment, while Grade 4 is life threatening.

Prevention

The main aim with GVHD is to prevent it becoming severe enough to require treatment. In allogeneic transplants the most common form of immunosuppression is cyclosporin, a potent immunosuppressant, which interferes with the function of T lymphocytes. The action of cyclosporin is reversible and dose dependent. When used in conjunction with methotrexate the severity of GVHD is less and survival is improved (Storb et al 1989). Cyclosporin is initially given intravenously at a dose of 3 mg/kg the day before infusion of stem cells. The dose is then adjusted according to blood levels and changed to an oral preparation as soon as this can be tolerated. Blood levels of cyclosporin must be monitored closely with pre-dose trough levels being measured every 2 days until levels are stable. Adverse effects of cyclosporin include renal impairment and liver dysfunction, hypertension, tremor, hirsutism and central nervous system disturbances. Cyclosporin is continued for at least 3 months after transplant.

Treatment

GVHD is usually treated by increasing the cyclosporin dose and giving high-dose corticosteroids. Monoclonal antibodies and thalidomide have also been used. Treatment is often complicated by infection and the use of steroids enhances the risks from immunosuppression. Up to 80% of allogeneic recipients will experience GVHD and it may be responsible for about 25% of the mortality seen after allogeneic transplants (Barrett & Treleaven 1992). Studies of people treated for leukaemia suggest that GVHD also has a graft versus leukaemia (or tumour) effect, indicating that patients who have a degree of GVHD are less likely to relapse from their disease than people who have no GVHD.

Graft rejection

The inability of the recipient's body to accept the graft is called rejection. This is not a common complication. The rejection usually occurs up to 4 months after the transplant and usually means that the graft has been destroyed by immunologically active cells in the host. Rejection may be treated by giving a back up infusion of autologous cells.

Veno-occlusive disease of the liver

Veno-occlusive disease (VOD) can occur 1–3 weeks following transplant and occurs in approximately 20% of transplants. Individuals with a previous history of liver disease are particularly at risk. VOD results from the obstruction or narrowing of the small hepatic veins and is a direct result of high-dose therapy. The individual experiences jaundice, hepatomegaly and ascites, depending on the degree of the occlusion. Despite aggressive therapy, including the use of tissue plasminogen activator and heparin, severe VOD often results in progressive liver failure and is almost uniformly fatal. However, Richardson et al (1998) report some success with the use of defibrotide, a drug usually used in vascular disorders.

Psychosocial aspects

Transplantation is a demanding and complex area, but as we struggle to understand the intricacies of the science we can imagine the difficulty patients may have in trying to gain a clear picture of what will, or might, happen to them. People understandably feel confused and anxious as they try to assimilate information and gain enough understanding to enable them to make a decision as to whether or not they should have a transplant. The reactions of friends and family are also extremely important, particularly when a donor is involved. Innovative patient education is of extreme importance – as well as time to allow people to explore all possibilities, thoughts and fears. Transplantation offers people the chance of long-term disease-free survival (which commonly the lay person terms a 'cure'). However, there are absolutely no guarantees of success and the risk (although nowadays greatly reduced) of dying in the process, or suffering long-term side-effects resulting in a reduced quality of life also need to be considered.

Survivors may experience 'survivor guilt' as they question why fellow patients died. Many people feel changed as a result of the transplant experience and feel they have a different perspective on life, with different priorities from their peers. Others still just want life to return to 'normal', but cannot quite remember what 'normal' is anymore. Hjermstad & Kaasa (1995) have reviewed the extensive literature available on quality of life post-transplant and suggest that more prospective studies with long-term follow-up are required to expand understanding of transplant-specific problems and the interventions that can be implemented (see Ch. 20).

 Case study 10.1

Betty, a 31-year-old secretary, had recently become engaged to her long-term boyfriend. They had set up home together and were busy planning a holiday when she started to feel unwell. She managed to carry on working, but her friends noticed that she was unable to enjoy life to the full and encouraged her to see a doctor. In July 1998 Betty was admitted to hospital with lethargy, shortness of breath, night sweats and weight loss. A chest X-ray revealed a widened mediastinum and globular heart and a subsequent CT scan showed a mediastinal mass. Guided biopsies proved this to be high-grade non-Hodgkin's lymphoma (stage IIB).

Betty was devastated, especially when she was told that the chemotherapy might affect her fertility. She was treated with two courses of combination chemotherapy, cyclophosphamide, doxorubicin, vincristine (Oncovin) and prednisolone (CHOP), but her chest X-ray showed progressive disease. The regimen was changed to expose her to a different group of drugs and she received two courses of dexamethasone, cisplatin and high-dose cytarabine (DHAP) to which she had an excellent response. Her stem cells were collected following the second course of chemotherapy, with G-CSF administered from day 5 after the end of the chemotherapy. Enough cells were collected from one apheresis session and it was decided to consolidate treatment with an autologous peripheral blood stem cell transplant. All pre-transplant investigations were

Continued

Case study 10.1 *Continued*

performed as an outpatient and Betty was admitted for transplant at the beginning of February 1999.

Betty tolerated chemotherapy very well and did not feel that it was significantly worse than her other treatments. However, the recovery phase of the transplant was a huge ordeal and far worse than she had anticipated. Very quickly after having had her cells returned she became neutropenic and was placed in protective isolation and almost immediately had terrible diarrhoea which made her feel extremely weak and very embarrassed. Her mouth became extremely sore and she was unable to eat at all and found drinking and talking difficult – at this stage she felt extremely isolated and alone. She was meticulous with her mouthcare but the pain became unbearable and she was given intravenous diamorphine which made her very sleepy. She was also pyrexial and required two lines of intravenous antibiotics. Blood and platelet transfusions were also required and she found all the interruptions extremely disturbing: she thought it was strange that she was 'isolated' when so many different people kept wandering in and out of her room.

Twelve days following transplant her cell count started to come up, her mouth felt far more comfortable and she was weaned off the diamorphine. Her temperature settled and she felt much better, although incredibly weak. The transplant team were pleased with her progress and happy to allow her home, but she was very concerned about leaving the security of the hospital especially as during the day when her fiancé was at work she would be on her own.

With as much community support as possible she left hospital on day 15 and was glad to have a list of contact numbers in case she needed help. She gradually recovered her strength and her progress was clearly seen on her weekly visits to the day unit. Three months after the transplant she appeared to be in complete remission, but did not seem at all happy. On careful questioning she admitted that the relationship with her fiancé was over as he felt too overburdened by all that they had been through and unable to cope any more. She felt more vulnerable than ever and was grateful that since her diagnosis she had been seeing a counsellor, who was helping her to come to terms with all her traumas.

Ambulatory transplants

Some units are currently considering the possibility of outpatient, or ambulatory, transplants. People would come to the transplant unit on a daily basis and only be admitted if it was considered necessary. This idea has developed as the toxicities associated with high-dose therapy are now managed more effectively and may be prevented by prophylactic therapy. Most studies investigating the practicalities of outpatient transplants are generated from the USA, such as that published by Meisenberg et al (1997) which considered total outpatient treatment and partial outpatient treatment for all types of transplant. It certainly appears to be a dynamic approach to reducing the costs associated with transplantation, but will doubtless need careful evaluation. One possible problem is the ability to readmit people when necessary into an appropriate transplant bed. It is also important to consider the effect this may have upon the primary health-care team, and whether this is an approach that patients would welcome.

REHABILITATION

Going home after the prolonged inpatient stay for transplant, although exciting and triumphal, can also be stressful. Advances in techniques and supportive care have led to earlier discharge dates. People often feel extremely vulnerable when leaving the hospital environment and most are reliant on a carer to help them adjust. Most patients feel enormous fatigue on discharge and need to be able to gradually increase their activities. Going home signifies the start of returning to their old lifestyle and people need encouragement to leave the sick role behind while taking sensible precautions to minimise further complications. Special advice is usually needed on several issues.

Diet

Patients may be advised to take care with food safety and follow the advice set down by the Ministry of Agriculture, Fisheries and Food. It is sometimes suggested that eating out should be avoided during the first month at home. A good fluid intake is encouraged and people may drink alcohol, although only in moderate amounts.

Socialising

During the first few weeks at home most centres recommend that socialising should not include visiting crowded, enclosed places such as cinemas, pubs and churches. Walks in the fresh air are encouraged and exercise should be gradually increased.

Sexual activities

A decrease in libido as well as fatigue may affect sexual relationships. As activity levels increase and people start to feel stronger the desire to become sexually active should return. Patients should be encouraged to discuss any concerns they have about resuming their sexual relationships.

Work

The date of returning to work varies between different people and depends on the type of job they have. People should return to work as soon as they feel ready and able to cope with it. Many people find returning on a part-time basis very helpful initially.

Although people are discharged from hospital more quickly they are expected to return regularly for checkups in the Outpatient Department. Some people find regular outpatients visits extremely tiring, especially those having to travel any great distance. Many units now have designated day-case areas where patients can be reviewed and receive treatments such as blood and platelet transfusions when needed. These areas have generally been developed and are led by the nursing team. The need for day-care facilities increases if patients are discharged earlier and will also be of great importance in facilitating ambulatory transplantation. Some units offer complementary therapies in this setting, and may also facilitate self-help or support groups for people in the post-transplant setting.

RELAPSE

People often remain under a cloud of fear as the possibility of relapse from their original disease remains ever present. Relapse can occur following any type of transplant, but is more common among autografts, and may occur at any time – but more usually within the first 2 years following transplant. Relapse following high-dose therapy is inevitably very disappointing; treatment options at this stage need careful consideration and will depend among other things upon the diagnosis, the extent of the disease, tolerance to treatment and willingness of the patient to undergo further treatment. Second transplants are given in some situations, although their usefulness is still under evaluation. A challenging aim of rehabilitation must be to help the patient live as fully as possible and not allow the fear of relapse to minimise their enjoyment of currently living without the disease.

IMPLICATIONS FOR PRACTICE

The multidisciplinary team (MDT) needs to work cohesively to ensure the expert care of this group of patients. In many areas nurses have emerged as the coordinators of this MDT approach. Lin (1994) describes the nurse's work in achieving continuity of care for patients in both the inpatient and outpatient setting in her combined role as nurse specialist and coordinator. Specialist courses for nurses working within this specialised field are well established, but Heron (1992) questions whether highly specialised nurses will be needed as transplantation becomes easier and more commonplace. Traditionally, transplants only occurred in specialist centres. But with the advent of ambulatory transplants will this still be essential? Guidelines regarding the facilities required for transplant patients were published by the British Committee for Standards in Haematology Task Force in 1995 and suggest that this expert level of care is definitely advised. However autologous transplants may take place in non-specialist areas and may commonly be carried out on oncology wards for people with solid tumours.

Nursing has a critical role in the field of transplantation, with the scope for nurses to acquire skills in new areas such as bone marrow aspiration, apheresis and central line insertion.

More importantly, nurses can ensure that people being transplanted receive in-depth education and sensitive and skilled care throughout the transplant process and beyond. If they make sure they have a solid understanding of the different aspects of transplantation, nurses should not hesitate to embrace this demanding area with enthusiasm.

DISCUSSION QUESTIONS

1. Is it necessary for all types of transplant to be carried out in specialist centres?

2. Is protective isolation really necessary for patients having BMT?

3. Are ambulatory transplants the obvious way of the future?

4. Should it become obligatory for all umbilical cords to be donated and stored?

5. What are the ethical implications of administering growth factors to healthy donors?

6. Do transplant survivors require long-term follow-up?

References

Apperley J, Girinsky T, Friedrich W, Goldstone A, Niethammer D, Rosti G 1998 Conditioning regimens. In: The EBMT handbook: blood and marrow transplantation. European School of Haematology, Paris, Ch. 8, pp 98–116

Barrett J, Treleaven J 1992 Bone marrow transplantation in practice. Churchill Livingstone, Edinburgh, pp 3–9

British Committee for Standards in Haematology Task Force 1995 Guidelines on the provision of facilities for the care of adult patients with haematological malignancies. Clinical Laboratory Haematology 17: 3–10

Campbell K 1997 Types of bone marrow and stem cell transplant. Nursing Times 93(7): 44–46

European Group for Blood and Marrow Transplantation 1998 The EBMT handbook: blood and marrow transplantation. European School of Haematology, Paris

Gluckman E, Rocha V, Boyer-Chammard A et al 1997 Outcome of cord blood transplantation from related and unrelated donors. New England Journal of Medicine 337(6): 373–381

Gratwohl A 1998 Organisational aspects. In: The EBMT handbook: blood and marrow transplantation. European School of Haematology, Paris, Ch. 2, pp 11–26

Heron D 1992 Talking about a revolution: growth factors and peripheral stem cell transplants are set to revolutionise leukaemia and bone marrow treatments. Nursing Standard 7(6): Leukaemia and Bone Marrow Transplant Nursing Suppl., 52–53

Hjermstad M J, Kaasa S 1995 Quality of life in adult cancer patients treated with bone marrow transplantation – a review of the literature. European Journal of Cancer 31A(2): 163–173.

International Society for Haemopoietic And Graft Engineering (Europe) 1997 Standards for blood and marrow progenitor cell collection, processing and transplantation, 1st edn

Kessinger A, Smith D M, Strandjord S E 1989 Allogeneic transplantation of blood derived T cell depleted hemopoietic stem cells after myeloablative treatment in a patient with acute lymphoblastic leukaemia. Bone marrow transplantation 4: 643–646

Lin E M 1994 A combined role of clinical nurse specialist and co-ordinator. Clinical Nurse Specialist 8(1): 48–55

Meisenberg B R, Miller W, McMillan R et al 1997 Outpatient high dose chemotherapy with autologous stem cell rescue for haematologic and non haematologic malignancies. Journal of Clinical Oncology 15(1): 11–17

Poe S S, Larson E, McGuire D, Krumm S 1994 A national survey of infection prevention on bone marrow transplant units. Oncology Nursing Forum 21(10): 1687–1694

Richardson P G, Elias A D, Krishnan A 1998 Treatment of severe VOD with defibrotide compassionate use results in response without significant toxicity in a high risk population. Blood 92(3): 737–744

Richman C M, Weiner R S, Yankee R A 1976 Increase in circulating stem cells following chemotherapy in man. Blood 47: 1031–1039

Russell J A, Poon M C, Jones A R, Woodman R C, Ruether B A 1992 Allogeneic bone marrow transplantation without protective isolation in adults with malignant disease. Lancet 339: 38–40

Sheridan W P, Begley C G, Juttner C A et al 1992 Effect of PBPC mobilised by filgrastim on patient recovery after high dose chemotherapy. Lancet 339: 640–644

Storb R, Deeg H J, Pepe M et al 1989 Methotrexate and cyclosporin versus cyclosporin alone for prophylaxis of GVHD in patients given HLA identical marrow grafts for leukaemia. Blood 73: 1729–1734

Surbeck D, Islebe A, Schonfeld B, Tichelli A, Gratwohl A, Hozgreve W 1998 Umbilical cord blood transplantation: acceptance of umbilical cord blood donation by pregnant patients. Journal Suisse de Medicine 128(18): 689–695

Further reading

Buchsel P C, Leum E W, Randolph S R 1996 Delayed complications of bone marrow transplantation: an update. Oncology Nursing Forum 23(8): 1267–1289
A review article looking at the complications that can arise months to years after transplantation and the associated morbidity and mortality. It is well researched, with relevant nursing diagnoses and interventions.

Burt R, Deeg H J, Lothian S T, Santos G W 1996 On call in … bone marrow transplantation. Chapman and Hall, New York
This book was written as a guide for medics, but is extremely useful as a quick reference, especially on treatments and investigations.

Decker W A 1995 Psychosocial considerations for bone marrow transplant recipients. Critical Care Nursing Quarterly 17(4): 67–73
This article provides a good overview of the factors to be considered to ensure the patient's well-being is at the centre of care.

Kusnierz-Glaz C R, Schlegel P G, Wong R et al 1997 Influence of age on outcome of 500 autologous bone marrow transplant procedures for haematologic malignancy. Journal of Clinical Oncology 15(1): 18–25
This useful research article indicates that age should be considered carefully before embarking on high-dose therapy.

Lin E M, Tierney D K, Stadtmauer E A 1993 Autologous bone marrow transplantation: a review of the principles and complications. Cancer Nursing 16(3): 204–213
This article was written by an experienced nursing team and concentrates on the autologous transplant patient.

Russell N H 1994 Peripheral blood stem cells for allogeneic transplantation. Bone Marrow Transplantation 13: 353–355
A useful text that highlights some of the specific issues and concerns of using stem cells rather than marrow for allogeneic transplants and looks at the effect this may have on the patient's outcome.

Soutar R L, King D J, 1995 Bone marrow transplantation. British Medical Journal 310: 31–36
A basic article which gives a good historical background of transplantation so far and highlights issues for the future.

Thompson C 1995 Umbilical cords: turning garbage into clinical gold. Science 268: 805–806
A very readable article, written for the general public, that indicates the pioneering nature of umbilical cord transplants.

Whedon M B, Wujcik D 1997 Blood and marrow stem cell transplantation: principles, practice and nursing insights, 2nd edn. Jones and Bartlett, Boston
This book is written by American nurses and doctors based at the Fred Hutchinson Cancer Centre in Seattle. It gives the American perspective on blood and marrow transplantation for both red and white cell disorders. It covers all aspects of BMT, with an emphasis on haematology nursing, including ambulatory care and fertility issues. Nurses working in haematology and BMT units will find this book extremely useful.

11 *Blood component support*

PAULA WILKINS

Key points
- Safety issues are paramount in transfusion of all blood components and products
- Checking procedures should always be strictly adhered to
- Most adverse transfusion events occur due to clerical errors and are avoidable
- Recipients should be closely observed for signs and symptoms of transfusion reactions.

INTRODUCTION

Successful blood component support is a relatively new concept. Although blood transfusion was experimented with during the 15th and 16th centuries it was during World War II that blood banking was launched into the modern era. In the 1960s sterile separation and storage of blood components led to the rapid expansion of blood transfusion and the development of a diversified, lifesaving branch of medicine.

The term blood transfusion refers to both transfusion of whole blood and its individual components. Less than 10% of all necessary transfusions require whole blood (Masouredis 1990). Whole blood once collected from a donor is 'fractionated' into its various components and red blood cells, platelets, plasma and plasma proteins are all used as vital supportive treatments in haemato-oncological disorders. Most treatment regimes cause severe myelosuppression, which is frequently a limiting

factor in effective treatment. Technological advances in transfusion medicine have allowed clinicians to treat haemato-oncological disorders with increasingly aggressive regimens while supporting the suppressed bone marrow with blood components, thus improving both morbidity and mortality.

However, transfusion of blood components is not without inherent risk and it is imperative that safety issues are addressed by everyone involved in the transfusion process. This chapter considers the use of blood components in the treatment of haemato-oncological disorders and associated safety aspects including management and prevention of adverse side-effects.

SAFETY ISSUES AND NURSING MANAGEMENT

Until the 1980s blood component support was seen as a relatively safe form of treatment. The advent of AIDS (acquired immune deficiency syndrome) and other infections such as hepatitis C which may be transmitted by blood transfusion, have highlighted its potential dangers and safety is paramount throughout the entire transfusion process.

Safety issues related to donated blood

Blood donation
Collecting blood from healthy donors is the first step in ensuring safety of blood components for

subsequent recipients and strict criteria are adhered to in pre-donation screening. This includes completion of an interview and questionnaire to identify 'high risk' donors.

Screening for infection

All blood donations in the UK are tested to detect the presence of infectious agents which could be transmitted to any future recipient. Infections transmitted by blood components may be bacterial, viral or parasitic (Table 11.1).

With donor selection and screening, the risk of transfusion-acquired infection is thought to be small (McClelland 1996). However, the safety of blood components cannot be guaranteed.

Virus inactivation processes

Fractionated plasma products such as immunoglobulins are derived from the pooled plasma of multiple donors, which increases the infection risk. Production processes remove or inactivate viruses, thereby increasing product safety.

Recently, concern has been expressed about the risk of transmitting new variant Creutzfeldt–Jakob disease (nvCJD) through transfusion of plasma products. Currently, the risk is theoretical, as there is no evidence that the disease can be transmitted by transfusion. However, no screening test capable of detecting nvCJD exists and the Department of Health (1998a) have decided as a precaution, to obtain all plasma used to manufacture blood products from outside the UK,

> until a reliable test is developed to detect nvCJD or, evidence is produced to prove that it cannot be transmitted by blood products or, that it can be destroyed in the manufacturing process.

Compatibility testing

Prior to transfusion both donor and recipient's blood are tested for compatibility as transfusion of incompatible blood can result in fatal transfusion reactions. There are a number of different blood group systems, with the most important being the ABO and rhesus groups.

ABO groups

The ABO group of an individual is determined by the presence of genetically inherited red cell antigens and plasma antibodies. Anti-A and Anti-B antibodies are present in the plasma of every individual who does not possess the corresponding antigen on their red cell membranes (Table 11.2). These plasma antibodies are capable of destroying transfused red cells of an incompatible ABO group and it is therefore imperative to ensure compatibility between donor and recipient blood groups to avoid a potentially fatal acute haemolytic transfusion reaction (AHTR).

Rhesus system

The rhesus D (RhD) antigen is most significant. Individuals whose red cells possess this antigen are rhesus positive and those without rhesus negative. RhD-negative individuals do not develop antibodies to the D antigen unless they are exposed to it. Exposure only occurs through pregnancy or transfusion of RhD-positive blood. Once antibodies have developed

Table 11.1 Infections transmitted by blood transfusion

Type of infection	Infectious agents
Viral	Hepatitis A, B, C Human immunodeficiency virus (HIV) Cytomegalovirus (CMV)
Bacterial May be introduced at collection or be endogenous	Pseudomonas, Achromobacters, Coliforms, Salmonella, E. coli, Syphilis
Parasitic	Malaria

Table 11.2 ABO blood groups

Blood group	Red cell antigens	Plasma antibodies
O	None	Anti-A/Anti-B
A	A	Anti-B
B	B	Anti-A
AB	A and B	None

they have no effect until an individual is exposed to the D antigen for a second time when the donor antigen and recipient antibody reaction can result in haemolytic disease of the newborn or a transfusion reaction.

Other antibodies

Previous blood transfusion and pregnancy may result in the development of other red cell antibodies capable of causing transfusion reactions. The multiple transfusions received by individuals with haemato-oncological disorders predispose them to development of red cell antibodies and subsequent difficulties in obtaining compatible blood for transfusion.

Human leucocyte antigen (HLA)

The cell membranes of leucocytes also possess antigens and individuals who have received multiple transfusions may develop HLA antibodies capable of destroying transfused cells. HLA-compatible blood components may therefore be required, especially for those receiving multiple platelet transfusions.

Measures taken to reduce transfusion-related complications

Individuals with haematological malignancies are particularly susceptible to transfusion-related complications because of the need for multiple transfusions and their immunocompromised status. The following measures are used to reduce complications.

Leucocyte depletion

It is now recognised that the transfusion of donor leucocytes in blood components may cause a number of clinical complications, including:

- non-haemolytic febrile transfusion reactions
- alloimmunisation to leucocyte antigens
- platelet refractoriness
- sensitisation to transplanted antigens in organ and bone marrow transplant (BMT) recipients, leading to graft rejection
- transmission of cell-associated viruses, such as cytomegalovirus (CMV) and human T-cell lymphotropic virus (HTLV-II)

- reactivation of latent recipient virus infection
- post-transfusion thrombocytopenia.

Until recently the decision to use leucodepleted blood rested with the individual clinician. However, in July 1998 the UK government decided that all donated blood should be leucodepleted to further reduce the risk of transmitting infection through transfusion (Department of Health 1998b). Leucodepletion is being implemented systematically and by the end of 1999 all donated blood will be routinely leucodepleted in the transfusion centre.

Irradiated blood components in haemato-oncology

Irradiated blood components are used to prevent transfusion associated graft versus host disease (TA-GVHD). This is a particular problem for severely immunocompromised individuals and occurs through engraftment of viable T lymphoctyes transfused with other blood components. The British Committee for Standards in Haematology (BCSH) Blood Transfusion Task Force 1996 guidelines recommend that blood components should be irradiated in the following circumstances:

- Individuals with acute leukaemia receiving HLA-matched platelets or blood components donated by first- or second-degree relatives. A shared HLA haplotype increases the risk of TA-GVHD.
- All adults and children with Hodgkin's disease of any stage.
- All individuals receiving purine analogue drugs: for example, fludarabine, cladribine, which cause profound lymphopenia, increasing susceptibility to TA-GVHD.
- All individuals undergoing autologous bone marrow or peripheral blood stem cell harvesting for 7 days prior to and during harvesting and from commencement of chemotherapy and radiotherapy conditioning until 3 months post-transplant or up to 6 months if the individual received total body irradiation.
- All individuals receiving allogeneic BMT from commencing chemotherapy and radiotherapy conditioning until withdrawal of

immunosuppressive therapy (usually 6 months or until lymphocytes are $>1 \times 10^9$/L). Irradiation needs to be continued for certain individuals, such as those with chronic GVHD.

■ All blood transfused to allogeneic BMT donors prior to or during harvesting to prevent TA-GVHD.

Cytomegalovirus-negative blood components

CMV is a herpes virus which in healthy people produces few symptoms but poses a severe infection risk for immunocompromised individuals and is an important cause of mortality in bone marrow transplant/peripheral blood stem cell transplant (BMT/PBSCT) (Hewitt and Wagstaff 1992). The following individuals should therefore receive CMV-negative blood components:

■ CMV-negative allograft recipients receiving a CMV-negative graft
■ CMV-negative autograft recipients
■ future potential transplant recipients who are CMV-negative
■ all newly diagnosed haemato-oncology patients until their CMV status is known (McClelland 1996).

Safety issues in administration

Many serious life-threatening AHTR and deaths associated with blood transfusion are avoidable and occur due to clerical error or non-adherence to hospital policy. In the UK, in the 2 years between November 1996 and November 1998, there were 191 incidents of transfusion of the incorrect blood component reported to the Serious Hazards of Transfusion (SHOT) Steering Group (Williamson et al 1998, 1999). As a result of these incidents, three people died and a further 29 suffered major morbidity. It is therefore vital that checks are made at every step in the administration process.

Prescription and ordering of blood components remains the doctor's responsibility, but many nurses are involved in the sampling and ordering process and it is important that they are aware of all the checks which should be made. The NHS executive circular 'Better Blood Transfusion' (NHSE 1998) requires all NHS Trusts to have agreed and disseminated local protocols for blood transfusion, based on guidelines and best national practice by March 2000. Further to this, the BCSH (1999) have produced guidelines for the administration of blood and blood components. As there is little evidence to prove the efficacy of specific procedures in blood ordering and administration these guidelines are based on current professional opinion. Given the expertise of members of the working group these guidelines should be accepted as best practice. Main areas of the checking procedure advocated by BCSH (1999) guidelines are outlined below.

■ Request forms should be clearly written and contain full patient details, including identification number, location of the patient, details of the blood component required, information about obstetric and transfusion history, the patient's diagnosis and reason for the request.
■ Only one patient should be bled at a time to minimise error. Patient details should be verified at blood sampling and the sample should be clearly labelled immediately after the blood has been added to the tube. A pre-labelled blood tube *must not* be used.
■ Collection and storage of blood components has been found to be a major source of identification error (Williamson et al 1998). Hospitals should have a policy for collection of blood and blood components from the blood bank or blood transfusion refrigerator and transport to the area of use. Blood should only be stored in blood transfusion refrigerators and should be transported in boxes specifically designed for this purpose. The person collecting blood must have documented patient identification details and withdrawals of blood from the refrigerator should be documented.
■ Administration of blood components and bedside identity checks are defined by local policy and vary across the UK. The BCSH (1999) recommend that hospitals should have a policy for administration of blood that identifies the staff responsible for

different aspects of the procedure: prescription of blood and blood components, inspection of the blood, patient bedside identity check and location of the blood transfusion compatability report form. The BCSH also recommend that one person (who must be a doctor or registered nurse) is responsible for the patient and blood component identity check at the bedside.

- The bedside identity check is crucial in preventing transfusion error and has been identified as the single most important cause of transfusion of the incorrect blood component (Williamson et al 1999). Given this information the need for standards for blood administration and strict adherence to policies and procedures cannot be overemphasised.
- No other infusion solution or drug should be added to blood components as they may cause clotting or red cell lysis.
- Infusion pumps may damage blood cells and should not be used.
- If blood is to be warmed only a machine specifically designed for this purpose should be used.

 Reflection point

Take a few minutes to consider the above points in relation to your own practice. Do you *always* go through all these checks prior to commencing a unit of blood or, occasionally, when you are busy or short staffed, do you omit some of these steps?

After thinking about this you will probably conclude that you always undertake the recommended checks. However, if you find that you do sometimes omit some of the steps consider what you should do to develop your practice and improve safety for the individuals you care for.

Observation of recipients during transfusion

Transfusion reactions can develop within 5–10 min of commencement of transfusion or up to 4 weeks after completion (Urbaniak 1990). However, severe reactions are most likely to occur within 15 min of commencing a unit of blood (BCSH 1999).

The optimum type and timing of observations is unclear and until recently local policy has dictated the frequency of observations throughout the transfusion, resulting in great variation throughout the UK. BCSH (1999) guidelines recommend that before starting each unit of blood and at the end of each transfusion episode baseline observations of temperature, pulse, respiration and blood pressure should be recorded. Temperature and pulse should be recorded 15 min after the start of each unit of blood. Observations taken during transfusion should be recorded separately to routine observations. Visual observation of the patient is important and the recipient should be monitored closely, especially during the first 15 min for signs of AHTR. Nurses should be alert for any abnormal signs, such as agitation, flushing, pain or a rash. Further observations during transfusion are at the discretion of each clinical area and need only be taken if the patient becomes unwell or shows signs of a transfusion reaction. It is, however, recommended that routine observation patterns are continued for unconscious patients.

Time limits for transfusions

Red cells should not be collected from the refrigerator more than 30 min prior to being transfused and transfusions should be completed within 5 hours of commencement, as rapid bacterial proliferation can occur at room temperature (McClelland 1996). Blood should be administered as quickly as possible, according to the recipient's blood volume, cardiac status and haemodynamic condition (Widman 1985).

Once the transfusion is completed, transfusion records must be kept in the recipient's medical notes. All empty blood bags should be discarded, according to hospital policy for disposal of clinical waste (BCSH 1999).

BLOOD COMPONENT SUPPORT

Whole blood

Whole blood consists of red and white blood cells, platelets and plasma and its use is restricted to replacement following massive blood loss.

Red blood cells

Packed red cells are the red cell mass remaining following removal of plasma. Red cells are used to increase tissue oxygenation when this is reduced due to anaemia or haemorrhage (Scottish National Blood Transfusion Service 1995).

Washed red blood cells

Washed cells are red cells washed in 0.9% sodium chloride in the transfusion centre. They are occasionally used to prevent transfusion reactions in individuals who have had previous transfusion reactions thought to be caused by antigens in donor plasma and a corresponding IgE or IgA antibody in the recipient's plasma.

Indications for blood cell transfusion

The two most frequent causes of anaemia in people with haematological malignancies are

- decreased red cell production, secondary to myelosuppressive therapy
- the primary disease process.

Most centres attempt to keep a patient's haemoglobin (Hb) level higher than 8 g/dl, and transfuse either when the level drops below this or sooner if the patient becomes symptomatic. The volume given is generally enough to increase the Hb level to 10–11 g/dl. Normally, transfused red cells survive for long periods in the recipient's circulation, less than 1% of the number transfused being destroyed each day (Mollison et al 1997), which explains the therapeutic success of red cell transfusions.

Blood should be transfused through a blood component administration set with an integral filter (170 μm) which removes microaggregates composed of leucocytes, platelets, fibrin strands and cellular debris. Additional filters may also be used depending on local policy. Administration sets should be changed at least 12 hourly to reduce the risk of infection (BCSH 1999).

Platelets

One unit of platelets is obtained from either a single aphereed unit (i.e. from a donor specifically donating platelets) or from platelet concentrates (i.e. from five donor units of blood). Each unit should be given over 30 min, using either a blood or platelet administration set (BCSH 1999). Platelets should not be collected and removed from the agitator before they are required and should be given as soon as possible to prevent platelet aggregation in the bag.

Platelet transfusions have great therapeutic value in both controlling and preventing haemorrhage, allowing chemotherapy to be given at optimum doses and for longer periods. Platelets are given therapeutically when spontaneous bleeding associated with thrombocytopenia occurs or prophylactically when the platelet count falls below a pre-determined level, to reduce the risk of spontaneous bleeding.

Some controversy exists as to the level at which prophylactic platelet transfusion should be administered. Traditionally, platelets have been transfused when levels have dropped to between 10 and 20×10^9/L depending on local policy. However, a consensus statement (Royal College of Physicians of Edinburgh 1997) suggests that a threshold of 10×10^9/L is safe for most individuals without additional risk factors.

Many individuals with haemato-oncological disorders will, however, possess additional risk factors which increase platelet consumption and exacerbate the potential for haemorrhage. These factors include fever, sepsis, concurrent administration of antibiotics, disseminated intravascular coagulation (DIC) and splenomegaly. Administration of antipyretics prior to transfusion may minimise platelet destruction in recipients with fever due to infection. For individuals with additional risk factors, platelet transfusion will be required at levels higher than 10×10^9/L, depending on clinical judgement and local policy.

Following transfusion, an average increase of 40×10^9/L in the recipient's peripheral platelet count should be seen after 1 hour and the half-life of platelets in the circulation is approximately 4 days (Hows & Brozovic 1992).

Refractoriness to platelets

Multiple transfusion of platelets from random donors can cause alloimmunisation to HLAs, leading to rapid destruction of transfused platelets, and the expected increment in platelet count may not be achieved. This is frequently referred to as being 'refractory' to platelets. Refractoriness is defined as a poor platelet increment on two consecutive occasions, i.e. where the corrected increment count is $<7.5 \times 10^9/L$ at 1 hour, in the absence of other factors known to increase platelet consumption (Hows & Brozovic 1992). Refractoriness increases the chance of spontaneous bleeding and may restrict administration of chemotherapy.

Preventative measures

- reduce donor exposure by only transfusing when absolutely needed, using single aphered units
- leucodeplete red cells and platelets.

Once refractoriness has developed, HLA-matched platelets, if available, should be administered to sustain an adequate platelet count and prevent or stop bleeding (Hows & Brozovic 1992).

Plasma therapy

Immunoglobulins are used in a variety of situations in haemato-oncology. Individuals with chronic lymphocytic leukaemia or multiple myeloma are unable to produce effective antibodies (see Chs 4 and 5) and, as a result, suffer severe recurrent infections that respond poorly to antibiotics. Regular infusions of immunoglobulins are given to reduce the frequency of infection. Immunoglobulins are also used in the treatment of post-transfusion purpura (PTP) and in conjunction with gancyclovir in the treatment of CMV.

Adverse reactions to immunoglobulins are rare and range from mild allergic reactions to severe anaphylaxis. (Management of these reactions is outlined later in Table 11.4.) Individuals should be closely observed therefore for signs of a reaction, and infusions should be administered slowly initially.

Reactions are more likely to occur if an individual has an infection; if infection is suspected, antibiotics should be commenced and immunoglobulin infusion may be delayed for 24–48 hours (Cochrane 1997).

The most common use of plasma components in haematological malignancies is with coagulation disorders such as DIC associated with the disease itself – for example, promyelocytic leukaemia (AML, M3) (see Chs 4 and 14) – or due to AHTR or septicaemic shock.

Therapeutic apheresis

Therapeutic apheresis is used to treat patients with many different conditions and involves the removal of whole blood or a particular component of blood to reduce symptoms caused by pathogenic factors in the blood. It can range from a simple venesection, where whole blood is removed in a similar way to that of donor blood donation, to a more complex treatment, where an apheresis machine is used to selectively remove particular blood cells and in some cases replace them with normal blood components or solutions of electrolytes (McClelland 1996). Examples of therapeutic apheresis in haemato-oncology are now discussed.

Plasma exchange

Plasma exchange is undertaken to remove factors which cause or exacerbate disease. The patient's plasma is removed and replaced by 4.5% albumin, normal saline or a combination of the two. Fresh frozen plasma (FFP) is used to correct any coagulation deficiencies towards the end of the procedure (McClelland 1996).

Indications

Plasma exchange is most commonly used to remove immunoglobulins in hyperviscosity syndromes, such as multiple myeloma and Waldenström's macroglobulinaemia. (See Ch. 5 for symptoms associated with hyperviscosity syndromes.)

Leucopheresis

Removal of white cells may help to alleviate the symptoms caused by the high white cell count while waiting for chemotherapy to take effect.

Indications
Hyperleukaemic leucostasis (WBC > 100 × 10^9/L).

Peripheral blood stem cell collection
The main use of apheresis procedures in haemato-oncology is stem cell collection prior to transplant. This is described in detail in Chapter 10.

Complications of therapeutic apheresis
Complications of therapeutic apheresis include

- hypovolaemia due to excessive fluid being removed
- hypocalcaemia
- vasovagal attacks
- anaphylactic reaction to FFP or rarely albumin
- air embolism from the apheresis machine (this is not usually possible unless the procedure is being manually modified)
- citrate toxicity from the anticoagulant used by the apheresis machine
- extracorporeal clotting, requiring recannulation of the vein.

TRANSFUSION REACTIONS

Case study 11.1

Richard is a 29-year-old man with recently diagnosed acute myeloid leukaemia. He has received his first course of induction chemotherapy and is now waiting for his blood counts to recover. He has been prescribed two units of red blood cells as his Hb is 7.6 g/dl. He commenced the transfusion 10 min ago. As you walk past his bed you notice he is short of breath, red in the face and clutching at his back.
What action would you take immediately?
What is the likely cause of this?
What can be done to prevent this from happening in the future?

Acute haemolytic transfusion reaction

Acute haemolytic transfusion reaction is the most serious transfusion reaction and is potentially fatal. The life-threatening nature of this reaction means that all acute reactions must be assumed to be haemolytic until proven otherwise. AHTR are usually caused by ABO incompatibility, and may be

- mild or severe
- immediate (after transfusion of just a few millilitres of blood) or delayed (3–10 days after transfusion)
- intravascular or extravascular.

Intravascular haemolysis
This is the most severe form of haemolytic reaction and fortunately relatively rare. Immediate life-threatening reactions are associated with haemolysis of donor red cells within the circulation as a result of complement-activating antibodies – nearly always, ABO antibodies.

When incompatible cells are transfused, antigens on donor red cells bind with the incompatible IgM antibody in the recipient's plasma, causing agglutination of red cells and activating complement (see Ch. 1). Complement proteins erode the red cell membrane, causing rupture with subsequent leakage of haemoglobin into the plasma and lysis of donor red cells. Other complement proteins contribute to the development of an inflammatory response, which results in the accumulation of leucocytes and the release of pyrogens, bradykinin and serotonin with associated vasodilation (Fig. 11.1).

Clinical features of intravascular haemolysis include:

- pain at the infusion site and along the vein
- feelings of anxiety, agitation or restlessness
- flushing, headache, urticaria, pyrexia, rigors
- vomiting
- pain in the lumbar region
- chest pain and shortness of breath
- hypotension and circulatory collapse.

Leakage of haemoglobin into the plasma leads to haemoglobinaemia and subsequent development of jaundice. Haemoglobinuria may

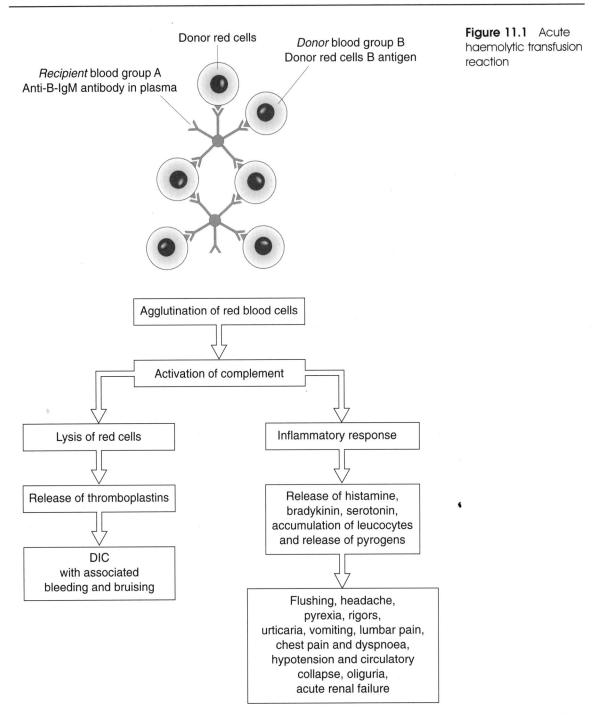

Figure 11.1 Acute haemolytic transfusion reaction

Recipient blood group A
Anti-B-IgM antibody in plasma

Donor red cells

Donor blood group B
Donor red cells B antigen

Agglutination of red blood cells

Activation of complement

Lysis of red cells

Release of thromboplastins

DIC
with associated
bleeding and bruising

Inflammatory response

Release of histamine,
bradykinin, serotonin,
accumulation of leucocytes
and release of pyrogens

Flushing, headache,
pyrexia, rigors,
urticaria, vomiting, lumbar pain,
chest pain and dyspnoea,
hypotension and circulatory
collapse, oliguria,
acute renal failure

also occur. Oliguria and renal failure may occur due to acute tubular necrosis as a result of poor renal perfusion due to hypotension. Furthermore, the release of thromboplastic substances during red cell lysis may activate the clotting cascade, resulting in DIC (Contreras & Mollison 1992, Bradbury & Cruickshank 1995).

Extravascular haemolysis
Extravascular haemolysis occurs in antibody reactions other than ABO incompatibilities.

Table 11.3 Non-acute haemolytic transfusion reactions

Type of reaction	Clinical features
Febrile non-haemolytic transfusion reactions (FNHTR) These account for over 90% of transfusion reactions and are caused by leucocyte antibodies binding to transfused leucocytes or platelets. The resulting antigen–antibody complex binds to and activates monocytes, which in turn release cytokines with pyrogenic properties (Dzik 1992). The febrile response occurs as a result of immunisation by leucocyte antibodies and is therefore common in those who have received multiple transfusions. Fifteen per cent of people experiencing FNHTR will have another with future transfusions (Westphal 1996). The febrile response is not usually serious, although it causes the recipient anxiety and discomfort	Fever and tachycardia Headache and flushing Chills and rigors In severe reactions hypotension, breathlessness and vomiting may be experienced
Febrile or non-febrile non-haemolytic allergic reactions These are the second most common type of transfusion reaction and usually occur due to hypersensitivity to donor plasma proteins. Reactions range from mild urticarial reactions initiated by IgE antibodies to severe anaphylactic shock initiated by IgA antibodies. Severity of the reaction is dependent on the level of antibody present in the recipient's plasma. Clinical features occur quickly after commencement of the transfusion as a result of histamine release, producing vasodilation and increased capillary permeability	Urticaria/rash Pyrexia and rigors Dyspnoea, wheezing and cyanosis Facial oedema and flushing Nausea and vomiting Tachycardia Chest pain Hypotension and shock
Bacterial reactions Bacterial contamination of blood resulting in septic shock (confirmed by blood cultures sent from the unit of blood) is rare. Clinical features occur within minutes of commencing the transfusion due to the release of bacterial endotoxins	Fever, chills and rigor Headache Backpain Nausea and vomiting Circulatory collapse Septicaemia DIC
Transfusion related acute lung injury (TRALI) A rare and potentially fatal transfusion reaction, TRALI occur rapidly after commencement of transfusion and are related to antileucocyte antibodies in donor plasma reacting with the recipient's leucocytes. Granulocytes aggregate in the pulmonary capillaries and the inflammatory response initiated by the antigen–antibody complex results in vasodilation and increased capillary permeability	Acute respiratory distress Cough Fever and chills Pulmonary oedema with no other signs of left heart failure Cyanosis

Continued

Table 11.3 continued

Type of reaction	Clinical features
Transfusion associated graft-versus-host disease (TA-GVHD) TA-GVHD is caused by transfusion of viable T lymphocytes to an immunocompromised recipient and the resulting reaction with the recipient's histocompatibility antigens. Although rare outside the BMT setting TA-GVHD is usually fatal. However, it may occasionally occur in individuals with haematological malignancy. Risk depends on the number and viability of transfused lymphocytes, the susceptibility of the recipient's immune system to their engraftment and the degree of immunological disparity (HLA) between donor and patient (BCSH 1996). TA-GVHD may develop) 1–4 weeks post-transfusion (Urbaniak 1990)	Similar to acute GVHD following BMT (see Chapter 10) Fever Maculopapular, erythematous skin rash Anorexia Nausea and vomiting Diarrhoea Hepatomegaly Abnormal liver function tests Pancytopenia
Post-transfusion purpura (PTP) A rare but potentially lethal reaction to transfusion of red blood cells or platelets due to the formation of platelet-specific alloantibodies, PTP reactions range from mild to severe thrombocytopenia with bleeding occurring 5–9 days after transfusion (McClelland 1996)	Purpura Bruising Bleeding
Post-transfusion circulatory overload Post-transfusion circulatory overload is most likely to occur in the elderly and in those with existing cardiac disease as a result of increased circulatory volume; pulmonary oedema may develop	*Clinical features are those of cardiac failure* Dry cough Dyspnoea Cyanosis Raised jugular pressure Fullness in the head
Iron overload Every unit of blood contains 250 mg of iron and the body has no mechanism for excreting excess iron. Regular frequent transfusions can lead to an increased body iron level which can cause hepatic cirrhosis, diabetes, hypoparathyroidism, cardiac failure, arrhythmias and eventually death. Iron overload may occur in those with chronic haematological malignancies or following BMT	

Table 11.4 Management of transfusion reactions

Type of reaction	Management
Acute haemolytic transfusion reaction (AHTR)	In the 'shock' phase, both blood pressure and renal perfusion need to be maintained. Hydrocortisone, an antihistamine and adrenaline 1 : 10 000 concentration may be administered and cardiac monitoring commenced. Intravenous fluids may be administered to maintain blood volume, and frusemide to induce diuresis. Fluid balance requires close monitoring and catheterisation may be required to monitor urine output A urine specimen may be requested for haemoglobin estimation Dialysis may be required if acute renal failure develops Close observation is required to detect signs of bleeding or bruising. Heparin or blood components may be required to treat disseminated intravascular coagulation (DIC) Psychological support is very important as the patient is likely to be extremely frightened
Febrile non-haemolytic transfusion reaction (FNHTR)	Once it has been established that this is not an AHTR, antipyrexials, steroids and antihistamines are given
Non-haemolytic allergic reactions	*Mild reactions* Slow rate of transfusion, antihistamine may be prescribed Observe for further reaction Oral antihistamines may be prescribed for those who have had previous mild urticarial reactions prior to transfusion
	Severe reactions Resuscitative measures and maintenance of airway required Immediate treatment required with intravenous antihistamines, adrenaline and hydrocortisone. Oxygen therapy is required for respiratory distress. Intubation and ventilation may be necessary in severe cases

Continued

Table 11.4 continued

Type of reaction	Management
Bacterial reactions	Treatment of shock and DIC as for AHTR and allergic reactions Blood cultures should be obtained Intravenous antibiotics
Transfusion related acute lung injury (TRALI)	Supportive resuscitative measures Oxygen therapy, high-dose steroids Pulse oximetry and blood gas levels should be monitored Intravenous fluids to maintain cardiac output and blood pressure Ventilation may be required to correct hypoxia
Transfusion associated graft versus host disease (TA-GVHD)	No specific treatment once TA-GVHD has developed Supportive measures as for acute GVHD post-BMT
Post-transfusion purpura (PTP)	High-dose steroids and intravenous immunoglobulins
Post-tranfusion circulatory overload	Management is that of cardiac failure. Reactions can be prevented by slow administration of packed red cells and administration of diuretics to susceptible individuals prior to transfusion
Iron overload	An iron-chelating agent (desferrioxamine) is administered either intravenously or subcutaneously during transfusion and may be administered subcutaneously 2–5 times weekly to prevent organ damage in those with chronic disorders

These reactions tend to be less severe than intravascular haemolysis and are frequently initiated by IgG antibody. IgG does not fully activate complement and red cells are ingested by macrophages in the liver and spleen rather than being lysed. Reactions may be delayed and symptoms are likely to be confined to fever although jaundice and haemoglobinuria may occur.

Delayed haemolytic reactions

Delayed haemolytic reactions tend to occur 5–10 days after transfusion, as a result of immunisation to an antigen through previous transfusion or pregnancy. Subsequent re-exposure to this antigen results in antibody production, inducing destruction of transfused red cells. Clinical features of delayed haemolytic reactions include:

- fever
- falling haemoglobin level

- jaundice
- haemoglobinuria (Contreras & Mollison 1992).

Other non-acute haemolytic transfusion reactions are shown in Table 11.3.

Management of transfusion reactions

If a transfusion reaction is suspected, the transfusion should be stopped immediately and medical advice sought. Observations of temperature, pulse, respirations and blood pressure should be recorded throughout the reaction with frequency being determined by the condition of the individual and local policy. The blood bank must be notified to ensure relevant samples are taken and investigations carried out to identify the cause of the reaction. The remainder of the unit of blood and the administration set should be returned to the blood bank with post-reaction blood samples. Management of transfusion reactions is shown in Table 11.4.

CONCLUSION

Successful blood component support has certainly improved the treatment options and success of many treatment modalities for patients with malignant haematological conditions. However, transfusion of blood components also carries potentially fatal risks and it is vital that all possible measures are taken to ensure their safety.

DISCUSSION QUESTIONS

1. An individual newly diagnosed with acute myeloid leukaemia has a haemoglobin of 7.6 g/dl and is scheduled to receive a red cell transfusion. He confides to you that he is concerned about the risks associated with transfusion of blood components and has decided not to go ahead with the transfusion. How would you manage this situation?

2. In your area of practice could anything further be done to improve safety for individuals receiving blood component therapy?

References

Bradbury M, Cruickshank J P 1995 Blood and blood transfusion reactions: 2. British Journal of Nursing 4(15): 861–868

BCSH 1996 British Committee for Standards in Haematology Blood Transfusion Task Force, Guidelines on gamma irradiation of blood components for the prevention of transfusion-associated graft-versus-host disease. Transfusion Medicine 6: 261–271

BCSH 1999 British Committee for Standards in Haematology Blood Transfusion Task Force, The administration of blood and blood components and the management of transfused patients. Transfusion Medicine 9: 227–238

Cochrane S 1997 Care of patients undergoing immunoglobulin therapy. Nursing Standard 11(41): 44–46

Contreras M, Mollison P L 1992 Immunological complications of transfusion. In: Contreras M (ed) ABC of transfusion, 2nd edn. BMJ Publishing Group, London, pp 41–44

Department of Health 1998a Press release; Committee on Safety of Medicines completes review of blood products. Department of Health, London

Department of Health 1998b Press release; Government advice on leucodepletion from Spongiform Encephalopathy Advisory Committee. Department of Health, London

Dzik W H 1992 Is the febrile response to transfusion due to donor or recipient cytokines. Transfusion 32: 594

Hewitt P E, Wagstaff W 1992 The blood donor and tests on donor blood. In: Contreras M (ed) ABC of transfusion, 2nd edn. BMJ Publishing Group, London, pp 1–4

Hows J M, Brozovic B 1992 Platelet and granulocyte transfusions. In: Contreras M (ed) ABC of transfusion, 2nd edn. BMJ Publishing Group, London, pp 14–17

McClelland B (ed) 1996 Handbook of transfusion medicine, 2nd edn. Blood Transfusion Service of the United Kingdom. HMSO, London

Masouredis S P 1990 Preservation and clinical use of erythrocytes and whole blood. In: Williams W J, Beutler E, Erslev A J, Lichtman M A Haematology, 4th edn. McGraw-Hill, New York, pp 1628–1647

Mollison P L, Engelfriet C P, Contreras M 1997 Blood transfusion in clinical medicine, 10th edn. Blackwell, Oxford

NHSE 1998 National Health Service Executive Health Service Circular HSC 1998/99, Better Blood Transfusion. Department of Health, London

Royal College of Physicians of Edinburgh 1997 Consensus Conference on Platelet Transfusion: Final Statement. Royal College of Physicians, Edinburgh

Scottish National Blood Transfusion Service 1995 Compendium of product information. SNBT, Edinburgh

Urbaniak S J 1990 Adverse effects of transfusion.

In: Ludlam C A (ed) Clinical haematology. Churchill Livingstone, Edinburgh, pp 449–459

Westphal R G 1996 Handbook of transfusion medicine, 3rd edn. American Red Cross, Washington, DC

Widman F K 1985 Technical manual, 9th edn. American Association of Blood Banks, USA

Williamson L M, Lowe S, Love E et al 1998 Serious Hazards of Transfusion (SHOT), Summary of Annual Report, 1996–1997. SHOT Office, Manchester

Williamson L M, Lowe S, Love E et al 1999 Serious Hazards of Transfusion (SHOT), Summary of Annual Report, 1997–1998. SHOT Office, Manchester

Further reading

Pamphilon D H 1995 Modern transfusion medicine. CRC Press, London
For those wanting a greater depth of knowledge.

McClelland B 1996 Handbook of transfusion medicine, 2nd edn. Blood Transfusion Services of the United Kingdom. HMSO, London
Essential reading for all areas dealing with blood component therapy. Covers all aspects of blood component therapy; easy to read.

Mollison P L, Engelfriet C P, Contreras M 1987 Blood transfusion in clinical medicine, 8th edn. Blackwell, Oxford
An in-depth book covering all aspects of transfusion medicine in great detail. Written for medical staff but in a very easy to understand format.

SECTION THREE
Nursing Issues

12 *Venous access*

HELEN HAMILTON

Key points
- Infection is the most serious and most common complication associated with intravenous therapy
- Assessment is vital in determining the most appropriate type of venous access for the individual
- A consistent approach to management of intravenous access devices is required to prevent complications

INTRODUCTION

All individuals with haemato-oncological disorders will require venous access at some time during the often protracted period of their treatment. Venous access is required to obtain blood samples and for the administration of blood products, antibiotics, chemotherapy and parenteral nutrition (PN). Experience has demonstrated that high-technology, expensive intravenous (IV) medication may be administered safely and effectively in the hospital and community setting over considerable periods of time by the haematology team, or in some cases by patients themselves. Careful examination, assessment and communication are crucial in achieving a cohesive team approach to meeting individual needs.

Both peripheral and central venous access are used to deliver IV preparations and suitable venous access sites and selection of catheters will be discussed. Infection is the most frequent and serious complication associated with IV therapy. Adherence to basic principles in the preparation of the individual, appropriate selection of access site, skilled operating techniques and prompt action when complications occur will provide a safe and effective approach for individuals receiving long-term IV therapies (Elliott et al 1994). The maintenance of IV cannulas is another important issue and, consequently, care of the IV site, choice of dressings and flushing of the catheter will also be examined.

PERIPHERAL VENOUS ACCESS

Peripheral venous access refers to gaining entry to the peripheral vascular system via a small vein in the hand, arm or foot and is regularly employed in the management of patients requiring intravenous medication. Peripheral venous access is only suitable for low-volume bolus dosages and infusions that will not knowingly cause thrombophlebitis or increase the risk of infection. Individuals with a haemato-oncological disorder are likely to require frequent blood sampling, prolonged treatment with antibiotics and chemotherapy, transfusion of blood products and possibly PN.

Frequent venepuncture rapidly becomes a dreaded event for many individuals and adds to the risk of thrombosed and painful peripheral vessels. Continued use of the peripheral route is likely to result in infection, thrombosis, phlebitis or simple absence of suitable peripheral vessels. The lack of available vessels, due to sclerosis following numerous venepunctures

Reflection point

Consider what measures may be taken to overcome needle phobia in an individual requiring frequent cannulation.

and the irritating effect on the endothelium of peripherally infused chemotherapy, is often the first criteria for the insertion of a central venous catheter (cvc). Therefore central venous access is usually considered more appropriate for this patient group, providing additional comfort for the individual and reliability for the health-care team.

CENTRAL VENOUS ACCESS

Central venous access refers to gaining access to one of the great veins of the neck or thorax, enabling infusions of high osmolarity such as PN and high-dose chemotherapy to be infused in a safe and controlled manner often over long periods of time. The indications for using central venous access are increasing constantly as many pharmaceutical preparations rapidly result in the development of thrombophlebitis and infection if administered peripherally. This may cause not only discomfort to the individual but serious and potentially life-threatening complications.

It is possible for central venous cannulae to remain patent and free from infection for months or even years. However, strict protocols incorporating every aspect of catheter management are required to achieve this. When protocols are not enforced, infection and other associated complications are inevitable.

Both short- and long-term venous access may be used for individuals with haemato-oncological disorders. To ensure correct and appropriate venous access, sound assessment must be undertaken by the nursing and medical team.

Assessment

The venous network of any individual and in particular one who may require intravenous therapies intermittently to sustain life, is very precious. Preservation and respect of these vessels should be a priority in the assessment process.

A detailed assessment of the individual's clinical status should be undertaken and the anticipated duration of treatment considered.

The insertion of a cvc for any therapy requires maximum stability of the individual's clinical condition and precise assessment will ensure the individual is sufficiently stable for this potentially high-risk procedure.

Areas of assessment may include:

- Individual patient's understanding of the forthcoming procedure and the associated, potential complications.
- Haematological status, particularly clotting ratios, must be within the recommended limits of the protocol, prior to an invasive procedure such as central venous catheterisation. Correction of an abnormal clotting profile must be done either with blood products or coagulant agents.
- Respiratory function – respiratory difficulty and/or failure may be present due to sepsis, sputum retention and/or electrolyte imbalance, in which case tunnelled central venous catheterisation may be contraindicated.
- Cardiovascular status – cardiovascular stability is desirable but not always possible when the insertion of a cvc is proposed. Careful assessment and intervention by the cardiology team will establish the underlying cause of the instability and arrhythmias and, in some cases, correction of biochemical abnormalities may resolve the problem.
- Infection profile – insertion of a permanent, tunnelled cvc may be inappropriate for the septic patient. Assessment may indicate that temporary venous access is advisable until the source of infection is located and treated.
- Vascular assessment aids in establishing the patency of the venous system. The presence of thrombosis, stenosis and anatomical anomalies should be noted. Careful visual examination may reveal the presence of a dilated collateral venous circulation of the chest wall, suggesting the presence of thrombosis or potential stenosis, as a possible result of previous central venous access or radiotherapy. Interventional radiology may aid in confirming the diagnosis and assist in the selection of an alternative cannulation site.
- Any known allergies should also be noted as skin cleansing agents, sedatives and certain

dressings may cause unnecessary discomfort and present possible complications at a later stage.

To an experienced operator, familiar with central venous catheterisation, assessment of these factors provides valuable information when considering the safest and most appropriate venous access for the compromised patient. Accurate assessment will aid in determining the method of insertion and type of venous access device to be used.

TYPES OF VENOUS ACCESS DEVICE

The estimated duration of IV therapy influences the selection of a venous access device. Box 12.1 shows categories of venous access device.

Box 12.1   Categories of venous access

- Short-term venous access
- Short–medium-term access
- Medium–long-term venous access

Successful use of any type of catheter depends entirely on scrupulous attention to aseptic technique, care and management of the access site, with staff education paramount in prompt recognition of catheter-related complications.

Short-term venous access

Peripheral venous access

The peripheral route is useful for the administration of some chemotherapy, antibiotic therapy and short-term peripheral PN; i.e. 2–3 days. Success in the use of the peripheral route relies on precise, detailed care and management of the cannula. Many advances have been made in improving peripheral cannula, thereby reducing the problems associated with thrombophlebitis and infection, both of which can lead to loss of valuable venous access. Cannula material, cannulation site, the duration of therapy and the type of fluid being infused

can influence the incidence of thrombophlebitis and infection.

- Use of Vialon cannulae have been shown to result in a lower incidence of thrombophlebitis than Teflon (Gaukroger et al 1988).
- Insertion of IV cannula over joint areas such as the wrist and elbow should be avoided as they are likely to result in an increased incidence of phlebitis (Consentino 1977) and extravasation if cytotoxic drugs are being administered.
- Multiple attempts at cannulation should be avoided as they increase the infection risk (Turnidge 1984), which emphasises the need for experience and skill in insertion.
- Cannula use should be restricted to its original purpose only.
- Regular inspection of the access site is important and any erythema developing around the cannulation site, pain or discomfort should be noted.
- Infection risk increases with the length of time a cannula is in place and it is recommended that they are replaced at least every 72 hours and preferably every 48 hours (Messner & Gorse 1987).
- Regular inspection of any venous access site, particularly when chemotherapy is being administered, is important and should be an integral part of the management protocol. Four- to six-hourly inspection of the site will enable the nursing team to assess the development of potential complications.
- Cannula should be firmly secured with sterile dressings as movement of the cannula can increase infection risk.

Medium-term venous access

Peripherally inserted central venous catheters (PICC)

When the peripheral route is inadequate and central venous cannulation is inappropriate, a PICC is a useful method of gaining central venous access. Use of a PICC may also minimise complications associated with peripheral cannula. PICCs are becoming increasingly popular possibly because of the ease of placement in appropriate patients, thus reducing the risk of causing serious complications in the high-risk individual where a subclavian or internal jugular approach may be contraindicated.

The majority of PICC lines are made of silicone or polyurethane, or a blend of both and their use has been developed very successfully in North America, particularly for individuals receiving chemotherapy, PN and long-term antibiotic therapy in the community.

A fine-bore PICC catheter is inserted into a vein in the antecubital fossa and advanced via the basilic, median cubital or cephalic vein into one of the great vessels of the thorax or neck. Once positioned (Fig. 12.1), the PICC rests at the junction of the superior vena cava and right atrium of the heart, reducing the risk of phlebitis or thrombus formation often associated with peripheral cannula (Ryder 1993).

The insertion protocol for PICC lines will vary in different hospitals. However, successful use of these catheters depend on the following criteria:

■ Careful patient examination and assessment, noting any evidence of arthritis associated with the elbow or shoulder which may prevent advancement of the catheter.
■ A normal platelet count is essential to ensure prompt coagulation following cannulation of a large vessel.
■ Appropriate patient selection, protection of the selected vein, avoiding unnecessary cannulation, which may result in the formation of scar tissue, sclerosis or generalised bruising, thus reducing the possibility of successful cannulation.
■ Avoidance of selecting a cannulation site adjacent to another infusion or an infected cannulation site.
■ Application of local anaesthetic cream to the proposed cannulation site 1 hour prior to the procedure will avoid distortion of the vein when intradermal or subcutaneous local anaesthetic is used.
■ Appropriate selection of catheter size; for example, if blood products are part of the treatment, use of a larger lumen catheter may reduce the risk of blockage. However, in general, the smallest viable lumen should be chosen, as phlebitis may result from use

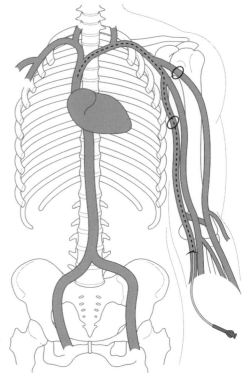

Key:

$\bigcirc$ Indicates superficial vein passing deep vein

Figure 12.1 Route of a peripherally inserted catheter (PICC) with the tip of the PICC located in the superior vena cava (SVC) (reproduced with permission of Bard Ltd). Accurate measurement for placement of PICCs can be achieved by adding the length of the patient's humerus and the length of the clavicle together. This measurement will demonstrate to the operator the required length of PICC to dwell within the venous system and result in the tip of the PICC residing in the optimal position of the lower third of the superior vena cava. Any external portion of the PICC will lie on the skin surface or be trimmed to meet individual patient requirements and fitted with a luer connection to facilitate either bolus or infusional administration (Lum 1999).

of too large a catheter, especially in women, whose veins are relatively small.
■ Experienced personnel performing the procedure.

Following insertion, it is advised that dressings be performed by two nurses to support the PICC throughout the procedure, reducing the risk of the catheter accidentally falling out.

Reflection point

Consider the implications of the UKCC Scope of Professional Practice in relation to PICC insertion.

A secure method of dressing is essential as suturing is not commonly used. A tubular, elasticated bandage will aid in protecting the PICC and reduce the risk of accidental damage or pulling of the catheter.

Troubleshooting PICC lines

Discomfort or redness at the PICC entry site normally indicates mechanical phlebitis. This may be overcome by elevation of the limb and applying warm compresses to the affected site, which will have the effect of dilating the vein and reducing friction of the catheter within the vein. Glyceryl trinitrate patches applied over the affected area may also aid in venous dilatation and relieve symptoms of swelling and discomfort. If the inflammation and discomfort do not resolve within 36 hours, however, the catheter may become an infection risk and should be removed.

- Regular measurement of the distance from cannulation site to the administration end of the catheter will ensure no movement or displacement of the catheter has occurred. This is particularly important if the catheter is to be used for chemotherapy and displacement could result in extravasation.
- Due to the fragile nature of the PICC catheter, care should be taken to avoid catheter kinking. To alleviate the risk of catheter rupture it is advised that only 10-ml syringes or larger are used for flushing PICC catheters, thus preventing excessive pressure when infusing therapies.

Case study 12.1 demonstrates the importance of assessing the individual's clinical condition prior to performing a high-risk procedure. Peripherally inserted cvc certainly have a place in such situations, providing necessary central venous access without placing the individual at risk of potentially life-threatening complications.

Case study 12.1

Janet, a 26-year-old photographer, presented to her GP with recurrent infection and exhaustion. Blood samples were taken and she was found not only to be grossly anaemic but also neutropenic. A preliminary diagnosis of acute myeloid leukaemia was made and she was admitted to the local haematology centre.

On admission, Janet was very unwell. Her cardiovascular state was unstable, she was tachycardic, febrile, lethargic and breathless on any exertion. Venous access was required for immediate infusion of blood products and temporary peripheral venous access was established in her hand. Blood products and crystalloid fluids were administered effectively, resolving Janet's hypovolaemic picture. However, she also required antibiotics and chemotherapy urgently.

Ideally, a multi-lumen central venous catheter was required; however, Janet's condition was too unstable for a long-term catheter to be placed safely using the conventional subclavian approach. Adopting the head down, Trendelenburg position, would increase Janet's respiratory distress and hyperventilation, therefore increasing the potential for pneumothorax. Her haematological status was also unstable, with an increased risk of haemorrhage if a subclavian approach was used.

Following transfusion of blood products, Janet's basilic and cephalic veins were visible and palpable in the antecubital fossae of both arms. After explanation and obtaining consent, it was decided to insert a peripherally inserted double-lumen, central catheter (PICC) via one of these vessels. Both Janet and the medical team appreciated that this would only provide relatively temporary central venous access, and once Janet's condition stabilised a more permanent cvc would be required.

Janet was prepared for the procedure. Further blood samples were taken to ensure a stable clotting profile and additional blood products were made available for the procedure. She was given information regarding the proposed procedure and gave written consent. Despite feeling very unwell, Janet was virtually unaware of the procedure and was in no way distressed. The

Continued

Case study 12.1 *Continued*

PICC was successfully inserted and remained *in situ* until the initial course of chemotherapy was completed. Subsequently, the catheter was removed and the tip sent for culture. No organisms were detected.

Two weeks later, following a brief spell at home, Janet was admitted for further intensive chemotherapy. To ensure maximum venous access for this prolonged treatment, a cuffed and tunnelled, double-lumen cvc was felt to be the most suitable venous access device for the delivery of chemotherapy and antibiotics. This was subsequently inserted percutaneously prior to commencing chemotherapy.

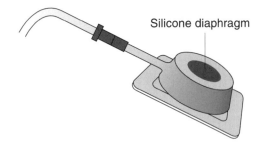

Silicone diaphragm

Subcutaneous port

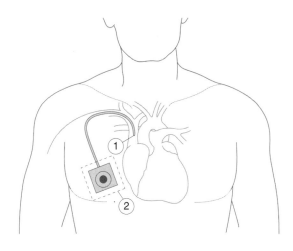

Key:

---- subcutaneous tunnel

1   Tip of catheter in superior vena cava

2   Subcutaneous pocket housing subcutaneous port

Figure 12.2   Subcutaneous port

Medium- to long-term venous access

Subcutaneous ports

These devices are subcutaneously implanted reservoirs placed either on the chest or abdominal wall and attached to a venous catheter lying in the vein. The port itself is made of either stainless steel, titanium or plastic with a self-sealing silicone membrane which can be accessed via a percutaneous puncture. The device is normally placed surgically, although with recent advances it is now possible to perform this procedure percutaneously.

The venous catheter is inserted into the superior vena cava usually via either the subclavian or cephalic vein with the tip of the catheter positioned at the junction of the superior vena cava (svc) and right atrium, in the same way as a conventional cvc. The position of the attached port should ideally be discussed with the individual concerned, particularly when the care of the port is to be their responsibility. However, it commonly lies in a subcutaneous pocket on the chest wall. The reservoir is accessed by a Huber needle, an angled needle which after puncturing the skin enters the resealable injectable membrane providing secure venous access for the duration of IV therapy.

Subcutaneous ports (Fig. 12.2) are a useful alternative for individuals who require a good

body image or have experienced infections with a conventional cvc. They are expensive but may be attractive to younger people who wish to swim, avoid any alteration in body image, and enjoy greater freedom of activity (Plate 8).

A smaller version of subcutaneous port is also available which can be implanted in the antecubital fossa or forearm, with the catheter inserted through the basilic or cephalic vein until the tip is positioned in the superior vena cava.

The same meticulous attention to aseptic technique applies to this type of venous access device. Infection is the most serious complication when using any type of long-term venous access device, but even more so when a subcutaneous port is the device of choice as prompt removal can be more difficult as surgical intervention is required.

Long-term venous access

When prolonged IV access is required, central venous catheters with single, double or triple lumen are commonly used. Multiple lumen catheters are frequently used for those undergoing intensive chemotherapy regimens and bone marrow/peripheral blood stem cell transplant (BMT/PBSCT) when various combinations of drugs, blood products and PN may require to be infused simultaneously. These catheters can be divided into two types, the Hickman-type catheter and the Groshong® catheter.

Hickman-type catheters

These catheters (Plate 7) are made of silicone with a Dacron/polyester cuff and are radio-opaque. Silicone elastomer is thought to reduce the incidence of catheter-related thrombus and infection (Jones & Craig 1972). Each lumen of the catheter has an external clamp which is opened to allow aspiration of blood or infusion of drugs and fluids. At all other times the clamp is kept closed to prevent air entry and backflow of blood.

The most commonly used insertion site is the subclavian vein. Following cannulation of the vein, a subcutaneous tunnel is created on the chest wall, below the clavicle through which the catheter is guided. The Dacron/polyester cuff is positioned in the subcutaneous tunnel and the catheter exits on the chest wall (Fig. 12.3). Over a period of 5–21 days the Dacron/polyester cuff fibroses within the subcutaneous tissue, creating a securing mechanism for the catheter. The time taken for fibrosis to occur varies and may be extended when steroid therapy is part of the treatment plan. To prevent dislodgement of the catheter prior to fibrosis formation, the catheter is secured to the skin by sutures. Local protocols

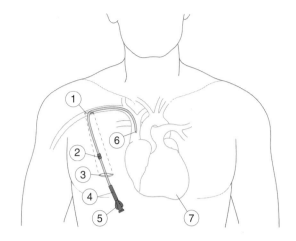

Key:
- - - - Subcutaneous tunnel
1   Clavicular incision
2   Dacron cuff
3   Skin exit site
4   Lumen
5   Luer connection
6   Catheter tip in superior vena cava
7   Heart

Figure 12.3 Position of a Hickman-type tunnelled, cuffed catheter, using percutaneous approach

for removal of securing sutures vary; however, a 3-week period usually allows time for fibrosis to occur.

This type of central venous catheter can also be inserted using a femoral approach, although this is not as popular with clients and the incidence of infection and thrombosis has been found to be higher (Stenzel et al 1989). However, if it is not possible to use the major veins of the upper thorax and neck, the femoral approach offers an alternative.

The Groshong® catheter

The Groshong catheter is also a cuffed tunnelled catheter made of rubberised silicone and may have single or multiple lumen. However, the Groshong catheter has no external clamp. The tip of the catheter contains the three-way Groshong valve, which remains closed unless negative or positive pressure is exerted upon it. The valve opens outwards to allow infusion and inwards for aspiration of blood. In principle the valve reduces fibrin formation at the tip of the catheter, potentially reducing the risk of thrombus formation and associated infection risk (Fig. 12.4).

The advantages and disadvantages of the varying types of venous access device are shown in Table 12.1 and the complications associated with cvc insertion are shown in Table 12.2.

The team approach to successful venous access

Research clearly demonstrates that a specific team dedicated to insertion of venous catheters, patient preparation and management will reduce potential post-insertion complications (Keohane et al 1983, Faubion et al 1986). The introduction of IV teams has been shown to decrease the incidence of catheter-related sepsis dramatically and to be significantly cost effective, by reducing the incidence of complications, minimising waste, avoiding unnecessary cannulation of peripheral or central vessels and standardising subsequent care of venous access devices (Hamilton 1995). However, if a dedicated team is not available, dramatic and rewarding improvement of catheter-related sepsis can be achieved by ensuring that all members of the health-care team involved with venous catheters adhere to the same strict local protocols (Elliott et al 1994).

MANAGEMENT OF VENOUS ACCESS DEVICES

Infection is the most serious complication associated with IV therapy but the most easily avoided if strict protocols are adhered to.

Infection control

Systemic infection is a serious limiting factor in the use of all IV devices. Skin flora is a major source of infection and good handwashing techniques are an important aspect of infection control but one which is frequently overlooked.

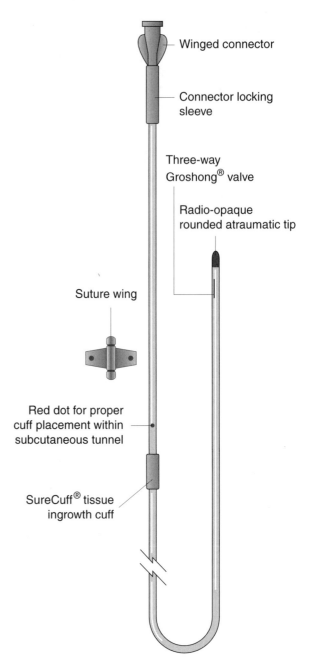

Figure 12.4 Groshong® valved single-lumen tunnelled, cuffed catheter (reproduced with permission of Bard Limited, Crawley, UK)

The IV administration system and IV fluids themselves represent a further source of infection. Reducing the number of times the

Table 12.1 Advantages and disadvantages of venous access devices

Venous access device	Advantages	Disadvantages
Peripheral cannula	Placement quick and easy in experienced hands Can be inserted by relatively inexperienced personnel Less risk of complications than cvc	Thrombophlebitis Limited use Frequent replacement required Single small lumen Risk of extravasation
PICC	Central venous access without the associated risks of the intraclavicular or jugular approach; e.g., pneumothorax, redirection into the neck, haemorrhage Cardiac arrhythmias and potential perforation of heart and svc avoided Acceptable body image Strong Limited risk of infection No risk of catheter compression between clavicle and first rib (pinch-off syndrome)	Risk of blockage due to small lumen Kinking can occur due to the fine lumen and material of the line Thrombophlebitis Thrombosis Accidental dislodgement May limit arm movement and restrict activities May require regular dressing and flushing
Subcutaneous ports	Decreased risk of infection No visual impact on body image No restriction on activities Long-term use Need less care when not in use No dressings required	Insertion and removal requires highly skilled surgical operator Inappropriate for needle-phobic individuals Thrombosis more prevalent Needle displacement and extravasation can occur
Hickman-type catheter	No venepuncture or cannulation required Easily accessed May be inserted percutaneously reduces theatre time and associated costs Relatively easy to remove Repair possible Can be left in place for several years	Highly skilled operator required for insertion May require general anaesthetic and theatre time Thrombosis Blockage Air embolism Pneumothorax Increased risk of infection with multi-lumen catheters Requires regular flushing May require regular dressings May have negative effect on body image
Groshong® catheter	As for Hickman-type catheter plus: Reduced risk of thrombus formation at catheter tip and associated infection risk Reduced risk of air embolus Reduced risk of blockage Repair possible No external clamps Flushing only required once per week	Similar to Hickman-type catheters

Table 12.2 Complications associated with central venous catheter insertion

Complication	Observation	Action
Haemorrhage Symptoms present during or persistently post-cvc insertion	Extent of bleeding Chart blood loss and consider replacement Assess cardiovascular status	Gain cardiovascular stability Pressure dressing Prompt medical assessment Possible surgical intervention
Bleeding into mediastinum or lung caused by malpositioning of cvc during insertion	Monitor cardiovascular and respiratory function Monitor conscious level As above	Urgent medical attention required Stop any infusion Urgent chest X-ray Prepare for chest drainage
Pneumothorax Symptoms present, during or immediately post-cvc insertion	Shoulder tip pain Dyspnoea Altered respiratory and cardiac function	Medical assessment Chest X-ray Monitor respiratory function Oximetry Prompt interpretation of X-ray Oxygen therapy if necessary Prepare for chest drainage Pain control
Latent pneumothorax Due to slow pleural leak manifesting symptoms 2–5 days post-insertion	Onset of pleuritic pain or dry recent cough Monitor as pneumothorax	As above Repeat chest X-ray Medical assessment Ensure chest drainage equipment available
Cardiac arrhythmias Caused by advancing Seldinger wire or the catheter and exciting electrical cardiac pathway	Irregular or abnormal cardiac rhythm Regular monitoring	Medical assessment Check position of cvc on recent X-ray ECG
Air embolism Introduced during insertion of catheter Caused by damage to catheter Loculated air in administration system	Collapse and loss of consciousness Monitor conscious status Monitor cardiovascular status	Seek urgent medical help Lay patient on left side, head lower than pelvis (Trendelenburg position) Ensure all connections are tightly secured in the administration system Operator must ensure cvc is primed with sodium chloride prior to insertion, thus avoiding the introduction of air
CVC redirection Occurs when cvc is incorrectly positioned. May occur on insertion or later, either spontaneously or caused by body movement	Monitor cardiovascular status, particularly when cvc tip in right ventricle, causing ventricular arrhythmias Associated swelling of neck and arm with malposition	Seek medical and radiological advice Review chest X-ray If repositioning is not possible, remove catheter

Table 12.2 continued

Complication	Observation	Action
Neurological damage to brachial plexus Uncommon complication caused by damage to nerve during cannulation or excessive infiltration of local anaesthetic	Monitor specific pain, particularly tingling fingers or facial tingling	Notify medical team Analgesia Re-assess chest X-ray
Catheter damage Caused by puncture of cvc or accidental damage	Monitor extent of damage and leakage from the catheter Consider signs and symptoms of air embolism Monitor vital signs to detect early infection	Protect damaged line, ensure patient safety, clamping with non-traumatic forceps clamp over gauze as close to the chest wall as possible Report damage to operator immediately Assemble repair kit and repair catheter if possible Consider reinsertion of cvc if damage too extensive to repair Exclude infection by performing blood cultures

administration set is changed reduces handling and is thought to reduce infection risk (Band & Maki 1979). These investigators suggest that changing administration sets every 48 hours is justified. However, comparison of changes at 48- and 72-hour intervals have shown no significant differences in infection rate, which suggests that administration sets can be left in place for up to 72 hours (Maki et al 1990). This does not apply to the administration of blood or PN, where administration sets should be changed every 24 hours.

Catheter hubs and the colonisation of these is a subject much debated. Sitges-Serra et al (1984, 1985, 1995) have conducted extensive research and are convinced that hub colonisation is the first step in the presentation of catheter-related sepsis due to coagulase-negative staphylococci. A variety of products have been manufactured to overcome the contamination of the cvc hub; however, despite the sophisticated nature of these devices contamination will still occur unless strict handwashing and aseptic techniques are adhered to.

Additionally, extension sets, three-way taps and multi-lumen central lines increase the infection risk (McCarthy et al 1987, Goodinson 1990) probably because the need for increased access corresponds with increased handling by health-care professionals. Needle-free, closed intravenous injection systems should be used wherever possible, reducing the risk of catheter contamination from skin flora.

Modern production of IV fluids usually entails central preparation under strict, aseptic conditions, therefore reducing the risk of contamination. However, all fluid containers should be checked to ensure sterility before use and the fluid should be checked for cloudiness or precipitation.

Bacterial filters have been shown to prevent infusion of bacteria and particulate material, although these will only be effective with a pore size of $0.22 \mu m$ or less. Infusion devices are necessary to drive infusions via this small pore filter, but they can reduce the incidence of phlebitis, pyrogenic reactions and particulate matter (Baumgartner 1986).

Bacteriological monitoring of the individual with a cvc is essential and should be performed routinely by the multidisciplinary team. Bacteriological investigations should be instituted if any evidence of infection is present, with the close cooperation of the microbiologist. A full infection screen should be arranged (see Ch. 13).

Regular blood cultures may be a useful guide as to the presence of organisms likely to cause overwhelming sepsis. Weekly microbiological monitoring of the exit site of the catheter may also provide early evidence of any exit-site infection. In the presence of sepsis, peripheral blood cultures should accompany a set from the catheter itself, demonstrating to the microbiologist where the heaviest growth of organisms has been located.

Catheter-related bacteraemia is defined as identification of the same organism in at least two blood cultures, obtained from at least two separate sites, at different times, plus evidence of colonisation of the catheter with the same organism (Weightman & Speller 1986, Elliott et al 1994, BCSH 1997).

Insertion/exit-site care

A variety of skin-cleansing agents have been used for both peripheral and central catheters, and some controversy exists over the most appropriate solution and the necessity of skin cleansing at dressing changes. Alcohol-based solutions – i.e. 70% isopropyl alcohol, chlorhexidine and povidone-iodine – are all effective in reducing bacterial contamination, if allowed to dry completely. Research to date suggests chlorhexidine as the most effective agent, although Maki et al (1991) demonstrate that a 2% aqueous solution of chlorhexidine is most effective but this solution is not available commercially in the UK.

Povidone-iodine ointment containing both antimicrobial and antifungal properties is sometimes applied to central line exit sites although there appears to be little evidence to support its effectiveness (Allen 1977).

Some units do not routinely practice skin cleansing after initial wound healing. Further research is required to establish the most appropriate practice in relation to skin cleansing.

Dressings

The type of dressing and the frequency of dressing change to reduce IV-related infection also remains controversial. Post-cvc insertion it would seem reasonable to suggest that unless excessive bleeding is noted the original dressing should not be disturbed for 24 hours. Where persistent oozing presents a problem, forming a pressure dressing, by adding padding to the original dressing, thereby encouraging clot formation, may be helpful. The site may then be redressed after 24 hours, taking care not to disturb any blood clots.

Following initial wound healing, some centres do not use dressings at all for cvcs. Where dressings are used, sterile gauze dressings and transparent dressings are most frequently cited and many studies have compared these dressings. For peripheral cannula it is suggested that either of these dressings can be used and left in place until the cannula is removed (Maki & Ringer 1987). For cvcs, sterile gauze dressings may require to be changed more frequently, as they are easily soiled and dislodged. Frequent dressing changes may contribute to the risk of infection. Transparent dressings have the advantage of providing clear observation of the catheter and require less frequent changing, making them more cost and time efficient. They are also reported as being safe, comfortable and cost effective for individuals undergoing bone marrow transplant (Shivnan & McGuire 1991). However, moisture retention under transparent dressings has been found to be associated with significantly increased rates of colonisation of micro-organisms and increased risk of infection if the dressing is left in place for longer than 48 hours (Maki & Will 1984, Conly et al 1989).

More recently, transparent dressings with increased moisture vapour permeability have been produced which do not appear to be associated with increased colonisation by micro-organisms if changed every 5 days (Maki 1991, Keenlyside 1992). However, studies of different dressings are difficult to compare as they have often been performed for different reasons and under different clinical conditions, which may affect the reported infection rate. Further research is required to determine optimum dressing type and frequency of dressing change. Additionally, individual skin sensitivity and comfort need to be taken into consideration when choosing a dressing.

This lack of consensus regarding dressings means that most haematology units will have their own dressing protocols. 'Principles of infection control associated with central line dressings' and 'Skin tunnelled catheters: guidelines for care' (Royal College of Nursing 1991, 1995) may be helpful to centres requiring such a protocol.

Flushing regimens

The optimum flushing regimen for maintaining patency and preventing thrombus formation in cvcs has also yet to be established (Kelly et al 1992). Catheters require flushing with 0.9% sodium chloride after aspiration of blood or following infusion of drugs, PN or blood. However, when not in use the recommended frequency of flushing varies from daily to weekly. There is also no consensus as to whether the flushing solution should contain heparin or simply be 0.9% sodium chloride. The concentration and amount of heparin contained in flush solutions may vary, and concern has been expressed about the iatrogenic effects of heparin. It would appear that for peripheral cannula 0.9% sodium chloride is as effective in maintaining patency as heparin solutions (Goode et al 1991). The use of heparin is also disputed in cvcs (Evans Orr 1993), although there is currently insufficient research evidence to support use of 0.9% sodium chloride only.

However, due to the adverse effects of heparin, it has been recommended that a flush should contain 5 ml of 5 units/ml when the catheter is not in use (Kelly et al 1992).

In the absence of clear research evidence, manufacturer's guidelines should be followed. The directions for Groshong catheters are clear, and weekly flushing with 0.9% sodium chloride is recommended. Similarly, Groshong PICC lines are maintained with a weekly flush of 10 ml of 0.9% sodium chloride (Oakley 1997). Open-ended PICCs appear to require flushing more frequently and the manufacturers' guidelines usually recommend heparinisation 4–6 hourly in the smaller PICC; i.e. 2 Fg (French gauge). PICC lines of 3 Fg and larger require heparinisation 12 hourly, whereas subcutaneous ports only require flushing every 4–8 weeks when not in use (Wickham 1990).

Blockage of the central venous catheter

Loss of vital central venous access due to catheter occlusion can be a frustrating and distressing experience both for the medical team and the patient. Regular flushing of cvcs will reduce the possibility of occlusion although blocked cvcs will still occur occasionally. The first sign of catheter occlusion is often the inability to aspirate blood from the catheter. Causes and treatment of cvc occlusion are shown in Table 12.3.

Venous access for the haematology client will be a 'life-line', often for months, and occasionally many years. It is therefore extremely important that the medical and nursing team involved in the individual's care provide information in a way that is clearly understood, allowing time for fears to be allayed and questions to be addressed.

Local information booklets can be a useful and an effective tool for those who wish to absorb the information provided, either independently, or with their family. A team approach to the ongoing care of a cvc is paramount, with guidelines and policies relevant to local protocol being made available for clients and staff.

Table 12.3 Causes and treatment of central venous catheter occlusion

Cause	Treatment
Blood clot	Use of fibrinolytic agents, e.g. urokinase
Precipitation of lipids used in parenteral nutrition	Instillation of 70% ethanol solution (Pennington & Pithie 1987)
Precipitation of drugs	Use of hydrochloric acid or sodium bicarbonate to alter pH have been reported but little information is available
Fibrin sheath surrounding catheter tip	Urokinase
Central venous catheter thrombosis occurring around catheter or within intima of vein	Symptom relief and lysis/stabilisation of clot. Catheter may have to be removed
Superior vena cava syndrome secondary to thrombosis	Thrombotic therapy, e.g. urokinase, streptokinase

CONCLUSION

No amount of sophisticated products will overcome the hazards associated with central venous access, in particular infection. Success in the safe and effective administration of treatment stems from a well-informed team, using simple effective protocols. Prevention of the hazards associated with IV therapy will be significantly reduced with the experience of a dedicated team whose meticulous attention to client preparation, siting of venous catheters, catheter selection and after care will pay dividends.

DISCUSSION QUESTIONS

1. What are the informational needs of an individual prior to central line insertion?
2. What teaching strategies should be available for the individual and his/her carer to ensure optimum care of their central venous catheter or PICC line?
3. How can a team approach to the management of intravenous access devices be developed and maintained?
4. What is the procedure in your unit for central line occlusion?
5. What systems are in place in your unit for detecting central line infection?
6. What is the evidence base for the intravenous protocols in your ward/department?

References

Allen J R 1977 The incidence of nosocomial infections in patients receiving parenteral nutrition. In: Johnston I D A (ed) Advances in parenteral nutrition. Proceedings of an international symposium, Bermuda, 16–19 May 1977. MTP, Lancaster, p 339

Band J D, Maki D G 1979 Safety of changing intravenous delivery systems at longer than 24-hour intervals. Annals of Internal Medicine 91: 173–178

Baumgartner T G, Schmidt G L, Thakker K et al 1986 Bacterial

endotoxin retention by in-line intravenous filters. American Journal of Hospital Pharmacy 43: 681–684

BCSH (British Committee of Standards in Haematology) 1997 Guidelines on the insertion and management of central venous lines. British Journal of Haematology 98: 1041–1047

Conly J M, Grieves K, Peters B 1989 Prospective randomised study comparing transparent and dry gauze dressings for central venous catheters. Journal of Infectious Diseases 159(2): 310–319

Consentino F 1977 Personnel-induced infusion phlebitis. Bulletin of the Parenteral Drug Association 3: 288–293

Elliott T S J, Farouqui M H, Armstrong R F, Hanson G C 1994 Guidelines for good practice in central venous catheterization. Journal of Hospital Infection 28: 163–176

Evans Orr M 1993 Issues in the management of percutaneous central venous catheterization. Nursing Clinics of North America 28(4): 913–919

Faubion W C, Wesley J R, Khalidid N, Silva J 1986 Total parenteral nutrition catheter sepsis; impact of a team approach. Journal of Parenteral and Enteral Nutrition 10: 642–645

Gaukroger P B, Roberts J G, Manners T A 1988 Infusion thrombophlebitis: a prospective comparison of 645 Vialon and Teflon cannulae in anaesthetic and postoperative use. Anaesthetic Intensive Care 16: 265–271.

Goode C J, Titler M, Rakel B et al 1991 A meta analysis of effects of heparin flush and saline flush: quality and cost implications. Nursing Research 40(6): 324–330.

Goodinson S 1990 Good practice ensures minimum risk factors,

complications of peripheral venous cannulation and infusion therapy. Professional Nurse 6(3): 175–177.

Hamilton H C 1995 Central lines inserted by clinical nurse specialists. Nursing Times 91(17): 37–39

Jones M V, Craig D B 1972 Venous reaction to plastic intravenous cannulae: influence of cannulae composition. Canadian Anaesthetists Society Journal 19: 491–497

Keenlyside D 1992 Every little detail counts. Infection control in IV therapy. Professional Nurse 7(4): 226–232.

Kelly C, Dumenko L, McGregor S E, McHutchison M E 1992 A change in flushing protocols of central venous catheters. Oncology Nursing Forum 19(4): 599–605

Keohane P P, Attrill H, Northover J, Jones B M J, Silk D B A 1983 Effect of catheter tunnelling and a nutrition nurse on catheter sepsis during parenteral nutrition. Lancet ii: 1388–1390

Lum P 1999 Techniques for optimising catheter tip position. Paper presented at 13th North American Vascular Access Network (NAVAN) Meeting, Orlando, Florida

McCarthy M C, Shives J K, Robison R J, Broadie T A 1987 Prospective evaluation of single and triple lumen catheters in total parenteral nutrition. Journal of Parenteral and Enteral Nutrition 11(3): 259–262

Maki D G (ed) 1991 A prospective, randomized, three-way clinical comparison of a novel, highly permeable,

polyurethane dressing with 206 Swan Ganz pulmonary artery catheters: Opsite 3000 vs Tegaderm vs gauze and tape. Effectiveness and tolerance as catheter dressings. Improving catheter site care. Royal Society of Medicine Services, New York

Maki D G, Ringer M 1987 Evaluation of dressing regimens for prevention of infection with peripheral intravenous catheters, gauze, a transparent polyurethane dressing and an iodophor-transparent dressing. Journal of the American Medical Association 258(17): 2396–2403

Maki D, Will L 1984 Colonization and infection associated with transparent dressings for central venous catheters: a comparative trial. Presentation at APIC, June, Washington, DC

Maki D G, Botticelli J T, Leroy M L, Thielke T S 1990 Prospective study of replacing administration sets for IV therapy at 48 vs 72 hour intervals – 72 hours is safe and cost effective. Official Journal of Canadian Intravenous Nurses Association 6(4): 12–16

Maki D G, Ringer M, Alvarado C J 1991 Randomised trial of povidone iodine, alcohol and chlorhexidine for prevention of infection associated with central venous and arterial catheters. Lancet 338: 339–343

Messner R L, Gorse F J 1987 Nursing management of peripheral intravenous sites. Focus on Critical Care 14(2): 25–33

Oakley C 1997 Peripherally inserted central venous catheters: the experience of a specialist oncology department. Journal of Cancer Nursing 1(1): 50–53

Pennington C R, Pithie A D 1987 Ethanol lock in the management of catheter occlusion. Journal of Parenteral and Enteral Nutrition 11(5): 507–508

Royal College of Nursing 1991 Infection Control Nurses' Association. Intravenous line dressings – principles of infection control. Royal College of Nursing, London

Royal College of Nursing 1995 Leukaemia and Bone Marrow Transplant Nursing Forum. Skin tunnelled catheters: guidelines for care, 2nd edn. Royal College of Nursing, London

Ryder M A 1993 Peripherally inserted central venous catheters. Nursing Clinics of North America 28(4): 937–971

Shivnan J C, McGuire D et al 1991 A comparison of transparent adherent and dry sterile gauze dressings for long term central catheters in patients undergoing bone marrow transplantation. Oncology Nursing Forum 18(8): 1349–1356

Sitges-Serra A, Puig P, Linares J, Farrero N, Jaurrueta E, Garau J 1984 Hub colonisation as the initial step in an outbreak of catheter related sepsis due to coagulase negative staphylococci during parenteral nutrition. Journal of Parenteral and Enteral Nutrition 8(4): 668–672

Sitges-Serra A, Linares J, Perez J L, Jaurrieta E, Lorente L 1985 A randomised trial on the effect of tubing changes of hub contamination and catheter sepsis during parenteral nutrition. Journal of Parenteral and Enteral Nutrition 9(3): 322–325

Sitges-Serra A, Linares J, Garau J 1995 Catheter sepsis. The clue is in the hub. Surgery 97(3): 355–357

Stenzel J P, Green T P, Fuhrman B P, Carlson P E, Marchessault R P 1989 Percutaneous femoral vein catheterisation: a prospective study of complications. Journal of Pediatrics 114: 411–415

Turnidge J 1984 Hazards of peripheral intravenous lines. Medical Journal of Australia 141(1): 37–40

Weightman N C, Speller D C E 1986 Pour plate blood cultures to detect bacteraemias related to indwelling central venous catheters. Journal of Hospital Infection 8(2): 203–204

Wickham R S 1990 Advances in venous access devices and nursing management strategies. Nursing Clinics of North America 25(2): 345–364

Further reading

Bard Access Systems (undated) Handbook of management of central venous access devices. Bard Ltd, Crawley, West Sussex, UK
Excellent well-presented booklet, advising sensible and safe practice. Obtainable from Bard Ltd Access Systems, Forest House, Brighton Road, Crawley, West Sussex, UK.

BCSH (British Commitee on Standards in Haematology) 1997 Guidelines on the insertion and management of central venous lines. British Journal of Haematology 98: 1041-1047
This article provides a review of the basic principles, plus relevant research for nurses involved in the care of patients with skin-tunnelled central venous catheters.

Gabriel J 1996 Care and management of peripherally inserted central catheters. British Journal of Nursing 5(10): 594-599
Janice Gabriel is probably the most experienced British nurse inserting PICC lines and troubleshooting such catheters used for haematology disorders. Any of her articles provide excellent, patient-focused advice on PICC lines.

Hamilton H, Fermo K 1998 Assessment of patients requiring IV therapy via a central venous route. British Journal of Nursing 7(8): 451-460
A nursing assessment of patients requiring central venous access encompassing detailed catheter selection.

Rostein C, Brock L, Roberts S R 1995 The incidence of first Hickman catheter-related infection and predictors of catheter removal in cancer patients. Infection Control and Hospital Epidemiology 16(8): 451–457

This article provides a sensible approach to management of catheter-related infections.

Wilson J A 1994 Preventing infection during IV therapy. Professional Nurse 9(6): 388–390, 392

A useful article that reinforces the issues of effective management of central venous catheters.

13 **P**revention of infection

SARAH HART

Key points
- Prevention of infection is a major challenge in the management of patients with haemato-oncological disorders
- Infection risk is directly related to the severity and duration of neutropenia
- Collaborative multicentre research is required to establish the most effective protective isolation practices
- Adherence to infection control policies and procedures is crucial
- Research and effective quality assurance systems are required to improve infection control practice

INTRODUCTION

The basic principles of infection control can be assisted by simple procedures such as handwashing. This chapter is intended to be a practical guide on the nursing management of haemato-oncology patients. The references, which include text-books, will provide readers with the opportunity to extend their knowledge.

Infection is a major concern in the management of haemato-oncology patients, as its occurrence can be frequent and potentially life threatening (Wade 1994). Young (1994) discusses seven studies that show infection as the primary cause of death for patients with haematological malignancy. A further retrospective study of 66 patients who underwent high-dose chemotherapy indicated that 94% experienced at least one febrile episode during the neutropenic stage of their illness and 48% developed microbiologically and/or clinically documented infections (Kolbe et al 1997). Prevention of infection has increased in importance since treatments such as bone marrow transplantation have led to steadily improving rates of long-term, disease-free survival for haemato-oncology patients (Bowden & Meyers 1994).

There are three major challenges to be considered in the prevention or reduction of the occurrence of infection:

1. Use of increasingly toxic treatments, including aggressive antineoplastic chemotherapy, radiotherapy and procedures such as bone marrow transplantation, cause profound immunosuppression (Meunier 1995).
2. Increase in antibiotic-resistant organisms means clinicians can no longer rely on limitless supplies of antibiotics when infections do occur (Chanock 1993).
3. Impaired immune response means the usual signs and symptoms of infection are reduced (Schimpff 1995).

These challenges substantially increase the difficulty in preventing, treating and detecting infection in individuals.

Factors which increase the infection risk for those with haematological disease include

- *Immunocompromise* due to underlying disease, notably those affecting the bone marrow, but also diseases such as chronic alcoholism and diabetes mellitus.
- *Immunosuppression* as a consequence of radiotherapy, chemotherapy or steroid

therapy, causes neutropenia, cellular and humoral immune dysfunction.

■ *Presence of colonising organisms* in those who are immunosuppressed. Colonising organisms of otherwise low pathogenicity can cause endogenous infection (Van Der Meer 1994, Schimpff 1995).

■ *Age*: extremes of age increase susceptibility to infection.

■ *Loss of skin and mucous membrane integrity* provide entry for micro-organisms.

■ *Antibiotic therapy*: the administration of broad-spectrum antibacterial agents produces a shift in microbial flora. In the presence of antibiotics, resistant micro-organisms have a selective advantage (Hart 1998) and the risk of fungal infections is increased (Chanock 1993).

■ *Poor nutrition* reduces the production of white blood cells required for immunity.

■ *Multiple invasive procedures*: breaching skin and mucous membranes with intravenous catheters, urinary catheters and biopsy needles, for example, provides entry for micro-organisms.

SOURCES OF MICRO-ORGANISMS

Infection can be grouped into two categories: exogenous, which refers to organisms originating outside or away from the patient's body; endogenous, which is attributed to organisms already present in or on the patient's body (Wade 1994). The detrimental effects of both can be limited by scrupulous cleanliness of the patient and environment. About 10% of patients acquire infections following admission to hospital (Hospital Infection Working Group 1995). As the incidence and severity of infection are inversely proportional to the degree of immunosuppression (Schimpff 1995), it can be expected that haemato-oncology patients will have an even higher incidence of infection. Bowden & Meyers (1994) point out that the more aggressive treatment regimens are associated with a higher incidence of and mortality from infection, although it is not always clear whether the increase in infection is related to the underlying illness or its therapy. It has been suggested that infection as the cause of death for patients with leukaemia is as high as 75–80% (Young 1994) (Plate 6 illustrates an infective episode in acute leukaemia). Adoption and adherence to good infection control principles is therefore vital in reducing the incidence of hospital-acquired infection (Hospital Infection Working Group 1995).

Schimpff (1995) reviewed infections in a group of cancer patients and found nearly all infections originated from endogenous organisms colonising the patient at or near the site of infection; one-third of these organisms were initially exogenous and had been acquired subsequent to hospital admission. For example, *Pseudomonas aeruginosa* can usually be found colonising the rectum prior to bacteraemia originating from a perianal cellulitis. Similarly, the oral cavity harbours many varieties of bacteria which do not cause problems in an immunocompetent person (Clarke 1993). Unfortunately; the mucositis which frequently accompanies cytotoxic therapy increases the pathogenicity of these organisms, which can lead to local and systemic infection (Allbright 1984, Campbell 1987) (see Ch. 16).

INFECTING ORGANISMS

Immunosuppressed patients can become infected with any pathogenic micro-organism capable of causing infection in healthy persons and are particularly susceptible to opportunistic micro-organisms which do not normally cause infections in healthy persons (Mims et al 1993). Susceptibility to these organisms means that infections are likely to occur in immunosuppressed individuals despite efforts to avoid infection. Measures taken to prevent infection are therefore aimed at minimising the risk from micro-organisms. All micro-organisms are important if they have the ability to be transmitted in the environment, cause infection and produce clinical infection. These may be bacterial, viral, protozoal, helminths or fungal. Some organisms cannot survive for long outside the body; for example, meningococcal meningitis can be carried harmlessly in the back of the throat of one person but when inhaled by a susceptible host causes significant infection. Other organisms have the ability to contaminate and survive in the environment prior to reaching a susceptible host. Examples of organisms and their vectors are shown in Table 13.1.

In the past, bacterial infections have been relatively easily treated with intravenous antibiotics. However, the emergence of antibiotic-resistant organisms has further increased the risk of serious infection by changing the balance of survival in favour of the resistant organism. Coliforms, which include *Klebsiella* and *Enterobacter*, are especially important as they have the ability to acquire resistance to many antimicrobial agents. They can be found in the environment and cause opportunistic infections and outbreaks of cross infection. Recent reports of methicillin-resistant *Staphylococcus aureus* (MRSA) acquiring vancomycin resistance (Williams et al 1997) emphasise the

Reflection point

Suzanne, a 40-year-old diabetic with acute myeloid leukaemia has been admitted for allogeneic bone marrow transplant. She has a skin-tunnelled venous catheter *in situ*, the exit site of which is growing MRSA. Identify the factors which make this patient especially susceptible to infection (see 'Suggestions for first reflection point' on p. 197).

importance of compliance with effective infection control policies.

Fungal infections tend to have a high mortality rate. Commonly identified pathogens include *Candida* and *Aspergillus*. In one study of bone marrow transplant patients a 75% mortality rate was reported for those infected with *Aspergillus* (Meyers 1990).

Table 13.1 Organisms and their vector

Vector	Organism
Food Undercooked chicken, eggs Raw fruit and vegetables	*Salmonella, Listeria, Bacillus* *Pseudomonas, Campylobacter*
Tap water	*Cryptosporidium, Pseudomonas, Legionella*
Stagnant water [unsterile humidification water, flower water, etc.]	*Pseudomonas*
Soil	*Aspergillus, Clostridium*
Plants and flowers	*Aspergillus, Pseudomonas*
Contaminated intravenous fluids	*Pseudomonas*
Showers, hand basins, baths, toilets	*Pseudomonas, Clostridium difficile,* Vancomycin-resistant enterococci
Bedding	*Staphylococcus aureus,* Vancomycin-resistant enterococci
Air	*Aspergillus*
Furniture, floors, beds	*Staphylococcus aureus, Staphylococcus epidermidis,* Vancomycin-resistant enterococci, *Clostridium difficile*

PRINCIPLES OF INFECTION CONTROL

Protective isolation

The risk of infection for the haemato-oncology patient is directly related to the severity and duration of immunosuppression. Neutropenia is a predictable result of cancer therapy and the exact level of neutrophils is a useful index of infection risk. The risk of infection rises as the neutrophil count falls, with a major increase with a rapidly falling count or when the count approaches zero (Wade 1994).

Protective isolation procedures have traditionally been used to reduce infection risk for the neutropenic patient. The need for protective isolation has long been debated. Poe et al's (1994) survey of 91 bone marrow transplant programmes in the USA found that all units used some type of protective environment, although practices varied considerably.

Protective isolation practices range from the use of purpose-built units with air-filtration systems and plastic isolators to single rooms on a general ward or shared rooms within a controlled environment on a general ward (Mallett & Bailey 1996). Protective measures taken within these environments also vary. In complete protective environments a clean aseptic approach may be taken, with staff wearing clean clothing and patients undergoing gut decontamination and receiving a clean diet. At the other end of the range, practices may be limited to common sense measures, such as handwashing and avoiding people with obvious infections. In between are a variety of practices, including wearing gloves, gowns and masks, and use of a modified or low-bacterial diet. Research data demonstrating the effectiveness of protective isolation practices are currently inconclusive (Nauseef & Maki 1981, Pizzo 1989).

Expensive to build, maintain and staff, protective isolation units have been seen to reduce infection (Buckner et al 1978). Yet, protective isolation only appears to affect long-term survival by reducing graft versus host disease (GVHD) (Storb et al 1983). According to Dunleavey (1996), the lack of evidence supporting the effectiveness of protective isolation

practices has resulted in many units abandoning these practices. However, there is some evidence to suggest that positive-pressure air-filtration systems may be effective in reducing the incidence of bacterial and fungal infections, especially aspergillus (Rhame 1991, Wade 1994).

The risk of infection when using single rooms and shared rooms on general wards depends on the general condition of the ward environment and the infectious status of the other patients. However, if protective isolation is to be effective it needs to be instituted on the admission of the patient, before the patient has the opportunity to become colonised with potentially pathogenic organisms from the hospital environment such as MRSA and vancomycin-resistant enterococci (VRE) (Wade 1994, Humphreys & Duckworth 1997, Weber & Rutala 1997).

There is a lack of data comparing cross-infection rates in single rooms with those in shared rooms. However, a small study investigating transmission rates of urinary tract infection indicated cross infection is reduced if catheterised patients are nursed in single rooms (Fryklund et al 1997).

A further study of infection rates comparing hospitalised patients in single rooms and patients who spent some time at home where food restrictions and antibiotic prophylaxis continued, found mortality data compared favourably (Russell et al 1992). This evidence combined with the incidence of hospital-acquired infection supports the need for further investigation into the benefits of early discharge.

Microbial suppression of the alimentary tract organisms with oral non-absorbable antibiotics has also been evaluated as a means of preventing infection (Storring et al 1977). Inconsistent results have been obtained from randomised trials and Wade (1994) outlines the disadvantages of these regimens, which include poor patient compliance, nausea and cost. However, their use may reduce infection rates during periods of profound and persistent neutropenia, significant mucosal disruption or recurrent perirectal infections.

Collaborative multicentre research is required to establish the most effective protective isolation practices, so that national guidelines can be developed. Psychological distress caused by protective isolation also needs to be addressed (Belec 1992) (see Ch. 19) and highlights the importance of attention to all aspects of patient care.

Barrier nursing

Carriers of infection and infected patients must be identified early. The potential for cross infection should be evaluated and barrier nursing commenced when necessary. For example, patients colonised with MRSA will need barrier nursing while patients who are compliant with good handwashing and have *Clostridium difficile* in their stool will not (Sanderson & Richardson 1997). Viral infections, such as shingles or chicken pox (herpes zoster) may be easily transmitted between individuals with haematological malignancies and patients with these conditions will require strict barrier nursing (Gurevich & Tafuro 1986). As with those in protective isolation, individuals being barrier nursed because of an infection will need support as they can feel stigmatised and lonely (Knowles 1993).

Protective clothing

The choice of protective clothing is decided by expected contact with infected patients, immunocompromised patients or to comply with universal blood and body fluid precautions.

Generally, if protective clothing is worn correctly for universal blood and body fluid precautions, additional protective clothing is not required. Plastic aprons provide a cheap impermeable barrier to micro-organisms and should be worn during close contact with infected, immunosuppressed patients or when blood and body fluids are present; they must be changed between patients. Gloves do not replace handwashing, and clean boxed gloves should be worn to protect the wearer from blood and body fluid contamination. Sterile gloves are only required during certain aseptic techniques. Caps and overshoes are not required. Masks and eye protection are rarely required, except to protect the wearer during

universal precautions or administering toxic drugs (Ayton et al 1984).

STRATEGY FOR THE PREVENTION OF INFECTION

Attention to the following points will reduce the risk of infection for haematological oncology patients.

Handwashing

Handwashing is the single most important procedure for preventing infection. Hands must be washed before and after patient contact. Rings and wristwatches must be removed and sleeves rolled up. Plain liquid soap is suitable for general tasks and removes transient organisms. Bactericidal detergent will remove both transient and resident organisms and should be used prior to aseptic techniques and providing care for immunocompromised patients. Bactericidal alcoholic handrub is a quick effective means of cleansing hands (Pereira et al 1997) and can be used when hands are clean and during aseptic techniques.

Reflection point

Review the handwashing techniques of yourself and your colleagues. Compare current practice with these guidelines.

Fit healthy staff and visitors

Staff caring for those who are immunosuppressed should be free from infection. Visitors should be advised of the potential for cross infection and the importance of informing ward staff if they are unwell or have been in contact with a contagious disease.

Patient education

Patient education is important so that individuals recognise signs of infection and are aware of the need to report these signs promptly. Education increases patient satisfaction and enhances compliance with prevention of infection practices (Richards 1998). Additionally, it empowers individuals to participate in their care while improving quality of care (Gaston-Johansson et al 1992).

Visitor education
Educated visitors are more likely to encourage the patient to comply with care.

Regular observations
Vital signs must be regularly monitored for signs of infection and the condition of the mouth and skin observed on at least a daily basis. Rectal infections in persons with haematological malignancies have been associated with mortality rates as high as 50% (Yeomans 1986). It is essential that rectal lesions are diagnosed and treated accurately and quickly and this emphasises the importance of patient education.

The body's normal reaction to infection is for tissue macrophages to be attracted to the area in an attempt to remove the organisms inducing an inflammatory response. Phagocytes (neutrophils and macrophages) are attracted to the site of inflammation by the process of chemotaxis, destroying the organism by phagocytosis (Klein 1990). In neutropenic patients this inflammatory response to infection is reduced and the normal signs of inflammation will be reduced or absent. Therefore every sign of infection must be treated as significant. Frequently, the only sign of infection is a pyrexia and there may be no obvious indication of the site of infection. In the presence of pyrexia a full infection screen should be undertaken in an attempt to identify the infecting organism. Microbiological samples should be collected, including bacteriological and viral cultures of blood, urine and sputum specimens, nasal and throat swabs and swabs from any suspicious lesions. A chest X-ray may also be performed. Septicaemic shock can develop rapidly in an immunosuppressed individual and may result in death. It is therefore imperative that broad-spectrum intravenous antibiotics are commenced immediately when signs of infection are detected.

Patient hygiene
Daily showers or baths and regular hair-washes should be encouraged to remove micro-organisms and improve patient comfort. Individuals must be provided with clean towels and disposable wash clothes. Baths must be cleaned carefully after each patient.

Mouth care
Mouth care will help keep the mouth and lips clean, moist and intact and will reduce pain and infection. Regular assessment of the mouth and oral care is essential (see Ch. 16).

Maintenance of body's natural defences
Care should be taken to minimise the potential for infection at venous access sites (see Ch. 12). Care should also be taken to maintain skin integrity, with attention to pressure areas if the individual has reduced mobility. Keeping finger and toe nails clean and short will also help to prevent individuals accidentally injuring themselves. Avoidance of constipation will reduce the possibility of damage to the rectal mucosa. If constipation does occur, use of suppositories and enemas should be avoided, again to prevent damage to the rectal mucosa.

Environmental cleanliness
Thorough daily cleaning using hot soapy water will remove most organisms; disinfectants are not generally required (Ayliffe et al 1992). Microbial contamination can be removed by thorough cleaning with soap and water, or destroyed by sterilisation or disinfection (Ayliffe et al 1992). Generally, equipment which penetrates skin, mucous membranes or sterile cavities should be sterile disposable or sterilised by autoclaving. Equipment which has contact with mucous membranes should preferably be sterilised by autoclaving but may be thoroughly cleaned and disinfected. Care must be taken to comply with the 1994 Control of Substances Hazardous to Health (COSHH) regulations when using disinfectants. Equipment that is only used on intact skin can be cleaned with detergent and water. On discharge, the room and furniture should be cleared and terminally cleaned. Use of a bleach solution is required when the patient is colonised with VRE (Kearns et al 1995). Communal ward equipment such as the refrigerator

and food blenders are reservoirs for infection and must be meticulously cleaned and maintained (Kiddy et al 1987, Smith 1991).

Restrict plants and flowers

Cut flowers and potted plants should be restricted in the rooms of immunosuppressed individuals as they are a reservoir for potential pathogens (Rogues et al 1997).

Aseptic techniques

Aseptic techniques must be adopted during all tasks that bypass the body's natural defence mechanisms and when handling equipment such as intravenous catheters (see Ch. 12). Aseptic techniques help to prevent contamination of wounds and other susceptible sites (Mallett & Bailey 1996).

Clean food

Raw fruit and vegetables, undercooked fish, eggs and meat are a potential infection risk (Pattison 1993). Food restrictions vary between units and may be dependent on the treatment being administered. Greater restrictions may be placed on those undergoing bone marrow transplants; however, in general, raw fruit and vegetables and foods known to carry bacteria such as soft cheeses should be avoided. Other foods should be well cooked for those who are immunosuppressed.

Drinking water and ice

These may be contaminated by incorrect handling by staff, patients or visitors and environmental factors such as dirty ice machines and contaminated taps (Wilson et al 1997). For especially immunosuppressed patients, such as bone marrow transplantation patients, drinking water and ice should be provided from boiled or filtered water.

Disinfecting bed pan washer

Mechanically clean and disinfect bed pans and urinals. All shared equipment must be heat treated between use.

Reliable hospital laundry

Used linen must be thermally disinfected to remove micro-organisms by a laundry which complies to the Department of Health's (1987) regulations. Clean linen should be transported and stored in a safe clean manner.

Discharge planning

Discharge planning of immunocompromised patients involves the medical and nursing team from the hospital and the community, as well as the significant family or friends who will be providing help and support in the community (Pfaff & Terry 1980). Once at home patients

---

 Case study 13.1

Joe is an 18 year old who was diagnosed with acute lymphoblastic leukaemia 12 months ago. During this time he has been treated with intensive chemotherapy and has spent prolonged periods of time in the isolation area of the haematology unit. Joe is currently receiving treatment as an outpatient in the day case unit.

Eight days after his latest chemotherapy treatment, Joe arrived on the unit unexpectedly one morning as he had developed a pyrexia. His temperature was found to be 38.9°C with a pulse of 110 and blood pressure of 110/70. A full blood count showed a haemoglobin of 9.8 g/L, white cell count of 0.7×10^9/L, an absolute neutrophil count of 0.04×10^9/L and a platelet count of 179×10^9/L.

Joe was admitted to an isolation room to protect him from further infection and screening was begun to establish the origin and causative agent of his infection. Blood was taken peripherally and from both lumen of Joe's central line for culture. Swabs were taken from the central line exit site for microscopy, culture and sensitivity. A throat swab and specimens of urine, faeces and sputum were also obtained for analysis. Joe was examined by the doctor and a chest X-ray performed. He was commenced on intravenous antibiotics as per hospital protocol for patients with a neutropenic septic episode. Joe's temperature and pulse were initially monitored 2 hourly until he became more stable, and his general condition was closely observed for signs of deterioration. Fluid intake and urine output were monitored to ensure adequate hydration and oxygen saturation levels were measured.

Blood counts were taken daily to check Joe's white count and renal and liver function. The source and causative organism for Joe's infection were never isolated. He became apyrexial after 24 hours, but continued to be closely observed throughout his admission. Remaining apyrexial, he completed 5 days of intravenous antibiotics and was discharged home.

need to be alert to signs and symptoms of infection so that they know to contact their doctor or the hospital immediately if problems occur. The risk of acquiring an infection in the community can be reduced by taking precautions when shopping, storing and preparing food and avoiding foods known to contain bacteria. While discharged patients can mix with other people they must avoid persons with colds, influenza and other infections. For these reasons it is sensible to avoid crowded pubs, theatres, shops or restaurants. Healthcare professionals should advise outpatients when they can mix more freely with people again, as this will depend on the underlying disease and treatment programmes. Animals are generally restricted from the clinical setting; caution should continue following discharge to contact with known, well cared for, fit pets.

MEANS OF IMPROVING INFECTION CONTROL PRACTICE

Research
Research allows the development of scientific knowledge-based nursing practice, by seeking ways to improve and standardise practice (Burns & Grove 1993). The demands placed on nurses working in the rapidly changing field of oncology means that clinical research to identify new and effective strategies to prevent infection is essential.

Standards
Standards can be used as the basis for measuring quality of care provided to patients and underpin effective infection control programmes (Infection Control Standards Working Party 1993, Luthert & Robinson 1993).

Audit
Audit is a systematic critical and continuing analysis of quality of care and use of resources to identify where improvements can be made (Millward et al 1993). Most aspects of infection control, such as mouth care, care of central lines, compliance to handwashing, can be audited. Following an audit project related to hospital-acquired infections, clinical guidelines

for the following six nursing tasks have been produced (Ward et al 1997):

- handwashing
- routine blood and body fluid precautions
- prevention of infection associated with central intravascular devices
- prevention of infection associated with short-term indwelling urethral catheters
- prevention associated with tracheal suction
- prevention of infection associated with nasogastric tubes.

These guidelines need to be extended to include specific issues related to the care of immunosuppressed patients, so that national standards can be produced.

Policies and procedures
Approved policies and procedures that are regularly reviewed and updated to take account of new research and high-dose chemotherapy regimes should be available for all infection control issues (Mallett & Bailey 1996). Compliance with infection control policies and procedures is variable. Moore (1997) stresses that reducing infection requires ongoing education of staff in view of the high turnover of nursing and medical staff. Houang & Hurley (1997) suggest education programmes based on psychological principles improve motivation and compliance; Teare & Peacock (1996) found that the introduction of an infection control link nurse system raised the profile of infection control by disseminating knowledge and changing behaviour and attitudes. Adoption of

 Suggestions for first reflection point

Factors which increase the patient's risk of infection
- diabetic
- disease of bone marrow
- previous treatment with chemotherapy and antibiotics
- allogeneic bone marrow transplant, necessitating the use of immunosuppressive drugs to prevent GVHD
- already colonised with a potentially pathogenic organism.

one or both of these strategies may help adherence to infection control policies.

CONCLUSION

This chapter has reviewed strategies that help to reduce the incidence of infection. While controversy surrounds the nursing management of the haemato-oncology patient, nurses need to be familiar with the principles and rationale for good infection control practices.

DISCUSSION QUESTIONS

1. Why are haemato-oncology patients especially susceptible to infection?

2. What elements of nursing care are most useful in preventing infection in immunocompromised patients?

3. Which clinical features indicate that protective isolation is required?

4. Which common infections seen on your ward require barrier nursing?

5. What are the strengths and weakness of protective isolation in your place of work?

6. How might infection control practices be improved in your place of work?

7. How can communication with the Infection Control Team be strengthened?

References

Allbright A 1984 Oral care for the cancer chemotherapy patient. Nursing Times 80(2): 40–42

Ayliffe G A J, Lowbury E J L, Geddes A M, Williams J D (eds) 1992 Control of hospital infection: a practical handbook, 3rd edn. Chapman and Hall, London

Ayton M, Babb J, Mackintosh C, Maloney M H 1984 Report of an Infection Control Nurses Association working party on ward protective clothing. The Infection Control Nurses Association, London

Belec R H 1992 Quality of life: perceptions of long term survivors of bone marrow transplantation. Oncology Nursing Forum 19(1): 31–37

Bowden R A, Meyers J D 1994 Infection complicating bone marrow transplantation. In: Rubins R H, Young L S (eds) Clinical approach to infection in the compromised host, 3rd edn. Plenum, New York, 23: 601–628

Buckner C D, Clift R A, Sanders J E 1978 Protective environment for marrow transplant recipients.

A prospective study. Ann Intern Med 89: 893–901

Burns N, Grove S K 1993 The practice of nursing research, 2nd edn. W B Saunders, Philadelphia

Campbell S 1987 Mouth care in cancer patients. Nursing Times 83(29): 59–60

Chanock S 1993 Evolving risk factors for infectious complications of cancer therapy. Hematology/Oncology Clinics of North America 7(4): 771–794

Clarke G 1993 Mouth care in the hospitalised patient. British Journal of Nursing 2(4): 221–227

Control of Substances Hazardous to Health (COSHH) Regulations 1994. HMSO, London

Department of Health 1987 Hospital laundry arrangements for used and infected linen. HC(87)30. HMSO, London

Dunleavey R 1996 Isolation in BMT: a protection or a privation? British Journal of Nursing 5(11): 663–668

Fryklund B, Haeggman S, Burman L G 1997 Transmission of urinary bacterial strains between patients with indwelling catheters – nursing in the same room and in separate rooms compared. Journal of Hospital Infection 36: 147–153

Gaston-Johansson F, Franco T, Zimmerman L 1992 Pain and psychological distress in patients undergoing autologous bone marrow transplantation. Oncology Nursing Forum 19(1): 44–48

Gurevich I, Tafuro P 1986 The compromised host: deficit-specific infection and the spectrum of prevention. Cancer Nursing 9(5): 263–275

Hart C A 1998 Antibiotic resistance: an increasing problem? British Medical Journal 316: 1255–1256

Hospital Infection Working Group 1995 Hospital Infection Control. Department of Health, London

Houang E T S, Hurley R 1997 Anonymous questionnaire survey on the knowledge and practices of hospital staff in infection control. Journal of Hospital Infection 35: 301–306

Humphreys H, Duckworth G 1997 Methicillin-resistant *Staphylococcus aureus* [MRSA]: a reappraisal of control measures in the light of changing circumstances. Journal of Hospital Infection 36: 167–170

Infection Control Standards Working Party 1993 Standards in infection control in hospitals. Department of Health, London

Kearns A M, Freeman R, Lightfoot N F 1995 Nosocomial enterococci resistance to heat and sodium hypochlorite. Journal of Hospital Infection 30: 193–199

Kiddy K, Josse E, Griffin N 1987 An outbreak of serious infections related to food blenders. Journal of Hospital Infection 36: 191–193

Klein J 1990 Defence against pathogens and parasites. In: Immunology. Blackwell, Boston, 13: 311–335

Knowles H E 1993 The experience of infectious patients in isolation. Nursing Times 89(30): 53–56

Kolbe K, Domkin D, Derigs H G, Bhakdi S, Huber C, Aulitzky W E 1997 Infectious complications during neutropenia subsequent to peripheral blood stem cell transfusion. Bone Marrow Transplantation 19(2): 143–147

Luthert J M, Robinson L 1993 The Royal Marsden Hospital Manual of Standards of Care. Blackwell Science, Oxford

Mallett J, Bailey C 1996 Manual of clinical nursing procedures, 4th edn. Blackwell Science, London

Meunier F 1995 Infections in patients with acute leukaemia and lymphoma. In: Mandel G L, Bennett J E, Dolin R (eds) Principles and practices of infectious diseases, 4th edn. Churchill

Livingstone, New York, 2 (288): 2675–2685

Meyers J D 1990 Fungal infections in bone marrow transplant patients. Seminars in Oncology 17(3): 10–13

Millward S, Barnett J, Thomlinson D 1993 A clinical infection control audit programme. Journal of Infection Control 24: 219–232

Mims C A, Playfair J H L, Roitt I M, Wakelin D, Williams R 1993 Medical microbiology. Mosby, St Louis

Moore A 1997 Hospital bugbear. The Health Service Journal 30 October 1–4

Nauseef W M, Maki D G 1981 A study of the value of simple protective isolation in patients with granulocytopenia. New England Journal of Medicine 304(8): 448–453

Pattison A J 1993 Review of current practice in clean diets in the UK. Journal of Human Nutrition and Dietetics 6: 3–11

Pereira L J, Lee G M, Wade K L 1997 An evaluation of five protocols for surgical handwashing in relation to skin condition and microbial counts. Journal of Infection 36: 49–65

Pfaff S J, Terry B A 1980 Discharge planning. Nursing Clinics of North America 15(4): 893–908

Pizzo P A 1989 Considerations for the prevention of infectious complications in patients with cancer. Review of Infectious Diseases II (suppl 7): 1551–1563

Poe S S, Larson E, McGuire D, Krumm S 1994 A national survey of infection prevention practices on bone marrow transplant units. Oncology Nursing Forum 21(10): 1687–1694

Rhame F S 1991 Prevention of nosocomial aspergillosis. Journal of Hospital Infection 18 (suppl A): 466–472

Richards T 1998 Partnership with patients. British Medical Journal 316: 85–86

Rogues A M, Quesnel C, Revel P, Saric J, Gachie J P 1997 Potted plants as a potential reservoir of fusarium species. Journal of Infection Control 35(2): 163–164

Russell J A, Poon M C, Jones A R, Woodman R C, Ruether B A 1992 Allogeneic bone marrow transplantation without protective isolation in adults with malignant disease. Lancet 339: 38–40

Sanderson P, Richardson D 1997 Do patients with clostridium need to be isolated? Journal of Infection Control 36(2): 157–158

Schimpff S C 1995 Infections in the cancer patient. In: Mandell G L, Bennett J E, Dolin R (eds) Principles and practices of infectious diseases. Churchill Livingstone, New York, 2(287): 2666–2686

Smith F 1991 Looking into the refrigerator. Nursing Times 87(38): 61–62

Storb R, Prentice R L, Buckner C D 1983 Graft-versus-host disease and survival in patients with aplastic anemia treated by marrow graft from HLA-identical siblings. Beneficial effect of a protective environment. New England Journal of Medicine 308: 302–307

Storring R A, Jameson B, McElwain T J, Wiltshaw E 1977 Oral nonabsorbed antibiotics prevent infection in acute non-lymphoblastic leukaemia. Lancet 2: 837–840

Teare E L, Peacock A 1996 The development of an infection control link-nurse programme in a district general hospital. Journal of Infection Control 34: 267–278

Van Der Meer J W M 1994 Defects in host mechanisms. In: Rubins R H, Young L S (eds) Clinical approach to infection in the compromised host, 3rd edn. Plenum, New York, 3: 33–55

Wade J C 1994 Epidemiology and prevention of infection in the compromised host. In: Rubins R H, Young L S (eds) Clinical approach to infection in the compromised host, 3rd edn. Plenum, New York, 2: 5–31

Ward V, Wilson J, Taylor L, Cookson B, Glynn A 1997 Preventing hospital acquired

infection. Clinical guidelines. Public Health Laboratory Service, London

Weber D J, Rutala W A 1997 Role of environmental contamination in the transmission of Vancomycin Resistant Enterococci. Infection Control and Hospital Epidemiology 18(5): 306–309

Williams D, Bergan T, Moosdeen F 1997 Arrival of vancomycin resistance in *Staphylococcus aureus*. Antibiotics Chemotherapy 1(2): 1

Wilson I G, Hogg G M, Barr J G 1997 Microbiological quality of ice in hospital and community. Journal of Hospital Infection 36: 171–180

Yeomans A C 1986 Rectal infections in acute leukemia. Cancer Nursing 9(6): 295–300

Young L S 1994 Management of infections in leukemia and lymphoma. In: Rubins R H, Young L S (eds) Clinical approach to infection in the compromised host, 3rd edn. Plenum, New York, 21: 551–575

Further reading

Ayliffe G A J, Lowbury E J L, Geddes A M, Williams J D (eds) 1992 Control of hospital infection. A practical handbook, 3rd edn. Chapman and Hall, London
This handbook provides practical guidance and information on effective ways of controlling infection, and is an interesting and useful guide for all health-care professionals.

Barrett J, Treleaven J (eds) 1998 The clinical practice of stem cell transplantation, Vols 1 and 2. Isis, Oxford
This book provides the latest information related to research, nursing and medical care of this rapidly expanding and changing treatment. It is a useful resource to health-care workers in the field of bone marrow transplantation.

British Committee for Standards in Haematology Clinical Task Force 1995 Guidelines on the provision of facilities for the care of adult patients with haematological malignancies (including leukaemia and lymphoma and severe bone marrow failure). Clinical and Laboratory Haematology 17: 3-10
This useful report defines four levels of care for the management of adult patients with haematological malignancies and marrow failure, outlining the extra specialist expertise, staffing and resources required to provide this care.

Horton R, Parker L 1997 Informed infection control practice. Churchill Livingstone, Edinburgh

This comprehensive book, with numerous useful references, addresses the control and prevention of infection in the hospital and the community, and provides a valuable resource for all health professionals.

Wilson J 1995 Infection control in clinical practice. Baillière Tindall, London
This book provides practical, relevant, readable, research-based information on the prevention and control of infection, and includes chapters on microbiology and immunology. This sound scientific information provides a basis for the formulation of standards of care in infection control.

14 Haemorrhagic problems

SHELLEY DOLAN

> **Key points**
> - Haemorrhagic problems may occur as a result of both disease and treatment
> - Haemorrhagic problems may be chronic and relatively easily controlled or acute and potentially life threatening
> - Thrombocytopenia is the commonest cause of bleeding in haemato-oncological disorders
> - Bleeding episodes can be extremely frightening for patients and their families
> - Infection can exacerbate spontaneous bleeding
> - Awareness of the factors which increase a bleeding tendency along with prompt recognition and management of bleeding is essential

INTRODUCTION

Nurses caring for the client with a haematological malignancy need to be prepared for problems associated with both the disease and resulting from treatment. Haemorrhagic problems may occur as a result of both disease and treatment. For example, an individual may present with thrombocytopenia when the bone marrow is invaded by neoplastic cells as in acute lymphoblastic leukaemia (ALL) (Sarzotti et al 1978) or their blood may be rendered pancytopenic by the marrow-ablative chemotherapy administered as treatment.

Haemorrhagic problems may be chronic and relatively easily controlled or, in a small percentage, acute and life threatening (Caudell & Bakitas Whedon 1991). The nurse caring for these patients needs to be aware of haemorrhagic complications and, as in other areas of haemato-oncology nursing, care will be focused on prevention and careful monitoring to ensure that any sign of bleeding is noted rapidly and treatment commenced promptly. It is essential that the patient and, where possible, the family are aware of the need to prevent bleeding problems. This chapter will therefore describe the haemorrhagic problems that may be encountered and their interdisciplinary management.

There are four causes of bleeding:

1. Low platelet count (thrombocytopenia).
2. Platelet dysfunction.
3. Erosion of a blood vessel.
4. Coagulation disorders, especially disseminated intravascular coagulation (DIC).

THROMBOCYTOPENIA

Thrombocytopenia is the commonest cause of bleeding in haemato-oncological conditions. It can occur for a number of reasons, the most common being invasion of the bone marrow by neoplastic cells and the effects of chemotherapy and/or radiotherapy on platelet production. Some cytotoxic drugs, especially carmustine and lomustine, have a delayed but prolonged effect on the bone marrow and severe thrombocytopenia may occur several weeks after treatment. Platelet count recovery may also be delayed. Platelets are also the last blood cell to recover following blood and marrow transplant (BMT) and in some cases thrombocytopenia may be prolonged. Other causes of thrombocytopenia in this population include:

- Autoimmune thrombocytopenia, which may occur in lymphoproliferative conditions such as lymphoma and the lymphocytic leukaemias, causing rapid destruction of platelets.
- An enlarged spleen occurs in some conditions, especially the chronic myeloproliferative disorders such as chronic myeloid leukaemia (CML). Platelets collect in the enlarged spleen, thereby reducing the number of circulating platelets.

Spontaneous bleeding may occur when the platelet count is lower than $100 \times 10^9/L$, although major haemorrhage is more likely when the platelet count is less than $20 \times 10^9/L$. However, the relationship between platelet count and spontaneous bleeding varies between individuals (Hughes-Jones & Wickramsinghe 1991). Spontaneous bleeding is also more likely with a rapidly falling platelet count than with a recovering one.

Thrombocytopenia and the risk of spontaneous bleeding may be increased by certain drugs and infection. Aspirin is known to cause an increased risk of bleeding by its effect on platelet aggregation and by prolonging bleeding time. Beta-lactam antibiotics such as penicillins and cephalosporins, which are frequently used intravenously to combat infection, have also been cited as a cause of prolonged bleeding time and impaired platelet aggregation. The incidence of haemorrhage with these drugs is difficult to ascertain but bleeding risk may be increased by renal failure, existing thrombocytopenia or DIC (Sattler et al 1986).

In infection, the release of bacterial endotoxins increases platelet consumption, and platelet counts may therefore fall rapidly, which further increases the risk of spontaneous bleeding.

Common bleeding episodes

A low platelet count is the single most important predictor of bleeding. Where the platelet count is low or there is a coagulopathy there is a predisposition to minor vascular bleeding from

Case study 14.1

John, a 48-year-old man, had been recently diagnosed with acute myeloid leukaemia. One evening towards the end of his induction chemotherapy he spiked a temperature of 38.5°C. John was seen by the doctor, a full infection screen was performed and antibiotics were commenced intravenously. That morning John's platelet count had been $30 \times 10^9/L$. During the night John's condition deteriorated. He became tachycardic, mildly breathless and was pale and clammy. The doctor was asked to see John again; while he was being examined, John complained of feeling nauseous. He had a massive haematemesis and, despite vigorous resuscitation efforts with transfusions of platelets, whole blood and fresh frozen plasma (FFP), died later that night. Analysis of a blood sample taken shortly before John's haematemesis showed a platelet count of $2 \times 10^9/L$.

the mouth, nose or any cutaneous lesion (Buschel & Bakitas Whedon, 1995). Nursing care should be aimed at reducing the potential for bleeding and management of bleeding when it occurs.

An awareness of the factors which increase the bleeding tendency is necessary along with prompt recognition and management of signs of bleeding. Care should be taken to prevent injury and avoid any procedures which may cause trauma. Individuals should be advised on oral care to prevent injury (see Ch. 16). Where the oral mucosa and vascular integrity may be further altered by infection this should be promptly treated by antimicrobial therapy, as prevention and treatment of infection is essential in minimising the potential for bleeding (Groenwald et al 1997).

Ingestion of aspirin-based or non-steroidal anti-inflammatory drugs (NSAIDs) should be advised against. Males should also be advised to use an electric razor for shaving and females are usually commenced on progesterone preparations such as norethisterone to suppress menstruation. Invasive procedures such as intramuscular and subcutaneous injections, and the administration of enemas and suppositories, should be avoided. Pressure should be applied to venepuncture sites for several minutes. If patients are bed-bound, care should be taken to avoid pressure damage to the skin.

Reflection point

Consider the information you give to patients and their relatives about preventing and recognising bleeding. Could this information be improved in any way?

Nurses should be constantly vigilant for signs of bleeding, and individuals and their families should be educated to recognise signs of bleeding and to report these promptly. The skin should be closely observed for bruising and petechiae, and any changes in the colour of urine or stools should be reported promptly (Plate 10 demonstrates severe bruising in thrombocytopenia).

Small bleeds can usually be managed by the application of pressure, topical clotting preparations, or the administration of blood products such as platelets or fresh frozen plasma (FFP) (see Ch. 11). However, epistaxis can be severe and nasal packing may be required. The following topical products have been used effectively in clinical practice but (with the exception of calcium alginate) more work is needed to prove their efficacy in clinical trials:

- local application of tranexamic acid
- vasoconstrictive agents – cocaine, adrenaline (epinephrine)
- ice crystals
- calcium alginate (Milford et al 1991).

Bleeding episodes, however small, can be extremely frightening for patients and their families and the value of good communication and support cannot be overemphasised.

In thrombocytopenia, platelet transfusions may be given prophylactically to reduce the bleeding potential (see Ch. 11).

Major upper gastrointestinal haemorrhage

Devastating upper gastrointestinal (UGI) haemorrhage can be caused by the presence of pre-existing lesions or ulcers, as the result of endothelial damage from chemotherapy or radiotherapy, GI tract infection, graft versus host disease (GVHD), or stress ulceration as the result of a critical illness (Buschel & Bakitas Whedon 1995).

One of the challenges to management of a UGI bleed is that even in severe cases there may be relatively few symptoms or clinical signs (Groeger 1991). If a transplant recipient has become shocked with haemodynamic changes suggestive of bleeding (e.g. tachycardia, lowered mean arterial pressure, sweating, pallor) then a UGI bleed should be suspected and eliminated. The cardinal signs of a UGI haemorrhage are melaena and, less commonly, haematemesis (Groeger 1991).

Investigations

- full blood count (FBC)
- clotting profile
- early endoscopic evaluation.

It should be noted that with advances in endoscopic procedures, especially with flexible videoscopic techniques, trauma to the vulnerable client is reduced; however, the procedure may still be avoided in the presence of a profound neutropenia.

The advantages of an early endoscopy are that secondary bleeds may be avoided and that discrete bleeding points may be identified (Crifiths et al 1979).

Treatment

As in all other haemorrhagic situations, if the patient is known/suspected to be actively bleeding, efforts should be directed at achieving cardiovascular stability and improving platelet numbers or clotting deficiencies.

Endoscopic treatment

If discrete bleeding points/lesions are identified, the following therapeutic options can be administered endoscopically:

- sclerosis with adrenaline (Edmunds & Laurence 1988)
- electrocoagulation (Laine 1987)
- laser photocoagulation (Laurence et al 1980).

Pharmacological therapies

Pharmacological therapies are divided into the prophylactic agents used largely to reduce gastric acid and maintain the intragastric pH at 7 or above and agents used during an acute bleed.

PREVENTATIVE STRATEGIES The following therapies have been shown in clinical trials to be useful in the prevention of UGI haemorrhage:

- cimetidine (Priebe et al 1988)
- ranitidine
- sucralfate
- omeprazole.

It should be noted that there are some trial data to show that cimetidine and ranitidine may inhibit platelet recovery in the thrombocytopenic patient (Mehta 1994). Their use should therefore be avoided during the transplant period.

PHARMACOLOGICAL THERAPIES DURING AN ACUTE BLEED *Vasopressin* has been shown in clinical trials to reduce the severity or longevity of an acute bleed. It can be used intravenously and should be given a brief therapeutic trial with careful haemodynamic monitoring, as the resulting vasoconstriction can cause cardiac arrhythmias.

These have been shown to reduce if coupled with an infusion of nitroglycerin (Gimson et al 1986).

Protamine sulphate, given intravenously, has been shown to reduce acute severe bleeding. Protamine sulphate can also cause cardiovascular (CVS) problems, particularly the lowering of mean arterial pressure; it is therefore essential that the drug is only used where continuous CVS monitoring is available.

Embolic therapy

If the client cannot undergo major surgery, embolisation of the artery supplying the UGI bleeding focus may be considered (Groeger 1991). This procedure is performed during arteriography by the injection of small pieces of gelatin sponge or an autologous clot through the catheter. There are obvious risks associated with this procedure and it can only be performed in a facility with the necessary expertise and equipment.

Formal laparotomy

If none of the above measures is possible, a formal laparotomy may be considered. Most individuals with a haematological malignancy, especially transplant recipients, present a severe perioperative risk because of their thrombocytopenia and or clotting abnormalities; they may also have concomitant problems, such as infection and reduced pulmonary or renal function (see Ch. 10). However, in some instances, where there seems to be no other choice, laparotomies have been performed successfully. In these situations, a consultant anaesthetist experienced in the care of immunocompromised patients should be present (Audit Commission 1997). Haematology experts will need to advise and provide appropriate blood product support for the operation. It is essential that immediate postoperative care is provided in a high-dependency area as this is a high-risk intervention.

Major lower GI bleeding

Bleeding from the lower gastrointestinal (LGI) tract may be caused by ischaemic ulceration, pseudomembranous colitis, or severe infection. When a client has received many antimicrobial agents there is a tendency to develop one of the multiresistant organisms such as methicillin-resistant *Staphylococcus aureus* (MRSA) or vancomycin-resistant *Enterococcus* (VRE); in the presence of bone marrow failure these infections may lead to bowel obstruction, severe infection leading to a translocation septicaemia and subsequent major bleeding (Mower et al 1986). Furthermore, typhilitis (inflammation of the caecum) probably occurs in about 10% of clients with leukaemia who are receiving acute anticancer therapy (Steinberg et al 1973).

Investigations

- FBC
- clotting profile
- plain X-ray of the abdomen
- computerised tomography (CT scan) of abdomen.

Treatment

As referred to earlier in the chapter, an important part of therapy is rapid aggressive treatment of infection. Although many patients have few symptoms, pain is frequently reported and should be adequately controlled using the World Health Organization (WHO) pain ladder as a guide to the use of appropriate analgesia (WHO 1990).

Angiography can be used, with administration of vasoconstrictive substances as described earlier. In the presence of severe LGI haemorrhage, a colonoscopy is a very difficult procedure and should only be attempted briefly.

Aggressive attempts should be made to control bleeding by the transfusion of platelets, packed red blood cells and clotting factors. Most acute massive bleeds from the LGI tract stop spontaneously with transfusion support: once the patient has been stabilised, further attempts should be directed at treating the cause of the bleed and preventing further occurrence. LGI surgery will only be used in the thrombocytopenic transplant recipient as a last resort and is reserved for bleeding which is continuous or massive in scale (Boley & Brandt 1986).

Haemorrhagic cystitis

Haemorrhagic cystitis (HC) is usually diagnosed early in the period after transplant when there are signs of engraftment but it may also arise acutely during conditioning therapy (Treleaven & Barrett 1996). HC is thought to be caused by acrolein, which is a metabolite of cyclophosphamide that causes ulceration and vasculitis of the bladder mucosa (Buschel & Bakitas Whedon 1995). Although cyclophosphamide is thought to be the major cause of HC, several other causative agents have been reported, including

- radiation (Goldstein et al 1968)
- busulphan (Millard 1981)
- doxorubicin (Ershler 1980)
- cytosine arabinoside
- etoposide (Blume et al 1987)
- acute and chronic GVHD (Ost et al 1987)
- adenovirus (Miyamura et al 1987)
- BK virus (Rice et al 1985).

The symptoms of HC are mild-to-severe pain which tends to be spasmodic in character, the worst pain often accompanying the passing of a blood clot.

Treatment

Preventative strategies are very important and consist of aggressive hydration and the administration of intravenous 2-mercaptoethane sulphonate sodium (mesna) during the period that cyclophosphamide is being given. Mesna is thought to work by forming an inactive complex with acrolein, it is widely reported in the literature to be very effective in the prevention of HC (Link et al 1981, Blacklock et al 1983).

If haemorrhagic cystitis occurs, good pain control is essential, as is careful monitoring of urea and electrolytes to observe for any sign of acute renal failure. Particular attention should be given to fluid balance, noting any reduction in urine output or signs of clot retention. If there is any sign of urinary retention, a triple-lumen urinary catheter should be inserted to allow continuous bladder irrigation. Bladder irrigation should be titrated until the urine flow is 'rose' coloured and may have to be continued for several days.

Full blood count and clotting profile should be carefully monitored, and if there is severe haemorrhage it is imperative that advice and support is sought from urological experts. In the rare circumstance that all other therapies fail, surgical intervention may be necessary (Andriole et al 1990).

Central nervous system haemorrhage

A bleed anywhere in the central nervous system (CNS) may represent a clinical catastrophe. It is therefore essential to implement preventative strategies if there is any suspicion of a CNS bleed. Preventative measures include

- prophylactic platelets and clotting factor transfusion prior to any invasive procedure such as lumbar puncture or where there is any suspicion of cerebral injury.
- pharmacological measures to prevent fitting during the pancytopenic period. This is particularly important where patients are likely to become prone to infection, severe fluid

shifts or where chemotherapy such as cyclophosphamide may cause cerebral irritation. In these cases patients should be treated with prophylactic antiepileptic drugs such as sodium valproate.

A major CNS bleed is fortunately rare, with infection, drug toxicity or disease being more common reasons for CNS disturbance (Treleaven & Barrett 1996). However, if there are changes in consciousness level or deterioration in the Glasgow coma scale, CNS haemorrhage must be excluded.

Treatment

Therapy for a major CNS bleed will depend upon the condition of the bone marrow and the clotting profile. In the presence of thrombocytopenia it is essential to transfuse platelets and carefully monitor consciousness levels using the Glasgow coma scale. Any deterioration in condition should be reported to medical colleagues immediately, as this may represent an acute rise in intracranial pressure (ICP). A sudden rise in ICP may be treated with diuretic therapy such as a mannitol infusion.

Surgical intervention such as an exploratory or decompressive craniotomy may be required but the possibility of surgery will depend on the level of thrombocytopenia.

PLATELET DYSFUNCTION

Platelet function may be affected by the effects of abnormal immunoglobulins in conditions such as myeloma (see Ch. 5).

EROSION OF BLOOD VESSELS

Erosion of blood vessels may occur as a result of tumour invasion or erosion due to infective processes and can result in rapidly catastrophic haemorrhage.

COAGULATION DISORDERS

A number of coagulation factor deficiences may occur with haematological malignancies. This may be more pronounced at the commencement of chemotherapy when there is rapid tumour lysis or at relapse where there is a large tumour burden (Rao & Rapaport 1987). DIC is probably the most commonly reported coagulation disorder.

Disseminated intravascular coagulation

DIC is a condition that results from a severe insult to the body and is always a secondary condition (Groeger 1991). It is characterised by the formation of microthrombi, activation of the fibrinolytic system, consumption of clotting factors and a variable degree of bleeding diathesis (Francis 1995). DIC can cause fulminant bleeding but also end-organ failure from the widespread thrombotic damage. DIC has been reported after a number of conditions, but the major causes in the haemato-oncology population are severe sepsis and acute promyelocytic leukaemia.

Aetiology of DIC with malignancy

Many types of malignant tumour express tissue factor (TF) on the surface of circulating monocytes (Rao 1992). In the patient with leukaemia, particularly acute promyelocytic leukaemia, TF seems to be released from the granules of the malignant promyelocytes (Gralnick & Abrell 1973). TF interacts with factor VII and there is a resultant formation of thrombin and deposition of fibrin. Platelets and blood coagulation factors are consumed during this process (Groeger 1991). The large mass of tumour cells in the leukaemic patient may result in a very aggressive DIC. A sudden release of TF from dying malignant cells accounts for the acute onset of DIC that is sometimes seen as chemotherapy begins. Early mortality rates due to haemorrhage in acute promyelocytic leukaemia have been reported to be between 10 and 20% (Rodeghiero et al 1990, Tallman & Kwaan 1992).

Aetiology of DIC with sepsis

In sepsis there are many ways that the haemostatic mechanism may be altered:

■ Stasis of blood can occur in any severe shock state, resulting in accumulation of activated clotting factors (Garcia-Barreno et al 1978).

- The acidosis associated with sepsis causes platelet numbers to fall and a decrease in fibrinogen with a prolonged prothrombin time (PT) and partial prothrombin time (PTT) (Dunn et al 1979).
- Bacteria may secrete the lipopolysaccharide endotoxin, activating the clotting mechanism. The secretion of endotoxin results in release of TF and factor VII, vascular injury, activation of platelets and Hageman factor, kinin generation, and complement activation (Leon et al 1982).
- Bacterial interaction with normal tissue may cause tissue breakdown and necrosis with resultant TF release.
- Factor XII activation, platelet aggregation and thrombocytopenia may result from the generation of antigen–antibody complexes (Rothberger et al 1977).

The mortality rate for DIC following severe sepsis in the haematology setting may be as high as 70–80% (Oh 1995).

Investigations

The clinical picture of DIC may be difficult to differentiate from the bleeding associated with general marrow failure; however, together with the history, the following laboratory tests will be diagnostic:

- PT
- activated partial thromboplastin time (aPTT)
- thrombin time (TT)
- platelet count
- fibrinogen assay
- antithrombin.

The major clotting defect found in acute DIC is a very low or absent fibrinogen level. The PT and aPTT are usually abnormal and often very prolonged. Fibrinogen degradation products (FDP) are also raised (Gross & Roath 1996).

Treatment

As DIC is always a secondary phenomenon and a complication of an underlying disease

process or trigger, the key to successful treatment is to eradicate the trigger, which will mean aggressive anticancer or antimicrobial therapy.

The next phase of treatment is designed to halt the process of intravascular coagulation. The administration of low-dose heparin has been shown to be beneficial (Bick 1993). However, its use in promyelocytic leukaemia is controversial. Antithrombin III concentrates may also be useful, and research continues in this area (Hanada et al 1985).

In the presence of acute promyelocytic leukaemia, all-*trans* retinoic acid (ATRA or tretinoin) may be a useful therapy. ATRA aids the development of promyelocytes into mature cells and has a direct effect on the TF synthesis of abnormal or dying malignant cells (Rickles et al 1993, Barbui et al 1998) and may therefore slow down or prevent the onset of DIC. ATRA is administered to individuals prior to the commencement of chemotherapy to induce remission and reduce the likelihood of DIC. Currently, study results vary in relation to the effect of ATRA on bleeding in promyelocytic leukaemia. Some studies have shown a reduction in early mortality from bleeding (Di Bona et al 1997) and shorter duration of coagulopathy (Fenaux et al 1993). Yet, statistical differences in the incidence of early fatal haemorrhage have not always been found (Fenaux et al 1993, Tallman et al 1997). However, it is noted that statistical differences in the number of haemorrhagic deaths are difficult to confirm due to the rareness of the disease (Barbui et al 1998).

In the presence of overt bleeding in DIC, transfusions of concentrated red cells, platelets and plasma volume expanders are given (Gross & Roath 1996). The prognosis from a fulminant DIC will depend very much on the efficacy of interventions for the primary disease.

Reflection point

In your area of practice what measures are utilised to prevent haemorrhagic problems?

CONCLUSION

As in many other areas of haematology nursing the emphasis on care with regard to haemorrhagic problems is on prevention, monitoring and rapid intervention. During the disease trajectory the 'bleeding risk' will alter and the interdisciplinary team needs to be informed and prepared for any of the clinical situations presented in this chapter. Some of the haemorrhagic risks will continue into the post-transplant setting and it is therefore essential that education and training is also provided for the patient/family, and the primary health care team in the community or referring unit.

With improvements in blood product support, non-invasive diagnostic facilities and relevant pharmacological therapy haemorrhage-associated morbidity and mortality has diminished. The haematology nurse is the key to good liaison in the interdisciplinary team that will ensure all clients have access to the highest standards of evidence-based practice.

DISCUSSION QUESTIONS

1. An individual has had a Hickman line inserted today and is bleeding from the exit site. What measures would you take to arrest the bleeding?
2. An elderly gentleman with myelodysplasia tells you that he takes an aspirin a day for his angina. What advice would you give him?

References

Andriole G L, Yuan J J, Catalona W J 1990 Cystotomy, temporary urinary diversion and bladder packing in the management of severe cyclophosphamide-induced haemorrhagic cystitis. Journal of Urology 143: 1006–1007

Audit Commission 1997 Anaesthesia and analgesia, The Audit Commission for Local Authorities and the National Health Service in England and Wales. Belmont Press, UK

Barbui T, Finazzi G, Falanga A 1998 The impact of all-trans-retinoic acid on the coagulopathy of acute promyelocytic leukaemia. Blood 91(9): 3093–3102

Bick R L 1993 Disseminated intravascular coagulation and related syndromes. In: Bennett J M et al (eds) Haematology, clinical and laboratory practice. Mosby–Year Book, St. Louis

Blacklock H, Ball L, Knight C, Schey S, Prentice G 1983 Experience with mesna in patients receiving bone marrow transplants for poor prognostic leukaemia. Cancer Treatment Reviews 10(suppl A): 45–52

Blume K, Forman S, O'Donnell M R 1987 Total body irradiation and high-dose etoposide: a new preparatory regimen for bone marrow transplantation in patients with advanced haematological malignancies. Blood 69: 1015–1020

Boley S J, Brandt L J 1986 Vascular ectasias of the colon. Digest of Dissertation in Science 31: 265–271

Buchsel P, Bakitas Whedon M 1995 Bone marrow transplantation: administrative and clinical strategies. Jones and Bartlett, Boston

Caudell K A, Bakitas Whedon M B 1991 Haematopoietic complications in bone marrow transplantation In: Bakitas Whedon M (ed) Bone marrow transplantation: principles, practice, and nursing insights. Jones and Bartlett, Boston, pp 136–159

Crifiths W J, Neumann D A, Welsh J D 1979 The visible vessel as an indicator of uncontrolled or recurrent gastrointestinal haemorrhage. New England Journal of Medicine 300: 1411–1415

Di Bona E, Castaman G, Avvisati G et al for the GIMEMA Group 1997 Hemostasis related early morbidity and mortality during remission induction treatment with or without all-trans-retinoic acid (ATRA) in acute promyelocytic leukemia. Blood 90 (Abstr Suppl 1): 331a

Dunn E L, Moore E E, Breslich D L, Colley P S 1979 Acidosis induced coagulopathy. Surgical Forum 30: 471–475

Edmunds S E J, Laurence B H 1988 Endoscopic sclerotherapy in nonvariceal GI bleeding. Journal of Gastroenterology and Hepatology 3: 355–361

Ershler W B 1980 Adriamycin enhancement of cyclophosphamide induced bladder injury. Journal of Urology 123: 121–122

Fenaux P, Le Deley M C, Castagine S et al (the European APL 91

Group) 1993 Effect of all-trans-retinoic acid in newly diagnosed acute promyelocytic leukaemia, results of a multicenter randomized trial. Blood 82: 3241–3249

Garcia-Barreno P, Balibrea J L, Aparicia P 1978 Blood coagulation changes in shock. Surgery, Gynaecology, Obstetrics 147(1): 6–12

Gimson A E, Westaby D, Hegarty J, Watson A, Williams R 1986 A randomised trial of vasopressin and vasopressin plus nitroglycerin in the control of acute variceal haemorrhage. Hepatology 6: 410–413

Goldstein A G, D'Escrivon J C, Allen S D 1968 Haemorrhagic radiation cystitis. British Journal of Urology 40: 758–763

Gralnick H R, Abrell E 1973 Studies of the procoagulant and fibrinolytic activity of promyelocytes in acute promyelocytic leukaemia. British Journal of Haematology 24: 89–93

Groeger J S 1991 Critical care of the cancer patient. Mosby–Year Book, St. Louis

Groenwald S L, Frogge M H, Goodman M, Yarbro C H 1997 Cancer nursing: principles and practice, 4th edn. Jones and Bartlett, Boston

Gross S, Roath S 1996 Haematology: a problem orientated approach. Williams & Wilkins, Baltimore

Hanada T, Abe T, Takita H 1985 Antithrombin III concentrates for treatment of disseminated intravascular coagulation in children. American Journal of Paediatric Haematology and Oncology 7: 3–13

Hughes-Jones N C, Wickramasinghe S N 1991 Lecture notes on haematology, 5th edn. Blackwell, Oxford

Laine L 1987 Multipolar electro-coagulation in the treatment of active upper GI tract haemorrhage: a prospective controlled trial. New England Journal of Medicine 316: 1613–1621

Laurence B H, Vallon A C, Cotton P B et al 1980 Endoscopic laser photocoagulation for bleeding peptic ulcer. Lancet 1: 124–130

Leon C, Rodrigo M J, Tomasa A et al 1982 Complement activation in septic shock due to Gram-negative and Gram-positive bacteria. Critical Care Medicine 10: 308–310

Link H, Neef V, Niethammer D, Wilms K 1981 Prophylaxis of haemorrhagic cystitis due to cyclophosphamide conditioning for bone marrow transplantation. Blut 43: 329–330

Mehta J 1994 Platelet inhibition following transplant. Leukaemia and Lymphoma 13: 179–181

Milford C A, Bleach N R, Sudderick R M, O'Flynn P E, Mugliston T A 1991 Calcium alginate as a nasal pack. Revue de Laryngologie, Otologie Rhinologie 112(3): 261–263

Millard R J 1981 Busulphan-induced haemorrhagic cystitis. Urology 18: 143–144

Mower W J, Hawkins J A, Nelson E W 1986 Neutropenic enterocolitis in adults with acute leukaemia. Archives of Surgery 121: 571–581

Miyamura K, Minami S, Matsuyama T et al 1987 Adenovirus-induced late onset haemorrhagic cystitis following allogeneic bone marrow transplantation. Bone Marrow Transplantation 2: 109–110

Oh T E 1995 Intensive care manual. Butterworths, Sydney

Ost L, Lonnquist B, Eriksson L, Ljungman P, Ringden O 1987

Haemorrhagic cystitis – a manifestation of graft versus host disease? Bone Marrow Transplantation 2: 19–25

Priebe H J, Skillman J J, Bushnell L S, Long P C, Silen W 1988 Antacid versus cimetidine in preventing acute gastrointestinal bleeding: a randomised trial in 75 critically ill patients. New England Journal of Medicine 302: 426–430

Rao L V M 1992 Tissue factor as a tumour procoagulant. Cancer Metastatic Review 11: 249–251

Rao L V M, Rapaport S I 1987 Studies of a mechanism inhibiting the initiation of the extrinsic pathway of coagulation. Blood 69(2): 645–651

Rice S J, Bishop J, Apperley J, Gardner S D 1985 BK virus as cause of haemorrhagic cystitis after bone marrow transplantation. Lancet 2: 844–845

Rickles F R et al 1993 All-trans retinoic acid (ATRA) inhibits the expression of tissue factor in human progranulocytic leukaemia. Thrombosis and Haemostasis 69: 107–110

Rodeghiero F, Avvisati G, Castaman G, Barbui T, Mandelli F 1990 Early deaths and anti-hemorrhagic treatments in acute promyelocytic leukemia – a GIMEMA retrospective study in 268 consecutive patients. Blood 75(11): 2112–2117

Rothberger R, Zimmerman T S, Spiegelberg H L, Vaughan J H 1977 Leucocyte procoagulant activity: enhancement of production in vitro by IgC and antigen–antibody complexes. Journal of Clinical Investigations 59: 549–557

Sarzotti H, Baron S, Klingboll G R 1978 Metastases in spleen and bone marrow suppresses the NK activity generated in the organs. International Journal of Cancer 39: 117–125

Sattler F R, Weitekamp M R, Ballard J O 1986 Potential for bleeding with the new beta-lactam antibiotics. Annals of Internal Medicine 105: 924–931

Steinberg D, Cold J, Brodin A 1973 Necrotising enterocolitis in leukaemia. Archives of Internal Medicine 131: 538–540

Tallman M S, Kwaan H C 1992 Reassessing the hemostatic disorder associated with acute promyelo-cytic leukaemia. Blood 79(3): 543–553

Tallman M S, Anderson J W, Schiffer C A et al 1997 All-trans-retinoic acid in acute promyelocytic leukamia. New England Journal of Medicine 337(15): 1021–1028

Treleaven J, Barrett J 1996 Bone marrow transplantation in practice. Churchill Livingstone, Edinburgh

World Health Organization 1990 Cancer pain relief and palliative care. WHO Technical Report Series, 804. WHO, Geneva

Nausea and vomiting

JAN HAWTHORN

Key points
- Nausea and vomiting are the most distressing side-effects of chemotherapy and radiotherapy
- Therapeutic agents and non-pharmacological supportive techniques are available to prevent or treat nausea and vomiting
- Nursing interventions aim to minimise the distress caused to patients by these unpleasant side-effects

INTRODUCTION

For patients, nausea and vomiting are the most distressing aspects of cancer treatments (Coates et al 1983). Despite the age of this reference and the advances in anti-emetic treatment, nausea and vomiting remain problematic for a significant number of patients (Osoba et al 1997). They may cause a variety of debilitating medical problems such as dehydration or poor nutrition and can lead to low morale, depression and poor compliance with treatment. Patients with haematological malignancies are often given aggressive and highly emetogenic chemotherapy regimens; those undergoing bone marrow transplantation (BMT) will receive toxic chemotherapy and/or total body irradiation on consecutive days. Poor anti-emetic control adds to the burden of such treatment and can make the whole experience even more distressing. It is important, therefore, that nurses take an active role in prevention of these untoward side-effects in vulnerable patients. This chapter seeks to outline what we know about the process of nausea and vomiting and to investigate appropriate treatments – both pharmacological and supportive – for chemotherapy- or radiotherapy-induced vomiting. Nursing interventions to minimise the risk of vomiting occurring and to ameliorate symptoms are also discussed.

WHY DO CHEMOTHERAPY OR RADIOTHERAPY CAUSE NAUSEA AND VOMITING?

Vomiting is essentially a protective mechanism to remove ingested poisons. Although chemotherapy is given for therapeutic purposes it is still essentially a 'poison' and hence it will activate the vomiting response.

Receptors in the gastrointestinal tract and a specialised area of the brain called the chemoreceptor trigger zone (CTZ) detect the presence of noxious substances in the gut, the blood or cerebrospinal fluid. Despite the name, the CTZ is thought to be less involved than the gut in chemotherapy-induced vomiting. Once these receptors are stimulated, signals are relayed to a region of the brain stem, the 'vomiting centre' which interprets the incoming message and coordinates the responses that lead to nausea and vomiting.

THE PROCESS OF NAUSEA AND VOMITING

Feelings of nausea are probably due to changes in the gut, especially the stomach, which stops its usual rhythmic squeezing movements and becomes flaccid and quiescent. The nauseated individual usually appears pale, cold and clammy, may be sweating, have tachycardia, and will be producing a lot of saliva.

Nausea is followed by retching – rhythmic movements of the respiratory and abdominal muscles (probably serving to move the stomach contents to the correct position to be expelled) – which usually culminates in vomiting, which is the active expulsion of the stomach contents through the mouth. The epiglottis moves to prevent stomach contents entering the airways. Sometimes, for example after eating contaminated food, vomiting brings immediate relief of the nausea. For the chemotherapy patient this is often not the case and nausea may persist unabated, in spite of actively vomiting, for several hours; such nausea is often more distressing to the individual than vomiting itself.

Risk of vomiting after treatment

Not every patient will be sick after cancer treatment. For chemotherapy, which is generally more emetic than radiotherapy, the most influential factor on the risk of vomiting is the drugs used. Table 15.1 lists the common chemotherapeutic drugs in classes of emetic potential. This table is only a guide; the dose and route of administration of drugs can alter their emetogenicity and combination therapy of several chemotherapeutic agents can enhance overall emetic potential.

Delayed emesis

After highly emetogenic chemotherapy the nausea and vomiting produced can continue for several days; this 'delayed emesis' can have a major impact on patients' morale and quality of life. Unfortunately, it does not respond so well to anti-emetics as acute symptoms but it is still important to maintain anti-emetic cover, particularly for vulnerable patients, in the 3–5 days following treatment.

Predisposing factors

Individuals also vary in responses to therapy. The factors which predict a greater emetic

Table 15.1 Emetic potential of cytotoxic drugs used in haemato-oncology (adapted from Lindley et al 1989, Merrifield & Chaffee 1989, Hesketh et al 1995, Allwood et al 1997)

Frequency of emesis	Agent
<10%	Vincristine Bleomycin Fludarabine 2-Chlorodeoxyadenosine 6-Thioguanine (po) Chlorambucil (po) Cyclophosphamide (po) Busulphan
10–30%	Methotrexate $< 250\,\text{mg/m}^2$ Mitomycin Vinblastine Vinorelbine Bleomycin Etoposide Mercaptopurine Melphalan Hydroxyurea
30–60%	Methotrexate 250–$1000\,\text{mg/m}^2$ Cyclophosphamide $\leqslant 750\,\text{mg/m}^2$ Doxorubicin 20–$60\,\text{mg/m}^2$ Mitozantrone Daunorubicin Idarubicin Ifosfamide
60–90%	Dacarbazine Cyclophosphamide $> 750 \leqslant 1500\,\text{mg/m}^2$ Doxorubicin $60\,\text{mg/m}^2$ Procarbazine (po) Amsacrine Methotrexate $> 1000\,\text{mg/m}^2$ Carmustine $\leqslant 250\,\text{mg/m}^2$ Cytarabine $> 1\,\text{g/m}^2$
>90%	Cyclophosphamide $> 1500\,\text{mg/m}^2$ Carmustine $> 250\,\text{mg/m}^2$ Streptozotocin Mechlorethamine

response to chemotherapy are

■ gender – women are more easily sick than men (Zook & Yasko 1983, Roila et al 1988)

- age – younger patients are more susceptible (Roila et al 1988, 1989)
- anxiety – anxiety exacerbates post-treatment symptoms (Andrykowski & Gregg 1992)
- course of treatment – emesis is more easily controlled following the first dose of chemotherapy or radiotherapy (Gralla et al 1981, Roila et al 1989)
- alcohol intake – a history of high alcohol intake reduces the likelihood of suffering nausea and vomiting after chemotherapy (D'Aquisto et al 1986)
- treatment setting – anti-emetic control is less efficient in outpatient settings than in hospital (Roila et al 1989).

Factors predicting a greater response to radiotherapy (Priestman 1988) are

- field size – the greater the field the more emesis
- site of irradiation – the abdomen is the most susceptible site; cranial or spinal irradiation for CNS involvement in acute lymphatic leukaemia (ALL) is also emetogenic; irradiation of the limbs rarely causes nausea and vomiting
- dose per fraction – higher dose rates cause more emesis
- age – children experience less sickness than adults
- anxiety – more anxious patients vomit more.

 Reflection point

What factors would alert you to check appropriate anti-emetics have been prescribed for an individual due to commence chemotherapy? Would you look for the same characteristics in someone due to commence radiotherapy?

Anticipatory nausea and vomiting

If patients have severe nausea and vomiting after treatment they can develop anticipatory symptoms, where certain elements of the treatment or surroundings become 'cues' that make them feel nauseous or actually vomit. Common cues are the treatment nurse or sight or smell of the hospital. Anticipatory symptoms can develop after only one pulse of chemotherapy, although it is more common after three or four pulses.

This phenomenon can remain with the patient for many years after treatment has ceased and anticipatory symptoms respond poorly to anti-emetics. It is important, therefore, to prevent emetic symptoms as much as possible from the outset of treatment and in particular to identify especially vulnerable patients who may need more potent anti-emetics. If anti-emetic control is efficient, anticipatory symptoms do not have the opportunity to become established.

TREATMENT OF NAUSEA AND VOMITING

Pharmacological

There are several anti-emetic drugs available to control nausea and vomiting induced by chemotherapy or radiotherapy (Table 15.2). The anti-emetic must be tailored to the type of treatment being given, and to the susceptibility of the individual patient. A crucial point to remember is that although nausea and vomiting can be treated it is usually better to adopt a prophylactic approach and give anti-emetics before treatment. Sedatives are often added to reduce anxiety, and may be all that is required by patients receiving drugs of a very low emetogenic potential.

The last decade has seen the introduction of a new class of anti-emetic drug – the 5-HT$_3$ receptor (the 3-receptor for 5-hydroxytryptamine on which drugs act) antagonist. These are probably the most potent single agent anti-emetics available for chemotherapy- and radiotherapy-induced emesis. They cost more than many other anti-emetics but are not more expensive when their superior efficacy and the savings on hospital costs (laundry, nursing time, etc.) are considered (Cunningham et al 1993, Goddard 1993). However, during the delayed phase of emesis produced by highly emetogenic chemotherapy, there is little difference in efficacy between these drugs and the combination of metoclopramide and dexamethasone (Jones et al 1992).

Table 15.2 Common anti-emetic regimens for chemotherapy or radiotherapy

Emetic potential of chemotherapy	Acute emesis	Delayed emesis
Very low	Lorazepam 1–2 mg po bd/tds	
Low	Prochlorperazine 12.5–25 mg iv q3–6 h	
	Metoclopramide 5–10 mg po tds	Dexamethasone 4 mg tds po for 3 days
Medium	Metoclopramide 30–100 mg iv + dexamethasone 4–8 mg iv	Metoclopramide 20 mg qds for 3 days + dexamethasone 4 mg tds po for 2 days
	Ondansetron 8 mg po bd	
	Granisetron 1 mg × 2 po or 2 mg po	
	Tropisetron 5 mg iv/po	
High/very high	Ondansetron 8 mg iv before chemo* then 8 mg iv × 2 2–4 hours apart or 32 mg iv	Ondansetron 8 mg po bd up to 5 days
	Granisetron 3 mg iv before chemo* repeated at 10 min interval up to 9 mg in 24 h	
	Tropisetron 5 mg iv before chemo*	Tropisetron 5 mg po up to 5 days
	*Add dexamethasone 8–20 mg for highly emetogenic chemo or high-risk subject	
	Metoclopramide 2 mg/kg q 2–4 h + dexamethasone 8 mg iv + lorazepam 1–2 mg	Metoclopramide 20 mg qds for 3 days + dexamethasone 4 mg tds po for 2 days
Radiotherapy		
Fractionated	Metoclopramide 10–20 mg q 6 h	
	Domperidone 20 mg po q 6 h	
	Ondansetron 8 mg po q 8 h	
TBI	Dexamethasone 6 mg iv 30 min prior to irradiation + ondansetron 6 mg iv	

This information is taken from the literature. The manufacturer's data sheet should always be consulted for full information.
NB. Anti-emetic regimens containing dexamethasone are not used for individuals receiving high-dose steroids as part of their cytotoxic regimen.
Abbreviations: bd, twice a day; chemo, chemotherapy; iv, intravenous; po, per oral; q, every; tds, three times a day; qds, four times a day.

Frequently a combination of anti-emetics is used to increase efficacy. Notable is the addition of dexamethasone, which increases the potency of most anti-emetics. Just how this steroid works is not known for certain. It is not used in patients where chemotherapy already involves high doses of steroids such as prednisolone, for example in ALL. It must be injected slowly to avoid perineal itching, burning or scrotal pain.

Side-effects of anti-emetics

A common problem with many anti-emetics is extrapyramidal reactions (EPRs). These are caused by dopamine receptor antagonists and consist of restlessness, akathisia (involuntary shaking of the limbs), torticollis (spasms of neck and facial muscles giving rise to twisting of the head) and oculogyric crises (spasm of the muscles causing eyeball movement). EPRs are possible side-effects of haloperidol, droperidol, prochlorperazine, chlorpromazine and high-dose metoclopramide. More common in younger patients and especially children, they are dose-related (Bateman et al 1989) and may be treated with benztropine, benzhexol or procyclidine. A better tactic may be to avoid dopamine receptor antagonists where possible, by using for example a 5-HT$_3$ receptor antagonist.

Non-pharmacological

Since anxiety exacerbates emetic symptoms any intervention that promotes relaxation can have a beneficial effect on emetic symptoms. Useful techniques are

- relaxation
- progressive muscle relaxation technique (PMRT)
- hypnosis
- guided imagery
- systematic desensitisation
- therapeutic touch
- aromatherapy and massage.

The basis of many of these techniques is relaxation. Relaxation may be induced by placing the subjects in a soothing environment, playing gentle background music or using a commentary (a complete script is given in Copley Cobb 1984). A more definite image may be introduced by using guided imagery. The therapist 'paints' a scene verbally so that the subject can visualise it in some detail; a simple cue can then allow the image to be recalled at a later date to aid relaxation (see Donovan 1980 for a complete script). In PMRT, patients are taught to tense the entire body and, moving slowly from feet upwards, they actively relax each section of their body. Aromatherapy and massage both involve physical contact with the nurse or therapist. Touching can be important in reducing anxiety and opening up lines of communication (Byass 1988), and by 'formalising' such contact it can be carried out without invasion of an individual's personal space. Even where formal relaxation procedures are not employed a calm and soothing approach from the nurse can do much to help patients.

Generally speaking these techniques alone cannot control nausea and vomiting. However, they do make a valuable contribution to patient comfort and well-being; patients receiving supportive interventions have reported feeling more unafraid, in control, hopeful, powerful and relaxed (Troesch et al 1993).

Acupressure

Another supportive technique for controlling nausea and vomiting is acupuncture or more usually acupressure (pressing the acupuncture point rather than inserting a needle). The acupressure point for emesis, the Nei-Kuan point, is on the inside of the wrist, three finger widths above the crease of the wrist joint between the two visible tendons. This point can be pressed either with a finger or a wrist band containing a small plastic stud positioned over the acupressure point. Clinical trials have shown some benefit for acupressure (Dundee et al 1989, Sadler 1989, Stannard 1989, Dundee & Yang 1990). It is non-invasive and often appreciated by patients since it gives them some feeling of control over their situation.

NURSING CONSIDERATIONS

When nursing patients who are likely to experience nausea and vomiting there are a few interventions that can help patient comfort.

- It is important to assess patients adequately before chemotherapy or radiotherapy is given. Patients who are particularly prone to vomiting or who will be receiving highly emetogenic treatment should be given anti-emetics prophylactically.
- Make sure that appropriate anti-emetics have been prescribed and are administered before treatment and on schedule afterwards.
- Position patients away from stimuli which may cause nausea and vomiting – the smell of food from the kitchens, other patients being sick, strong odours.
- Try to provide some privacy – most patients find being sick in public quite embarrassing. Screens or curtains are useful.
- Reassure the patient that it is normal – and quite acceptable – to be sick, but that there are treatments that they can be given to control symptoms.
- Have a vomit receiver and tissues to hand – but perhaps out of sight.
- Monitor whether anti-emetics are being successful. It may be useful to keep a chart to document the amount of emesis a patient is experiencing, but avoid constant questioning about nausea and vomiting – it could act as an emetic stimulus.
- If anti-emetics are inadequate, discuss this with the medical staff and consider changing dose, changing drug or adding supportive techniques.
- Fizzy drinks, especially soda water or ginger ale, can help relieve nausea. Dry toast helps some people.
- Try to soothe/relax the patient by contact, verbal comments, music, etc., as appropriate.
- Where vomiting is prolonged the patient's fluid and electrolyte balance should be monitored as dehydration and electrolyte imbalance can be serious problems (Nolan 1985).

Reflection point

Review the non-pharmacological strategies currently used within your clinical area. Are there strategies which could be developed further?

Case study 15.1

Marion is a 37-year-old lady with a recurrence of Hodgkin's disease. She was originally diagnosed 7 years ago and treated at another hospital. Marion gave a history of severe emesis during her previous chemotherapy regimen.

During pre-chemotherapy assessment, Marion was very anxious about the recommencement of chemotherapy after her previous encounter, when she had lost 3 stones in weight due to nausea and vomiting. Marion also gave a history of emesis during pregnancy 12 years earlier. An anti-emetic regimen was discussed with Marion, which included the use of a 5-HT$_3$ receptor antagonist for 3 days followed by 7 days of a substituted benzamide together with the use of a relaxation tape (progressive muscle relaxation). Marion was taught the relaxation technique and informed how to contact staff on the unit if she encountered any problems. She was given an outpatient appointment for 10 days post-treatment.

Marion encountered no problems during her chemotherapy and was very pleased with the anti-emetic regimen.

- If patients are being treated as a day case or being discharged make sure that they or their carer understands about delayed symptoms.

Patient education is always an important part of the nursing process. Anxiety will exacerbate symptoms, so a proper explanation of what is about to happen and investing time in trying to calm and reassure the patient is usually worthwhile. Nurses should be realistic, but not alarmist, about the likelihood of nausea and vomiting occurring. For radiotherapy patients it may be less frightening to be given a 'tour' of the radiotherapy apparatus before they are left alone in the treatment room.

CONCLUSION

It is important for nurses to try and ameliorate emetic symptoms as much as possible for patient comfort and to aid compliance with treatment. Within the constraints of time it is important to try and provide a calm and soothing atmosphere. Anti-emetics should be monitored, given in the correct dose and on time. Prophylactic anti-emetics should always be given to those patients about to receive highly emetogenic procedures. Day-case patients, or those being discharged should have sufficient anti-emetics to cover the period when delayed symptoms may occur.

DISCUSSION QUESTIONS

1. What are the physiological processes of nausea and vomiting?

2. What are the main predisposing factors to nausea and vomiting in an individual with a haemato-oncological disorder?

3. Which anti-emetics are most effective in highly emetic drug regimens?

4. What would lead you to suspect that an individual is suffering anticipatory vomiting?

5. What pharmacological and non-pharmacological interventions would you use in an individual suffering from anticipatory vomiting?

References

Allwood M, Stanley A, Wright P 1997 The cytotoxics handbook, 3rd edn. Radcliffe Medical Press, Oxford

Andrykowski M A, Gregg M E 1992 Development of anticipatory nausea: a prospective analysis. Journal of Consulting Clinical Psychology 53: 447–454

Bateman D N, Darling W M, Boys R, Rawlins M D 1989 Extra-pyramidal reactions to metoclopramide and prochlorperazine. Quarterly Journal of Medicine 264: 307–311

Byass R 1988 Soothing body and soul. Nursing Times 84(24): 39–41

Coates A, Abraham S, Kaye S B et al 1983 On the receiving end – patient perception of the side-effects of chemotherapy. European Journal of Clinical Oncology 19: 203–208

Copley Cobb S 1984 Teaching relaxation to cancer patients. Cancer Nursing 7: 157–161

Cunningham D, Gore M, Davidson N, Miocevich M, Manachanda M, Wells N 1993 The real cost of emesis – an economic analysis of ondansetron vs metoclopramide in controlling emesis in patients receiving chemotherapy for cancer. European Journal of Cancer 29A: 303–306

D'Aquisto R W, Tyson L B, Gralla R J 1986 The influence of a chronic high alcohol intake on chemotherapy-induced nausea and vomiting. Proceedings of the American Society of Clinical Oncology 5: 257

Donovan M I 1980 Relaxation with guided imagery: a useful technique. Cancer Nursing 3: 27–32

Dundee J W, Yang J 1990 Prolongation of the anti-emetic action of P6 acupuncture by acupressure in patients having cancer chemotherapy. Journal of the Royal Society of Medicine 83: 360–362

Dundee J W, Ghaly R G, Fitzpatrick K T J, Abram W P, Lynch G A 1989 Acupuncture prophylaxis of cancer chemotherapy-induced sickness. Journal of the Royal Society of Medicine 82: 268–271

Goddard M 1993 The real cost of emesis. European Journal of Cancer 29A: 297–298

Gralla R J, Itri L M, Pisko S E et al 1981 Antiemetic efficacy of high-dose metoclopramide: randomized trials with placebo and prochlorperazine in patients with chemotherapy-induced nausea and vomiting. New England Journal of Medicine 3055: 905–909

Hesketh P J, Beck T, Grunberg S M et al 1995 A proposal for classifying the emetogenicity of cancer chemotherapy. Seventh International Symposium Multinational Association of Supportive Care in Cancer (MASCC), Luxembourg 20–23 September, Abstract

Jones A L, Lee G J, Bosanquet N 1992 The budgetary impact of 5-HT$_3$ receptor antagonists in the management of chemotherapy-induced emesis. European Journal of Cancer 29A: 51–56

Lindley C M, Bernard S, Fields S F 1989 Incidence and duration of chemotherapy-induced nausea and vomiting in the outpatient oncology population. Journal of Clinical Oncology 7: 1142–1149

Merrifield K R, Chaffee B J 1989 Recent advances in the management of nausea and vomiting caused by antineoplastic agents. Clinical Pharmacy 8: 187–199

Nolan E M 1985 Nausea, vomiting and dehydration. In: Jacobs M, Geels W (eds) Signs and symptoms in nursing interpretation and management. Lippincott and Co, Philadelphia

Osoba D, Zee B, Pater J, Warr D, Latreille J, Kaiser L 1997 Determinants of postchemotherapy nausea and vomiting in patients with cancer. Journal of Clinical Oncology 15(1): 116–123

Priestman T 1988 Radiation-induced emesis. Clinician 6: 40–43

Roila F, Tonato M, Basurto C et al 1987 Antiemetic activity of high

doses of metoclopramide combined with methylprednisolone versus metoclopramide alone in cisplatin-treated cancer patients: a randomised double-blind trial of the Italian Oncology Group for Clinical Research. Journal of Clinical Oncology 5: 141–149

Roila F, Tonato M, Basurto C et al 1989 Protection from nausea and vomiting in cisplatin-treated patients: high-dose metoclopramide combined with methyl prednisolone versus metoclopramide combined with dexamethasone and diphenhydramine: a study of the Italian Oncology Group for Clinical Research. Journal of Clinical Oncology

7: 1693–1700

Sadler C 1989 Can acupressure relieve nausea? Nursing Times 85(51): 32–34

Stannard D 1989 Acupressure prevents nausea. Nursing Times 85(4): 33–34

Troesch L M, Rodehaver C B, Delaney E A, Yanes B 1993 The influence of guided imagery on chemotherapy-related nausea and vomiting. Oncology Nursing Forum 20: 1179–1185

Zook D J, Yasko J M 1983 Psychological factors: their effect on nausea and vomiting experienced by clients receiving chemotherapy. Oncology Nursing Forum 10: 76–81

Further reading

Hawthorn J 1995 Understanding and management of nausea and vomiting. Blackwell Science, Oxford
This book (which won an award in the BMA Medical Book Competition) is one of the most comprehensive texts on nausea and vomiting. It gives a complete account of the physiology of nausea and vomiting and discusses the pharmacology and use of anti-emetic drugs. It also contains a discussion of the nursing approach to controlling nausea and vomiting, including alternative therapies. The book covers all types of nausea and vomiting; however, it is more oriented towards oncology nurses.

Stannard D 1989 Acupressure prevents nausea. Nursing Times 85(4): 33–34
This article places a nursing perspective on the use of acupressure, a useful alternative technique, which can by applied without specialist training.

Copley Cobb S 1984 Teaching relaxation to cancer patients. Cancer Nursing 7: 157–161
This article is useful because it actually provides concrete instructions for nurses on how to teach patients to relax, including a script for the reader to follow.

16 *Oral care*

HELEN PORTER

Key points
- Development of oral complications can be life threatening
- Oral care is an essential, skilled nursing intervention
- Assessment is an essential part of the oral care process
- Evidence-based protocols for effective oral care in the immunosuppressed individual are an indication of good practice

INTRODUCTION

For the individual with a haemato-oncological disease, oral problems can be a cause of immense pain and discomfort. There may be loss of function and local infection, which may lead to serious systemic problems. Development of oral complications can initiate life-threatening complications such as systemic sepsis that may not be resolved with aggressive medical, nursing and dental interventions (Madeya 1996). Causality is multifaceted, including the disease itself and treatment with its specific side-effects. Clients with haematological malignancies develop oral complications more often than those with solid tumours (Madeya 1996). Oral care, therefore, is an essential skilled nursing intervention. The nurse must be able to identify which clients are at risk, adopt preventative measures, detect changes in the oral cavity early and initiate prompt appropriate therapy. To do this the nurse must possess in-depth knowledge of all aspects of oral care.

THE HEALTHY ORAL CAVITY

The functions of the oral cavity are:

- ingestion of food and water
- communication
- breathing (with the nasal cavity) (Lippold & Winton 1972).

The oral cavity also plays a role in the general well-being of the person. It is lined with moist stratified epithelium consisting of 15–20 layers of cells (Hinchliffe & Montague 1988). These cells rapidly replicate and are replaced every 7–10 days. Within the oral cavity are the specialised structures of dentition, the tongue and the salivary glands. Approximately 1000–1500 ml of saliva is produced daily. Saliva is a complex fluid which protects the oral cavity and facilitates nutrition and taste. The oral cavity has a variety of functions which can be acutely affected by haemato-oncology disorders, their treatment and other associated problems.

THE EFFECT OF HAEMATO-ONCOLOGY DISORDERS ON THE ORAL CAVITY

Haemato-oncology disorders can cause problems from local disease infiltration, immuno- and myelosuppression, and associated coagulopathies.

Leukaemia
Neutropenia and thrombocytopenia render the client at risk from oral infection and bleeding. Spontaneous bleeding of the gums is a common feature at diagnosis. Gum hypertrophy and infiltration with leukaemic cells is a feature of acute myeloid leukaemia (AML) M4 and M5

(FAB classification) (Hoffbrand & Pettit 1993), whereas individuals with AML M3 may develop disseminated intravascular coagulation (DIC), leading to bleeding problems (see Chs 4 and 14).

Lymphoma

Loss of immunocompetent T cells leads to reduced cell-mediated immune reactions (Hoffbrand & Pettit 1993). Therefore, although individuals may not be neutropenic at diagnosis, their immune function will be impaired (see Ch. 6). Individuals may also have local infiltration of tissue with lymphoma. Where bone marrow involvement is evident, neutropenia and thrombocytopenia may occur.

Myeloma

Deficient antibody production and neutropenia may lead to persistent infections. Abnormal plasma proteins interfere with platelet function and coagulation and may lead to bleeding. In individuals with amyloid the tongue may become abnormally enlarged.

All treatment used in haemato-oncology can have an adverse effect on the oral cavity and improved treatment for cancer may go hand in hand with significant destruction of normal tissue (Kenny 1990).

The effects of chemotherapy on the oral cavity

Many cytotoxic drugs used in the treatment of haematological malignancies will cause mucositis. Antimetabolites (e.g. cytosine arabinoside, methotrexate) and antitumour antibiotics (e.g. daunorubicin, doxorubicin) are most frequently associated with mucositis (Madeya 1996). The extent of damage is generally dose-related. Damage will usually occur 5–7 days after treatment and may take 2 to 3 weeks to heal in the non-myelosuppressed individual (Dose 1995). Systemic chemotherapy will inhibit the replication of the oral mucosa, causing the epithelium to become thin and friable and both traumatic and atraumatic lesions can develop. Xerostomia can also be caused by chemotherapy, although chemotherapy-associated salivary gland injury is usually transient.

Changes in composition and salivary flow rates are possible, with decreased whole saliva rates, amylase and IgA levels but increased lysozyme being reported in a study of outpatients receiving chemotherapy (Main et al 1984).

The effect of radiotherapy on the oral cavity

Radiotherapy may be administered locally, e.g. cranial and mantle, or to the whole body, e.g. TBI (total body irradiation) or total nodal (see Ch. 9). Radiation causes atrophy of the oral mucosa due to inhibition of cellular renewal. It may also cause fibrosis to the structures of the oral cavity and can cause bone and dentition changes, including an accelerated rate of dental caries, a slow rate of growth of dentition and bone, and decreased osteoclastic and osteoblastic activity.

Xerostomia is a dryness of the mouth caused by a reduction or absence of saliva. Radiation directed at the parotid or submandibular glands will result in a marked decrease in salivary flow. A change in the organic and inorganic composition of saliva, such as decreased electrolytes and immunoproteins (Dudjak 1987) and increased acidity (McIlroy 1996), results from inflammatory and degenerative changes.

Xerostomia may lead to functional changes, such as impaired taste, difficulty in forming a food bolus, local immunosuppression and speech problems. Radiation-induced mucositis usually occurs at the treatment range of 2.5 Gy (Dudjak 1987), with changes becoming permanent after 40 Gy (Sonis 1993).

The effect of immunosuppression on the oral cavity

Immunosuppression resulting from either the disease process or from chemotherapy-induced myelosuppression will render the client at risk from infection. The risk of infection increases the longer the period of immunosuppression. Alteration in the normal microflora caused by salivary changes or systemic antibiotic or steroid therapy will also increase the risk.

Local superimposed infection in the oral cavity may be bacterial, viral or fungal. Damage to mucosal integrity allows oral pathogens to enter the circulation and may lead to systemic sepsis and life-threatening infection. Infection may arise from existing commensal organisms or from introduced pathogens (Porter 1994). Common oral pathogens include the following.

Bacteria

In immunocompromised clients 70% of severe bacterial infections are Gram-negative (*Pseudomonas aeruginosa, Klebsiella, Escherichia coli*), the remaining 30% are gram positive infections (*Staphylococcus aureus, Staphylococcus epidermidis, Enterococcus*).

Reflection point

Identify patients that you have cared for that have developed systemic sepsis in addition to oral infection and discuss whether you can identify a link between these two sites.

Fungi

Candida albicans and *Aspergillus. Candida* usually presents as pseudomembranous candidiasis, acute atrophic candidiasis, chronic atrophic candidiasis, chronic hyperplastic candidiasis or candidal cheilosis (Ventafridda et al 1993).

Viruses

Herpes simplex and herpes zoster are characterised by single or multiple clusters of small vesicles (Madeya 1996) appearing commonly on the lips or in the mouth. Immunosuppression may cause reactivation of the latent virus in patients who have had previous infection.

Other causes of problems in the haemato-oncology client

As well as the disease and its treatment there are a number of other factors that predispose an individual with a haemato-oncological disease to develop oral complications.

Graft versus host disease (GVHD) may be a significant problem in allogeneic transplantation (see Ch. 10). Oral GVHD occurs in over 80% of cases of chronic GVHD and resembles lesions in connective tissue disorders with mucosal erythema, atrophy, ulceration and lichen planus-like lesions (Schubert & Sullivan 1990). Many of the drugs used in treatment will also cause xerostomia. These include tricyclic antidepressants, antihistamines, anticholinergics, anticonvulsants, beta-blockers, diuretics, opiates and hypnotics. In the individual with xerostomia, vomiting can cause specific problems. The normal nausea and vomiting process involves hypersalivation prior to vomiting. This ensures protection of the mucosa and dentition from the acidic contents of the stomach. If there is no saliva to act as a buffer the client becomes more susceptible to developing mucositis and dentition damage.

Reduced nutritional intake secondary to mucositis may increase the severity of the mucositis due to decreased cellular renewal and migration (Madeya 1996). Vitamin deficiencies can also lead to oral problems. Riboflavin deficiency can lead to lesions in the mucocutaneous surfaces of the mouth (angular stomatitis, cheilosis and glossitis) and vitamin C deficiency can lead to bleeding gums (Department of Health 1991).

Effect of mucositis on therapy

Systemic chemotherapy regimens may be altered as mucositis develops. Drug doses may be adjusted, omitted or delayed if there is significant mucositis. This may lead to less than optimal therapy with a potentially negative effect on the individual's prognosis.

ASSESSMENT OF THE ORAL CAVITY

Patient assessment forms the basis of all nursing care interventions. Assessment is an essential part of the oral care process and should begin before therapeutic intervention to provide a baseline from which to measure change (Beck 1979). Assessment tools can help the nurse to identify the severity of oral complications and should be simple and quick to use (Porter 1992). A number of tools have been developed to enable thorough assessment of the oral cavity. When choosing a tool, ease of use, applicability to the client population and

Reflection point

What factors would you take into consideration when deciding on which oral assessment tool to implement on your ward/department?

Reflection point

Consider the effect that severe mucositis may have on a patient's sense of well-being and their body image.

proven reliability and validity are important factors to consider (Porter 1994). Assessment tools may be descriptive or numerical.

A number of oral assessment tools have been specifically developed for the haemato-oncology population. One example is the OAG (oral assessment guide) developed by Eilers et al in 1988. This tool was developed in the bone marrow transplant setting and has shown itself to be useful in clinical practice by a number of authors (Graham et al 1993, Holmes & Mountain 1993, Feber 1995). It is a nurse-administered scoring system consisting of the following eight categories:

- voice
- swallow
- lips
- tongue
- saliva
- mucous membranes
- gingiva
- teeth or dentures.

The assessment tool allows a score of 1 to 3 for each category, with 1 being normal and 3 indicating severe problems.

AIMS OF ORAL CARE

Daeffler (1980) describes the aims of oral care as to

- keep the mucosa clean, soft, moist and intact, thus preventing infection

- keep the lips clean, soft, moist and intact
- remove food debris and dental plaque without damaging the gingiva/peridontium
- alleviate pain and discomfort, thus enhancing oral intake
- prevent halitosis and freshen the mouth.

Trenter-Roth & Creason (1986) include the psychosocial importance of oral care, relating the condition of the mouth to body image and the ability of the client to communicate effectively both verbally and by facial expression.

Oral care

When planning oral care thought must be given to the psychological effects of oral problems. Mucositis can be an extremely distressing symptom, with both structural and functional effects. The mouth is important in expressing emotion and in intimate acts such as kissing. Dysfunction will effect patients' perception of body image and their sense of well-being.

The administration of oral care can be subdivided into frequency of care, oral tools and oral care agents and solutions. Unfortunately there is little research within the haemato-oncology setting to guide clinical practice. The nurse must identify the specific care needs of the client and formulate a care plan to meet them. Changes in the oral cavity can occur rapidly and so the frequency of assessment and care must be adapted to the individual. A variety of oral care tools are available, including toothbrush, foam sticks, waterpics and gauze swabs. The specific problems of thrombocytopenia and coagulopathy must be considered when choosing between toothbrushes and other tools: although the toothbrush is the better tool for removing plaque and debris, it may cause mucosal damage.

Oral care may also involve novel approaches to the prevention of mucositis. Oral cryotherapy where ice chips are sucked reduces the blood flow to the oral mucosa during administration of chemotherapy. Mahood et al (1991) showed a significant reduction in the severity of mucositis in clients receiving 5-fluorouracil (5FU) when cryotherapy was used. Although 5FU is predominantly used in gastrointestinal cancers this method of prophylaxis has also been shown to

Reflection point

Mr Jones is receiving craniospinal radiotherapy in conjunction with his induction chemotherapy for acute lymphoblastic leukaemia. What risk factors does he have for developing oral complications and what oral care should be initiated?

have some efficacy in preventing melphalan-induced stomatitis (Meloni et al 1996).

Pain relief

The sensation of burning is often the first indication of mucositis and may be present without any visible abnormality. As mucositis progresses the patient may experience severe pain. The degree of pain may vary throughout the day as the patient experiences different

Case study 16.1

Anne is a 35-year-old woman with Hodgkin's disease. She is in remission and has recently undergone high-dose chemotherapy with an autologous peripheral blood stem cell transplant.

Anne has good oral hygiene techniques and visits her dentist regularly. The oral assessment guide (Eilers et al 1988) was used with Anne twice a day and she used a prophylactic regimen of chlorhexidine mouthwash and topical antifungal mouthwash after meals and before going to sleep at night, allowing 30 minutes between the two mouthwashes.

Five days after her chemotherapy commenced, Anne developed severe mucositis, which was treated with Oramorph 1 hour before each meal, first thing in the morning and last thing at night. She was unable to brush her teeth because of the pain and foam sticks and gauze swabs were gently used to clean her mouth every 2 hours. After a further 7 days Anne's mucositis improved, allowing her to recommence a soft diet and clean her teeth with a soft toothbrush. The Oramorph was discontinued but continued use of chlorhexidine mouthwash was encouraged.

stressors such as eating, drinking and performing oral hygiene. The experience of pain will decrease compliance with mouth care and reduce the oral intake of food and fluids. Oral pain will also have a detrimental effect on the patient's quality of life. Although the experience of oral pain is well documented there is a dearth of information regarding guidance on appropriate, effective analgesia.

The choice of analgesia may be limited by the side-effects of drugs (e.g. bleeding with aspirin) and potential problems with routes of administration (e.g. risk of infection with per rectum analgesia in the myelosuppressed client and the risk of bleeding and bruising with skin punctures). In severe pain, intravenous opiates may offer relief. Patient-controlled analgesia allows patients to determine when and how much analgesia they receive (Macintyre & Ready 1996). As the intensity of acute pain is rarely constant, the patient can titrate the amount of analgesia delivered according to increases and decreases in pain.

GUIDELINES FOR GOOD PRACTICE

There is a paucity of research to determine good practice based on strong evidence. However, when reviewing the available literature it is possible to identify guidelines. These should always be used in conjunction with the individual assessment of patients and their particular needs and problems. The following guidelines reduce the potential for the development of oral complications and are based on information already outlined in this chapter.

Oral assessment

The oral cavity should be assessed at least daily using an assessment tool tested for reliability and validity. Where severe mucositis develops this should be increased to twice daily.

Frequency of care

Oral care should be performed at least four times a day (e.g. after meals and before sleep). This should be increased to 2 hourly in patients with severe mucositis and with xerostomia.

Table 16.1 Oral care agents

Patient's oral need care	Agent	Action	References
Cleansing/ antimicrobial	Chlorhexidine	Broad-spectrum antimicrobial activity, prevents dental plaque formation, sustained release from mucosal surfaces	Beck & Yasko 1993 Ferretti et al 1987 Walker 1988 Raybould et al 1994
	Iodine	Antiseptic and antibacterial	Walker 1988
Desloughing	Sodium bicarbonate	Dilutes mucus, loosens debris and raises the pH	Walker 1988
Prevention of mucositis	Allopurinol	Inhibition of enzyme orotidylate decarboxylase, which lessens the production of toxic metabolites of 5FU	Sonis & Clark 1991 Van Der Vliet et al 1989
	Prostaglandin E2	Protects against cell breakdown by protecting DNA from radiotherapy	Porteder et al 1988
	Vitamin E	Phytochemical, stabilising function on membranes, antioxidant	Wadleigh et al 1992
Protection of mucosa	Sucralfate	Coating and protection of mucosa	Barker et al 1991
	Carbenoloxone	Anti-inflammatory, increases mucosal blood flow, raises level of local cytoprotective prostaglandins	Poswillo & Partridge 1984
Antifungal	Amphotericin B Nystatin	Topical antifungal agent Antifungal antibiotic	Finlay 1995 Campbell 1995 Barkvoll & Attamandal 1989
	Miconazole	Topically acting azole, effective against *Candida* and Gram-positive cocci	Wray & Bagg 1997
	Itraconazole	Orally absorbed antifungal azole	Hay & Clayton 1987
	Fluconazole	Orally absorbed antifungal azole	Brammer 1990
Antiviral	Acyclovir	Inhibits herpes virus replication	Saral 1990
Xerostomia	Artificial saliva	Buffers acidity and lubricates the mucous membranes	Heals 1993 Kusler & Rambur 1992
	Pilocarpine	A parasympathetic agent that stimulates any remaining salivary gland function	Greenspan & Daniels 1987 Singal et al 1995
Miscellaneous	Fluoride	Incorporates into enamel, enhances remineralisation and inhibits bacterial metabolism	Mushanoff et al 1981 Sullivan & Fleming 1986

Oral care agents

Care should be taken to choose the appropriate agent for the specific need, e.g. antimicrobial or desloughing (Table 16.1). In patients at risk of secondary infection, chlorhexidine gluconate provides broad spectrum antimicrobial activity. Chlorhexidine is known to stain teeth although the stains can be removed by dentists. Topical antifungal agents are also of value in this patient group but care must be taken to leave an interval of 15–30 min between administering chlorhexidine mouthwash and nystatin solution to ensure the efficacy of each agent.

Oral care tools

The toothbrush should be used to remove debris and prevent plaque formation. For individuals who find this painful, in nurse-administered oral care or in thrombocytopenic patients a foam stick is a suitable alternative in order to minimise trauma.

CONCLUSION

Delivery of effective oral care is a skilled nursing activity, involving assessment, goal-setting, care delivery and evaluation (Porter 1994). The needs of the haemato-oncology patient are complex but it is essential that oral care is given priority to ensure the individual's well-being and to minimise the associated morbidity and mortality. The nurse also needs to be proactive in research and audit to continually optimise patient care.

DISCUSSION QUESTIONS

1. What are the physical manifestations of the different types of oral infection that you have seen?
2. What characteristics of the patient population on your ward/department make them at risk of developing oral complications? What oral care should be initiated?
3. What is the evidence base for the oral care protocol in your ward/department?

References

Barker G, Loftus L, Cuddy P 1991 The effects of sucralfate suspension and diphenydramine syrup plus kaolin-pectin on radiotherapy induced mucositis. Oral Surgery, Oral Medicine, Oral Pathology 71(3): 288–293

Barkvoll P, Attamandal A 1989 Effect of nystatin and chlorhexidine digluconate on *Candida albicans*. Oral Surgery, Oral Medicine, Oral Pathology 67: 279–281

Beck S 1979 Impact of a systematic oral care protocol on stomatitis after chemotherapy. Cancer Nursing 2: 185–199

Beck S, Yasko J 1993 Guidelines for oral care, 2nd edn. Sage, Crystal Lake, IL

Brammer K W 1990 Management of fungal infection in neutropenic patients. Haematology and Blood Transfusion 33: 546–550

Campbell S 1995 Treating oral candidiasis. Nurse Prescriber 1(5): 12–13

Daeffler R 1980 Oral hygiene measures for patients with cancer II. Cancer Nursing 3: 427–432

Department of Health 1991 Report on health and social subjects 41. Dietary reference values for food energy and nutrients for the United Kingdom: Report of the panel on dietary reference values of the committee on medical aspects of food policy. HMSO, London

Dose A M 1995 The symptom experience of mucositis, stomatitis, and xerostomia. Seminars in Oncology Nursing 4: 248–255

Dudjak J 1987 Mouth care for mucositis due to radiation therapy. Cancer Nursing 10: 131–140

Eilers J, Berger A M, Peterson M C 1988 Development, testing and application of the oral assessment guide. Oncology Nursing Forum 15(3): 325–330

Feber T 1995 Mouth care for patients receiving oral irradiation. Professional Nurse 10(10): 666–670

Ferretti G, Ash R, Brown A, Largent B, Kaplin A, Lillich T T 1987 Chlorhexidine for prophylaxis against oral infections and associated complications in patients receiving bone marrow transplants. Journal of the American Dental Association 114(4): 461–467

Finlay I 1995 Oral fungal infections. European Journal of Palliative Care 2(2) (Suppl 1): 4–7

Graham K M, Pecoraro D A, Ventura M, Meyer C C 1993 Reducing the incidence of stomatitis using a quality assessment and improvement approach. Cancer Nursing 16(2): 117–122

Greenspan D, Daniels T 1987 Effectiveness of pilocarpine in post radiation xerostomia. Cancer 59: 1123–1125

Hay R J, Clayton Y M 1987 Treatment of chronic dermatophytosis and chronic oral candidosis with itraconazole. Rev Infect Dis 9 (Suppl 1): 114–118

Heals D 1993 A key to well-being: oral hygiene in patients with advanced cancer. Professional Nurse 8(6): 391–398

Hinchliffe S, Montague S 1988 Physiology for nursing practice. Baillière Tindall, London

Hoffbrand A V, Pettit J E (eds) 1993 Essential haematology, 3rd edn. Blackwell Science, Oxford

Holmes S, Mountain E 1993 Assessment of oral status: evaluation of three oral assessment guides. Journal of Clinical Nursing 2: 35–40

Kenny S A 1990 Effect of two oral care protocols on the incidence of stomatitis in hematology patients. Cancer Nursing 13(6): 345–353

Kusler D L, Rambur B A 1992 Treatment for radiation induced xerostomia: an innovative remedy. Cancer Nursing 15(3): 191–195

Lippold A J C, Winton F R 1972 Hearing and speech. Human physiology. Churchill Livingstone, Edinburgh, pp 443–464

Macintyre P E, Ready L B 1996 Acute pain management: a practical guide. W B Saunders, London

McIlroy P 1996 Radiation mucositis: a new approach to prevention and treatment. European Journal of Cancer Care 5: 1153–1158

Madeya M 1996 Oral complications from cancer therapy: part 1 – physiology and secondary complications. Oncology Nursing Forum 23(5): 801–807

Mahood D, Dose A, Loprinzi C et al 1991 Inhibition of fluorouracil induced stomatitis by oral cryotherapy. Journal of Clinical Oncology 9: 449–452

Main B E, Calman K C, Ferguson M M 1984 The effect of cytotoxic therapy on saliva and oral flora. Oral Surgery, Oral Medicine, Oral Pathology 58: 545–548

Meloni G, Capria S, Proia A, Trisolini S M, Mandelli F 1996 Ice pops to prevent melphalan induced stomatitis. Lancet 347: 1691–1692

Mushanoff O, Gedalia I, Daphni L 1981 Fluoride acquisition of surface enamel of human teeth in vivo following toothbrushing with amine-fluoride toothpaste. Journal of Dentistry 9: 144–149

Porter H J 1992 Oral care for BMT patients. Nursing Standard 7(6): 54–55

Porter H J 1994 Mouth care in cancer. Nursing Times 90(14): 27–29

Porteder H, Rausch E, Kment G, Watzek G, Matejka M, Sinzinger H 1988 Local prostaglandin E2 in patients with oral manifestations undergoing chemotherapy and radiotherapy. Journal of Craniomaxillo-Facial Surgery 16: 371–374

Poswillo D, Partridge M 1984 Management of recurrent aphthous ulcers: a trial of carbenoxolone sodium mouthwash. British Dental Journal 157(2): 55–57

Raybould T P, Carpenter A D, Ferretti G A, Brown A T, Lillich T T, Henslee J 1994 Emergence of gram negative bacilli in the mouths of bone marrow transplant recipients using chlorhexidine mouthrinse. Oncology Nursing Forum 21(4): 691–695

Saral R 1990 Management of acute viral infections. In: National Cancer Institute Monographs No 9. Consensus development conference on oral complications of cancer therapies: diagnosis, prevention and treatment, pp 107–110

Schubert M M, Sullivan K M 1990 Recognition, incidence and management of oral graft versus host disease. In: National Cancer Institute Monographs No 9. Consensus development conference on oral complications of cancer therapies: diagnosis, prevention and treatment, pp 135–143

Singal S, Mehta J, Rattenbury H, Trealeaven J, Powles R 1995 Oral pilocarpine hydrochloride for the treatment of refractory xerostomia associated with chronic graft versus host disease. Blood 85 (letter): 1147–1148

Sonis S T 1993 Oral complications of cancer therapy. In: DeVita V, Hellman S, Rosenberg S (eds) Cancer: principles and practice of oncology. Lippincott, Philadelphia, pp 2385–2394

Sonis S, Clark J 1991 Prevention and management of oral mucositis induced by antineoplastic therapy. Oncology 5: 11–18

Sullivan M D, Fleming T J 1986 Oral care for the radiotherapy treated head and neck cancer patient. Dental Hygiene 60: 112–114

Trenter-Roth P, Creason J 1986 Nurse-administered oral hygiene: is there a scientific basis? Journal of Advanced Nursing 11(3): 323–331

Van Der Vliet W, Erlichman C, Elhakim J 1989 Allopurinol mouthwash for prevention of fluorouracil-induced stomatitis. Clinical Pharmacy 8: 655–658

Ventafridda V, Ripamonti C, Sbanotto A, De Conno F 1993 Mouth care. In: Doyle D, Hanks G W C, MacDonald N (eds) Oxford textbook of palliative medicine. Oxford Medical Publications, Oxford, pp 434–445

Wadleigh R, Redman R, Graham M, Krasnow S, Anderson A, Cohen M 1992 Vitamin E in the treatment of chemotherapy-induced mucositis. American Journal of Medicine 92: 481–484

Walker C 1988 Microbial effects of mouthrinses containing antimicrobials. Journal of Clinical Periodontology 15: 499–505

Wray D, Bagg J 1997 Pocket reference to oral candidosis. Science Press, London

Further reading

Adams R 1996 Qualified nurses lack adequate knowledge relating to oral health, resulting in inadequate oral care of patients on medical wards. Journal of Advanced Nursing 24(3): 552–560
This article gives a comprehensive review of the extent of knowledge and current practice of oral care. Although this study was carried out in medicine the themes and findings can be compared with the haematology setting.

Buschel P C, Whedon M B 1995 Bone marrow transplantation. Administrative and Clinical Strategies. Jones and Bartlett, Boston
This text includes a comprehensive chapter relating to oral complications during bone marrow transplantation and gives advice on appropriate therapeutic intervention and assessment.

Coleman S 1995 An overview of oral complications of adult patients with malignant haematological conditions who have undergone radiotherapy or chemotherapy. Journal of Advanced Nursing 22(6): 1085–1091
This article gives a comprehensive overview of complications of patients with haematological malignancies and relates these to the theory practice gap and therefore implications for practice.

Griffiths J, Boyle S 1993 Colour guide to holistic care: a practical approach. Mosby–Year Book Europe, London
An opportunity to see visual representations of oral complications.

Pearson LS 1996 A comparison of foam swabs and toothbrushes to remove dental plaque: implications for nursing practice. Journal of Advanced Nursing 23(1): 62–69
A clear example of nursing research evaluating an integral part of oral care practice.

17 | Nutritional issues

MAGGIE GRUNDY

Key points
- Multiple factors contribute to malnutrition
- Nutritional state should be assessed at diagnosis and at regular intervals throughout the disease trajectory
- Malnutrition is not an inevitable consequence of the disease and treatment
- Nutritional support should involve all members of the multidisciplinary team

INTRODUCTION

Malnutrition is a well-recognised problem associated with all forms of cancer and its treatment. It has been associated with a poor prognosis and response to treatment, enhanced treatment side-effects and a reduced quality of life (Harvey et al 1979, De Wys et al 1980). A variety of factors suggest that individuals with haematological malignancies, especially leukaemia and lymphomas, may be at increased risk of developing malnutrition. Nutritional assessment and management are therefore a vital component of care. This chapter outlines the factors contributing to malnutrition, and discusses issues associated with nutritional assessment and management.

FACTORS CONTRIBUTING TO MALNUTRITION

Numerous factors have been implicated in the development of malnutrition and their interrelationships are complex and unclear. An increased basal metabolic rate (BMR) has been suggested as one cause of malnutrition (Knox et al 1983). BMR has not been shown to be consistently raised in all individuals with cancer but does appear to be consistently raised in individuals with leukaemia and lymphoma (Waterhouse et al 1951, Watkin 1961). The reasons for this are unclear, but the disseminated nature of these diseases, frequent infections and the associated pyrexia may be contributory factors. Additionally energy expenditure is raised during the process of bone marrow transplant (BMT) (Aker et al 1983).

Abnormalities of glucose, fat, protein and electrolyte metabolism are also thought to be major contributors to weight loss in the presence of adequate protein and calorie intake, although the mechanisms underlying these metabolic disturbances remain incompletely understood (O'Regan et al 1977, Heber et al 1986).

Calorific intake may be exceeded by energy requirements as a result of illness- or treatment-induced anorexia and the body's catabolic response to illness (Bistrian 1977). The cause of anorexia is thought to be multifactorial and, again, is incompletely understood.

Anorexia may be exacerbated as a result of both the disease and adverse effects of treatment (see Chs 8, 9 and 10). Any of the following problems may be experienced and impact on food intake:

- mucositis
- xerostomia
- dysgeusia (abnormal taste)
- nausea and vomiting
- indigestion
- diarrhoea
- constipation
- malabsorption of nutrients
- anorexia
- early satiety

- food aversion
- complete food abstinence.

Individuals undergoing BMT may experience oral and gastrointestinal complications of increased severity due to the effects of graft versus host disease (GVHD) or aggressive treatment regimens (see Ch. 10).

Psychological factors have also been shown to affect appetite during various stages of the disease and treatment, especially

- at the time of initial diagnosis
- between diagnosis and the commencement of treatment
- at the time of relapse of the disease

and related to periods of pain and discouragement (Holland et al 1977, Padilla 1986).

Individuals with haematological malignancies may experience prolonged periods of protective isolation when neutropenic following chemotherapy or BMT. This is likely to increase psychological discomfort, which may further reduce appetite and food consumption. Protective isolation also removes the social contact which normally accompanies meal times and this has been proposed as an additional factor affecting appetite (Perry 1992).

DIETARY RESTRICTIONS

In BMT a range of dietary restrictions may be used to reduce the potential for bacterial infection from food.

Sterile and low microbial diets

The use of these diets varies between centres. However, they are usually recommended during the period of post-transplant neutropenia. Three categories of diet exist: sterile, low microbial and modified hospital diets which are specific to a particular institution (Bakitas Whedon & Wujcik 1997).

Sterile diets
All food is either irradiated or autoclaved to eradicate all bacteria and their spores. These diets require special facilities to sterilise food and are expensive. These methods may also alter the nutritional value and taste of some foods and they are now rarely used.

Low microbial diets
Certain foods are excluded from the diet to reduce the ingestion of pathogens. These include uncooked fruit and vegetables, cold meats, uncooked or semi-cooked eggs, soft cheeses or unpasteurised milk products, yoghurt and cream, uncooked spices, and all foods in multi-serving packs such as jams and sauces.

Modified hospital diets
These diets are not strictly low microbial as they allow dairy products, spices, nuts and other pathogen-containing foods although they exclude most raw fruits and vegetables.

There is currently insufficient research to determine whether these diets affect an individual's food intake. The effectiveness of the diets in reducing infection also requires further investigation.

IMPORTANCE OF MAINTAINING NUTRITIONAL STATUS

Individuals with good nutritional status have demonstrated an improved response to chemotherapy and an ability to tolerate higher doses of cytotoxic drugs (Copeland & Dudrick 1975, Copeland et al 1975). The success of treatment may therefore be significantly influenced by nutritional state, and the importance of maintaining nutritional status cannot be overemphasised. It is also considerably more difficult to restore nutritional status than to maintain it (Shils 1979).

There can be no doubt that nurses are well aware that individuals with haematological malignancies are at high risk of developing malnutrition. However, despite the wealth of available research, it has been suggested that people are frequently judged well or poorly nourished on the basis of a quick glance or the subjective opinion of individual nurses (Butler 1980, Ramstack & Rosenbaum 1990 – p 195). Identification of patients at risk appears to be at best haphazard and individuals may have lost significant amounts of weight before they are considered poorly nourished. Nurses, as the health professionals that have the most contact with patients, have a major responsibility for initial assessment of patients and, in collaboration with dieticians and doctors, for assisting in the maintenance and restoration of nutritional status.

ASSESSMENT OF NUTRITIONAL STATUS

Nutritional assessment is an important aspect of care and is said to be the first step in the prevention and treatment of malnutrition (Blackburn & Bistrian 1976). Methods of nutritional assessment can be divided into three categories: subjective, anthropometric and biochemical methods (Table 17.1).

Many of the above methods of assessment are either impractical for use by nurses or are inappropriate for individuals with a haematological malignancy. Dietary history is a good means of determining current intake although it should be remembered that the illness and treatment may have altered an individual's normal eating pattern. Other methods of determining intake including 24-hour recall and weighed dietary intake are problematic. Reporting of food intake has been found to be inaccurate, with consumption being both under- and overestimated (Holmes & Dickerson 1991). The individual's memory, ability to convey estimates of quantity, degree of motivation and the persistence of the interviewer are all considered to be contributory factors in the success of 24-hour recall

(Acheson et al 1980). An individual with a haematological malignancy who is feeling tired and unwell and may have poor concentration is unlikely to be a good candidate for this method of assessment.

Weighing of food, although considered to be the gold standard for assessing nutritional intake, is time consuming and may change patterns of consumption as usual practices may be changed to simplify the measurement process (Marr 1971).

Many of the biochemical and haematological tests, such as measurement of serum albumin or transferrin and lymphocyte levels, are inappropriate for individuals with haematological malignancies as they are affected by sepsis, administration of blood products and the myelosuppressive and immunosuppressive effects of the disease (Bistrian 1984, 1986, Long 1984 – p 18, Curtas et al 1989).

There is currently no standard method for assessing nutritional status. It is, however, crucial that assessment is undertaken. The British Association for Parenteral and Enteral Nutrition has recommended guidelines for first-line nutritional screening which could be employed in initial assessment, and used as a baseline for determining subsequent changes (Lennard-Jones 1995). These recommendations suggest asking the following four questions:

- Have you unintentionally lost weight recently?
- Have you been eating less than usual?
- What is your normal weight?
- How tall are you?

Additionally, individuals should be weighed and their height measured and recorded. Body

Table 17.1 Methods of nutritional assessment

Subjective	Anthropometric	Biochemical
Clinical examination	Height	Creatinine/height index
Dietary history	Weight	Nitrogen balance
Dietary intake	Triceps skinfold thickness	Visceral transport protein
	Upper arm muscle	levels (e.g. serum
	circumference	albumin, transferrin)
		Total lymphocyte count

mass index (BMI) can be calculated using a simple formula to establish the possibility of malnutrition:

$$BMI = \frac{Weight\ (kg)}{Height\ (m^2)}$$

It has been suggested that a BMI of between 20 and 24.9 kg/m^2 is desirable. A BMI of less than 20 kg/m^2 indicates malnutrition is possible.

Weight loss should always be regarded as significant. However, weight gain is not necessarily an indication of improving nutritional status. Various factors may influence weight gain, including fluid retention, organomegaly and the effects of drugs such as corticosteroids and norethisterone.

Weight needs to be measured and recorded serially. Additionally, factors affecting individual's ability to eat and drink and their food consumption require to be systematically assessed throughout the disease trajectory to detect indicators of malnutrition.

The likelihood of malnutrition increases with the length of hospitalisation (Weinsier et al 1979). Individuals with haematological malignancies are often hospitalised for long periods and changes in eating patterns and nutritional status may occur, especially, when receiving aggressive chemotherapy and/or BMT. Individuals may only have a few days at home between periods of hospitalisation. If weight is lost in hospital it may not be regained prior to the subsequent pulse of chemotherapy, leading to a pattern of rapid weight loss.

Additionally, for up to 1 year following BMT, a number of problems affecting nutrition may occur, including infection, GVHD and drug toxicities (Aker et al 1983). These individuals therefore require ongoing nutritional assessment and support in the outpatient setting.

Factors affecting food intake must be accurately identified so appropriate interventions can be initiated. Both patients' and nurses' perceptions of factors affecting intake should be considered as they have been shown to differ. Some factors are reported more frequently by patients than nurses and vice versa. For example, nausea and early satiety are likely to be reported more frequently by patients, whereas anorexia may be

noted by nurses or relatives but go unnoticed by the patient himself (Holmes & Eburn 1989, Armes et al 1992, Grundy 1994). Nurses have a vital coordinating role in communicating information to other members of the multidisciplinary team so that appropriate nutritional support can be provided.

 Reflection point

Consider the following questions in relation to your own clinical practice:

- Is everyone weighed on admission and at regular intervals during their hospital stay?
- Where is weight recorded?
- Are weight changes communicated to all members of the multidisciplinary team?
- Is there a standard framework for nutritional assessment which all nurses in your area use?
- How often is this assessment undertaken?
- Are you always aware of the amount and types of foods your patients are eating?

The optimum time for nutritional assessment has yet to be established. After reviewing the above points you may want to discuss this issue in more detail with your colleagues in order to determine an appropriate assessment schedule for your area.

INTERVENTIONS

Reduced food intake is a common occurrence for individuals with haematological malignancies. However, various strategies can be employed in an attempt to reduce symptoms and improve food consumption (Table 17.2). Table 17.2 highlights the need for different interventions for different problems and emphasises the importance of accurately identifying the reasons for an individual's low food intake.

Decreased food consumption and weight loss are frequently of great concern to both patients and their relatives and information should be provided regarding appropriate interventions.

Many individuals find that their appetite is greatest in the morning and decreases as the

Table 17.2 Interventions (adapted from Lees 1996, Holmes 1997)

Factors affecting food intake	Interventions
Sore mouth	Practise frequent oral care and analgesia (Difflam mouthwashes, prior to meals may be helpful) Avoid sharp foods such as crisps Avoid acidic, spicy and salty foods Provide a soft or liquid diet, including high-protein, high-calorie drinks and soups Serve food at room temperature; foods which are very hot or cold can irritate
Dry mouth	Use artificial saliva or sugar-free chewing gum Reduce dryness of food using sauces or gravy Sip water frequently with meals Sucking ice-pops/ice lollies or frozen orange segments may help
Taste changes (Dysgeusia)	These are individual and suggestions need to be adapted to each person Individuals should be encouraged to stick to foods that taste good to them Brushing teeth regularly may help *Bitter, metallic taste*: use plastic cutlery and non-metal cooking pots Add herbs and spices to food *Sweet taste*: add sharp flavours – use vinegar, lemon juice, pickles *Taste loss:* use herbs and spices Serving food piping hot so steam may be smelt may help to stimulate appetite if all sense of taste is lost
Nausea and vomiting	Administer anti-emetics at least 30 min prior to meal times Avoid fried and greasy foods Serve small amounts Dry foods, such as toast, may be better tolerated Carbonated drinks may help Avoid cooking smells; cold foods may be better tolerated
Diarrhoea	High fluid intake; avoid hot and milky drinks Administer antidiarrhoeal agents Avoid high-fibre foods likely to stimulate bowel movements
Constipation	High fluid intake Administer laxatives as prescribed High-fibre diet if tolerated, but difficult if anorexia/early satiety being experienced
Anorexia and early satiety	Offer small, frequent meals Offer food when the individual feels hungry Provide snack foods and supplements which are high in calories but of low quantity Use both sweet and savoury liquid food supplements Increase calorific value of foods by adding milk, cream, butter, icecream, sauces, mayonnaise, sugar or glucose supplements to soups, cereals, puddings and drinks Avoid drinks close to meal times, especially carbonated ones

Reflection point

Are you always aware of the specific factors affecting an individual's food intake?

day progresses with the best meal of the day being breakfast. Many hospitals operate a system of ordering meals 24 hours in advance. This system may be inappropriate for those with nutritional problems as they are unlikely to be able to decide what they will feel like eating that far ahead. Negotiations with the hospital kitchen may be necessary to ensure the flexibility to enable individuals to eat when they feel hungry. The amount and type of foods eaten require to be clearly documented and communicated to everyone involved in an individual's care so that everyone has the same information and care is consistent. De Vries et al (1982) note that individuals with acute leukaemia may suffer from total food abstinence because of their aggressive chemotherapy regimens and this is certainly a problem following BMT. However hard nurses try, individuals frequently have absolutely no inclination to eat and oral intake is unlikely to meet their increased energy demands.

Oral intake is frequently insufficient to maintain nutritional status and total parenteral nutrition (TPN) will be required to supplement this for some individuals receiving aggressive chemotherapy regimens and most individuals following transplant (De Vries et al 1982). TPN should not be seen as the panacea to all nutritional problems as, following BMT, weight loss has been shown to continue despite TPN (Layton et al 1981). However, without TPN, nutritional depletion would be even greater. Individuals should also be encouraged to eat as much as they feel able to while TPN is being administered and oral nutrition should be re-established as soon as possible to preserve gut function and immunity. Individuals with intestinal GVHD following allogeneic transplant may require extended periods of TPN to rest the gut before oral feeding is gradually reintroduced (McDonnell Keenan 1989).

Case study 17.1

Steve, a 21-year-old student recently diagnosed with acute lymphoblastic leukaemia, had lost 1 stone (6.35 kg) in weight in the 4 weeks prior to diagnosis. Both Steve and his parents were concerned about his weight loss. His parents tried to tempt him with his favourite foods but Steve had no appetite. He was seen by the dietician, who suggested that he eat small high-calorie snacks at frequent intervals during the day and suggested ways in which he might increase his calorie intake.

Steve did try to eat but his chemotherapy caused nausea, early satiety and a metallic taste, all of which was compounded by a dry mouth. Steve developed an almost total food abstinence and required total parenteral nutrition (TPN) during his induction chemotherapy. Nineteen days after commencing chemotherapy, Steve started to regain his appetite and started to eat small amounts.

CONCLUSION

Numerous factors predispose the individual with a haematological malignancy to malnutrition. The condition also has multiple effects, making maintenance of nutritional status a priority in care. However, nutritional assessment and support for these individuals is far from simple and straightforward. Further research is required to establish the best means of assessing nutritional condition and the optimum time and frequency of assessment. Despite these difficulties it is imperative that nutritional condition is assessed throughout the disease trajectory so a baseline can be established and problems addressed as they occur. Lack of attention to this important aspect of care may compromise an individual's response to treatment and their quality of life.

DISCUSSION QUESTIONS

1. How can the role of the nurse and the dietician complement each other in order to enhance patient care?
2. How could nutritional assessment and support be improved in your clinical area?

References

Acheson K J, Campbell I T, Edholm O G, Miller D S, Stock M J 1980 The measurement of food and energy intake in man – an evaluation of some techniques. American Journal of Clinical Nutrition 33: 1147–1154

Aker S N, Lenssen P, Darbinian J, Cheney C L, Cunningham B 1983 Nutritional assessment in the marrow transplant patient. Nutritional Support Services 3(10): 22–37

Armes P J, Plant H J, Allbright A, Silverstone T, Slevin M L 1992 A study to investigate the incidence of early satiety in patients with advanced cancer. British Journal of Cancer 65: 481–484

Bakitas Whedon M, Wujcik D 1997 Blood and marrow stem cell transplantation: principles, practice and nursing insights, 2nd edn. Jones and Bartlett, Boston

Bistrian B R 1977 Nutritional assessment and therapy of protein-calorie malnutrition in the hospital. Journal of the American Dietetic Association 71: 393–397

Bistrian B R 1984 Nutritional assessment in the hospitalised patient: a practical approach. In: Wright R A, Heymsfield S Nutritional assessment. Blackwell Scientific Publications, Boston, pp 183–206

Bistrian B R 1986 Some practical and theoretic concepts in the nutritional assessment of the cancer patient. Cancer 58: 1863–1866

Blackburn G L, Bistrian B R 1976 Nutritional support: resources in hospital practice. In: Schneider H Nutritional support of medical practice. Harper and Row, New York

Butler J H 1980 Nutrition and cancer: a review of the literature. Cancer Nursing 3: 131–136

Copeland E M, Dudrick S J 1975 Cancer: nutritional concepts. Seminars in Oncology 2(4): 329–335

Copeland E M, MacFadyen B V, Lanzotti V J, Dudrick S J 1975 Intravenous hyperalimentation as an adjunct to cancer chemotherapy. American Journal of Surgery 129: 167–173

Curtas S, Chapman G, Meguid M M 1989 Evaluation of nutritional status. Nursing Clinics of North America 24(2): 301–313

De Vries E G E, Mulder N H, Houwen B, De Vries-Hospers H G 1982 Enteral nutrition by nasogastric tube in adult patients treated with intensive chemotherapy for acute leukaemia. American Journal of Clinical Nutrition 35: 1490–1496

De Wys W D, Begg C, Lavin P T et al 1980 Prognostic effect of weight loss prior to chemotherapy in cancer patients. American Journal of Medicine 69: 491–497

Grundy M 1994 Patients' and nurses' perceptions of the factors affecting nutritional intake in patients with acute leukaemia. Unpublished MSc Dissertation, University of Surrey

Harvey K B, Bothe A, Blackburn G L 1979 Nutritional assessment and patient outcome during oncological therapy. Cancer 43: 2065–2069

Heber D, Byerley L O, Chi J et al 1986 Pathophysiology of malnutrition in the adult cancer patient. Cancer 58: 1867–1986

Holland C B, Rowland J, Plumb M 1977 Psychological aspects of anorexia in cancer patients. Cancer Research 37: 2425–2428

Holmes S 1997 Cancer chemotherapy: a guide for practice. Asset Books, Leatherhead, pp 222–250

Holmes S, Dickerson J W T 1991 Food intake and quality of life in cancer patients. Journal of Nutritional Medicine 2: 359–368

Holmes S, Eburn E 1989 Patients' and nurses' perceptions of symptom distress in cancer. Journal of Advanced Nursing 14(10): 840–846

Knox L S, Crosby L O, Feurer I D, Buzby G P, Miller C L, Mullen J L 1983 Energy expenditure in malnourished cancer patients. Annals of Surgery 197: 152–162

Layton P B, Gallucci B B, Aker S N 1981 Nutritional assessment of allogeneic bone marrow recipients. Cancer Nursing 4(2): 127–134

Lees J 1996 Nutrition. In: Tschudin V (ed) Nursing the patient with cancer. Prentice Hall, London

Lennard-Jones J E 1995 Screening by nurses and junior doctors to detect malnutrition when patients are first assessed in hospital. BAPEN, London

Long C L 1984 Nutritional assessment of the critically ill patient. In: Wright R A, Heymsfield S Nutritional assessment. Blackwell Scientific Publications, Boston, pp 15–26

McDonnell Keenan A M 1989 Nutritional support of the bone marrow transplant patient. Nursing Clinics of North America 24(2): 383–393

Marr J W 1971 Individual dietary surveys: purposes and methods. World Review of Nutrition and Diet 13: 105–164

O'Regan S, Carson S, Chesney R W, Drummond K N 1977 Electrolyte and acid–base disturbances in the management of leukaemia. Blood 49(3): 345–353

Padilla G V 1986 Psychological aspects of nutrition and cancer.

Surgical Clinics of North America 66(6): 1121–1135

Perry F 1992 Assessing and meeting the nutritional needs of patients receiving an autologous bone marrow transplant – art or science? In: Cancer nursing changing frontiers, nutrition in the 90s the changing perspective, Proceedings of weekend symposium, 7th International Conference on Cancer Nursing. Scutari Projects, Harrow, Middlesex, pp 14–18

Ramstack J L, Rosenbaum E H 1990 Nutrition for the chemotherapy patient. Bull Publishing Co, Palo Alto, California

Shils M E 1979 Nutritional problems induced by cancer. Medical Clinics of North America 63(5): 1009–1025

Waterhouse C, Fenninger L D, Keutmann F H 1951 Nitrogen exchange and calorific expenditure in patients with malignant neoplasms. Cancer 4: 500–514

Watkin D M 1961 Nitrogen balance as affected by neoplastic disease and its therapy. American Journal of Clinical Nutrition 9: 446–460

Weinsier R L, Hunker E M, Krumdieck C L, Butterworth C E 1979 A prospective evaluation of general medical patients during the course of hospitalisation. American Journal of Clinical Nutrition 32: 418–426

Further reading

Holmes S, Dickerson J W T 1987 Malignant disease: nutritional implications of disease and treatment. Cancer and Metastasis Reviews 6: 357–381
This article provides a comprehensive overview of the metabolic disturbances which occur as a result of cancer and the effects of chemotherapy and radiotherapy.

Holmes S 1997 Cancer chemotherapy: a guide for practice. Asset Books, Leatherhead, pp 222–250
This book contains a comprehensive chapter on nutritional care for the individual receiving chemotherapy.

White G 1998 Nutritional supplements and tube feeds: What is available? *International Journal of Palliative Nursing* 4(4): 176–183
A good overview of nutritional supplements is given in this article.

18 *Fertility issues*

EVELYN DANNIE

Key points
- Gonadal failure and sexual impairment are side-effects of both chemotherapy and radiotherapy
- Both men and women are affected
- A number of strategies are available for maintaining fertility post-treatment
- Patients should be advised of appropriate strategies prior to commencing treatment
- Advice should be given on contraception during treatment

INTRODUCTION

The use of high-dose chemotherapy/radiotherapy in the treatment of haematological malignancies results in a number of serious side-effects which can potentially interfere with any of the body's cellular, anatomical, physiological, behavioural, social and reproductive functions (Sherins 1993).

Gonadal failure and sexual impairment are late side-effects of blood and marrow transplant (BMT) (Kolb et al 1989, Vose et al 1992). Such late effects are often of low priority at the time of treatment but are permanent and inevitable consequences of high-dose alkylating agents and/or total body radiation (TBI) (Sanders et al 1983, Dannie et al 1994). The low priority afforded this side-effect may previously have been related to the high mortality and morbidity rates associated with transplant procedures. However, with survival curves now showing a gradual rise (Gratwohl et al 1993, Marks et al 1993) quality of life post-BMT has become increasingly important and fertility is a major concern for survivors and their partners.

Infertility is important not only because of its long-term physical, psychological and emotional consequences but also because the prospect of infertility has led some patients to refuse the treatment most likely to cure their disease or adversely influenced their decision to enter clinical trials.

This chapter will review the effects of chemotherapy/radiotherapy on gonadal function and discuss strategies for reducing these effects and maintaining fertility post-treatment. The role of hormone replacement therapy (HRT) and specific nursing issues will be addressed.

EFFECTS OF RADIOTHERAPY AND CHEMOTHERAPY ON GONADAL FUNCTION

Radiotherapy

Males

Damage to the testes caused by radiotherapy is well documented. Spermatogenesis can be affected by even small doses of radiotherapy, resulting in oligo-azoospermia approximately 50 days post-treatment and much earlier with larger doses. Recovery of spermatogenesis depends on the total dose administered and the mode of administration, such as a single total dose or several fractionated doses. High doses result in permanent sterility, although there is some considerable variation in susceptibility between individuals (Speiser et al 1972, Lushbaugh & Casarett 1976, Chatterjee et al 1994). In one study of 32 men with leukaemia treated with TBI prior to BMT, only two recovered spermatogenesis 6 years after transplant (Sanders et al 1983). In contrast, of 72 men with aplastic anaemia without TBI in their preparative transplant regimes, 65% had normal sperm counts and some had fathered children naturally (Sanders et al 1988).

Females

Premature ovarian failure occurs commonly following radiotherapy. Gonadal toxicity varies between individuals and sensitivity is related to the dose, type and duration of treatment, age and the development stage of the germ cell (Gradishar & Schilsky 1989). Advancing age and TBI appear to be correlated to ovarian failure. Single doses of radiation will often induce menstrual irregularities in women of all ages. However, less than 60% aged between 15 and 40 will be infertile, whereas in those aged 40 and over 100% will be infertile (Baker et al 1972). The main characteristics of ovarian failure are

■ ovarian fibrosis
■ primodial follicle destruction
■ elevated follicle-stimulating hormone (FSH) and luteinising hormone (LH) levels
■ low oestradiol levels
■ amenorrhoea
■ menopausal symptoms, including
   oestrogen deficiencies
   hot flushes
   vaginal dryness
   vaginitis
   dyspareunia
   decreased libido
   vaginal epithelial atrophy
   vaginal stenosis
   sexual dysfunction.

Chemotherapy

Several chemotherapeutic agents profoundly influence male and female gonadal function particularly the alkylating agents. Some of these agents are shown in Table 18.1.

Effects of chemotherapy on males

Alkylating agents are more likely to induce permanent infertility than other cytotoxic agents

Table 18.1 Chemotherapeutic agents associated with infertility (adapted from Gradishar & Schilsky 1989)

Drugs and risk of infertility	
Male	**Female**
Definite infertility	
Chlorambucil	Cyclophosphamide
Cyclophosphamide	Nitrogen mustard
Nitrogen mustard	Busulphan
Busulphan	L-Phenylalanine
Procarbazine	
Nitrosoureas	
Probable infertility	
Doxorubicin	Etoposide
Vinblastine	
Cisplatin	
Cytosine arabinoside	
Etoposide	
Unlikely infertility	
Methotrexate	Methotrexate
6-Mercaptopurine	6-Mercaptopurine
Vincristine	
Fertility risk unknown	
Bleomycin	Doxorubicin
	Bleomycin
	Vinca alkaloids
	Nitrosoureas
	Cisplatin
	Cytosine arabinoside

(Wang et al 1980) and both the mature and immature testes are at risk (Shalet et al 1981). The testes are very sensitive to chemotherapy, with the germinal cells within the seminiferous tubules being directly affected. Testicular biopsies in patients treated by chemotherapy show aplasia of the germinal epithelium with normal Sertoli's and Leydig's cells, which is reflected in a reduced sperm count with normal testosterone levels (Fairley et al 1972).

The characteristics of gonadal dysfunction in men and commonly reported problems are listed below:

■ testicular germ cell aplasia
■ reduced testicular volume

- atrophic seminiferous tubules
- oligospermia
- azoospermia
- elevated FSH and LH levels
- testosterone deficiencies
- permanent sterility
- depressed libido
- sexual dysfunction
- erectile difficulties
- premature ejaculation.

Effects of chemotherapy on females

A great number of different chemotherapeutic agents have been associated with ovarian failure (see Table 18.1). In addition to alkylating agents such as busulphan and cyclophosphamide (Udall et al 1972), combination therapy used for Hodgkin's disease causes permanent infertility in 70% of patients, regardless of age (Chapman & Sutcliffe 1981). More recently, drugs such as etoposide have also been reported to cause ovarian toxicity (Choo et al 1985).

As with radiation, the process of follicular growth and maturation of oocytes are affected; ovarian fibrosis results, with follicular destruction. This is clinically manifested by menstrual irregularity and eventual amenorrhoea, with increased levels of FSH and LH and lowered levels of oestradiol, resulting in symptoms of the menopause and sexual dysfunction (Quigley & Hammond 1979).

Additionally, chemotherapy and radiotherapy cause damage to the uterine endometrium and the ability of the endometrium to proliferate in response to hormonal stimulation may be lost. This may affect both embryo implantation and the ability to carry a pregnancy to full term (Gonen et al 1989, Rio et al 1994, Apperley & Reddy 1995).

The most important risk factor for ovarian failure is age at treatment (Fig 18.1). Recovery of gonadal function is often reported in younger women but sadly only the occasional pregnancy (Sanders et al 1996). However, it appears that women who recover gonadal function will suffer the menopause at an earlier age than women in the normal population (Horning et al 1981).

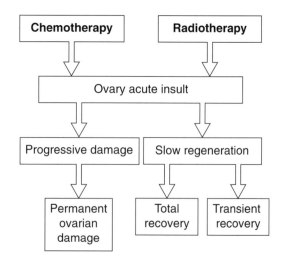

Figure 18.1 A model of ovarian failure and possible recovery following chemotherapy/radiotherapy

RECOVERY OF GONADAL FUNCTION AFTER HIGH-DOSE CHEMOTHERAPY/RADIOTHERAPY

Severe gonadal damage can be identified immediately after high-dose chemotherapy/radiotherapy although recovery can occur with time (Giri et al 1992). The chance of recovery is influenced by a number of issues, including

- sex of the recipient
- age at BMT
- nature and doses of drugs and irradiation.

After cyclophosphamide alone, 60–70% of male and female transplant patients had normal gonadotrophin levels 6 years post-BMT compared to only 20% of those whose conditioning regimens included TBI (Sanders et al 1983). However, it is important to note that normal gonadotrophin levels do not necessarily indicate a return of fertility (Chatterjee et al 1994).

Late recovery of spermatogenesis up to 14 years following treatment has been reported (Watson et al 1985). A number of factors are identified not only for causing infertility but also for influencing the chances of recovery of spermatogenesis. These are shown in Table 18.2.

Reflection point

The distressing short- and long-term side-effects of chemotherapy/radiotherapy are further exacerbated by premature ovarian failure and infertility. Consider the consequences of gonadal failure in both males and females. How could you prepare, educate and support a patient and his/her partner at this time?

The role of hormone replacement therapy (HRT)

The majority of women who develop ovarian failure will experience distressing menopausal symptoms. Some women also perceive loss of their femininity, resulting in lack of confidence, self-esteem and depression. Because of the rapidity of the onset of the menopause, 70% of women will suffer vasomotor symptoms as well as a number of other equally important and more permanent problems (Fig. 18.2) (Studd & Whitehead 1988, Dannie et al 1994).

In recent years HRT has been recognised as a successful method of treating distressing menopausal symptoms. It is used routinely in women suffering ovarian failure as a result of chemotherapy/radiotherapy treatments. The aim of HRT is to restore oestrogen levels to near normal, minimising symptoms and short- and long-term sequelae such as osteoporosis, heart disease and cerebral vascular accidents.

Table 18.2 Factors affecting recovery of gonadal function

Male	Female
Age	Pubertal status
Underlying disease	Age at diagnosis
Type of drugs used	Fertility status
Nature of the drug	pre-treatment
Total cumulative dose	Disease status
Duration of administration	Nature, dose and
Radiotherapy (site, dose,	duration of
mode of administration	chemotherapeutic
and duration)	agents used
	at diagnosis
	Nature and dose of
	chemotherapeutic
	agent used in
	transplant
	conditioning
	Dose, site and
	mode of
	administration
	of radiotherapy
	Type of transplant

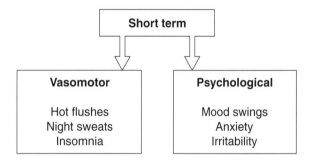

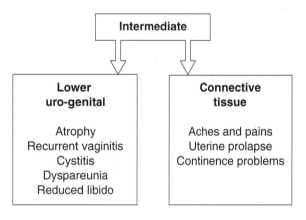

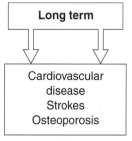

Figure 18.2 Symptoms of the menopause

Additionally, it may help to improve uterine function, enabling endometrial proliferation in response to exogenous hormones for successful embryo transfer.

Treatment should commence at the onset of symptoms and for women who are asymptomatic gonadotrophin levels should be monitored, and therapy begun when levels suggest ovarian failure. Menopausal symptoms such as night sweats may be similar to symptoms of chronic myeloid leukaemia (CML) and other haematological disorders. Therefore HRT must be commenced as soon as possible to prevent confusion between menopausal symptoms and signs of disease relapse (Goldman 1990, Chiodi et al 1991).

Premature menopause is associated with premature ageing, HRT can help to restore physical and mental well-being as well as reducing morbidity and mortality associated with osteoporosis and heart disease. It should be recommended for all suitable patients, and commenced as soon as possible. However, HRT is not suitable for all women. The side-effects and contraindications can be just as distressing for some women as the symptoms of the menopause itself. It is therefore important that each woman is assessed individually and provided with full counselling and an explanation of the benefits and side-effects.

A variety of differing preparations are available including oral, transdermal, subcutaneous and vaginal. The use of HRT varies widely between institutions and each patient must be assessed individually to determine the suitability of preparations and their associated risks. Products should be prescribed for maximum benefit, comfort and minimal risk. Careful follow up is essential to monitor benefit, record side effects, and recommend different preparations as clinically indicated. Side-effects and contraindications of HRT are shown in Table 18.3.

Education for the woman and her family will encompass a number of issues but information given must be clear and simple. Nurses should be aware of the potential problems of treatment and its side-effects. They should take the lead in initiating and encouraging discussion, as patients may be embarrassed to do so. The nurse's role should also encompass advice on physical, emotional and sexual well-being.

Table 18.3 Side-effects and contraindications for HRT

Common side-effects of HRT	Contraindications for HRT
Breast tenderness	Breast cancer
Fluid retention	Known or suspected
Leg cramps	pregnancy
Nausea and vomiting	Active liver disease/
Vaginal discharge	abnormal liver
Gastrointestinal symptoms	function
Headache	Endometrial cancer
Acne	Vaginal bleeding of
Depression	unknown cause
Irritability	Venous thrombosis
	Hypertension
	Gallstones
	Benign breast
	disease

Reflection point

Consider the questions you might be asked by a woman who has been advised about the likelihood of premature menopause following treatment and is concerned about the effects these symptoms might have on her relationships. How would you respond to these questions?

STRATEGIES FOR MAINTAINING FERTILITY

Currently, gonadal failure cannot be prevented but a number of strategies are available to enable patients undergoing chemotherapy/radiotherapy the possibility of parenthood after treatment (Winston & Handyside 1993, Rio et al 1994). For men it is possible to cryopreserve sperm, for female patients it may not be as easy. A number of techniques have been used to preserve fertility during gonadotoxic treatment (Morris & Shalet 1990): these include embryo cryopreservation in women with a regular partner, and oocyte and ovarian cryopreservation as a possible future option for women without a regular partner and young girls.

Other strategies for maintaining fertility have included oophoropexy, which involves surgical intervention to place the ovaries midline behind the uterus (Sherins 1993), and the development of chemotherapy combinations to include dose limitation of alkylating agents which retain efficacy against the disease and less gonadal toxicity (Viviani et al 1985).

Strategies for maintaining fertility post-treatment are

- sperm banking
- testicular shielding
- embryo cryopreservation
- oocyte and ovarian cryopreservation
- oophoropexy
- dose limitation of alkylating agents
- substitution of drugs for less toxic substances
- combined oestrogen/progesterone contraceptive pill
- gonadotrophin-releasing hormone (GnRH) analogues.

Some of these strategies require delaying the commencement of chemotherapy; others require surgical intervention, taking account of the patient's general condition and disease status; whereas, others utilise different doses or toxicity of drugs in an attempt to reduce gonadal toxicity. However, whichever type of strategy is used, a substantial proportion of patients will remain at risk of infertility. Therefore the treatment option must be agreed by the patient, be effective against the disease and must not compromise the therapeutic outcome (Gradishar & Schilsky 1989, Apperley & Reddy 1995).

Sperm banking

It is important that the patient is referred for sperm banking at the time of diagnosis as semen from men pre-treated for cancer or haematological malignancies may reveal a low sperm count and inadequate sperm motility (Redman et al 1987).

If possible, sperm should be stored on three separate occasions and at 48-hour intervals. Often patients have not been referred if they have already started treatment, because of the likelihood of obtaining an inadequate specimen. However, it appears recent chemotherapy may not affect the quality of sperm, as sperm contained in an ejaculate began their maturation process 3 months earlier and are highly unlikely to be adversely affected by recent chemotherapy. Theoretically patients can be referred early in their treatment, when their condition has been stabilised. However these men must be counselled and prepared for the possibility of sperm counts being low and of poor quality, thereby reducing the chances of achieving a subsequent pregnancy (Apperley & Reddy 1995). The evidence for teratogenicity is severely limited and clearly the best approach is to refer the patient as early as possible after diagnosis (Whedon & Wujcik 1997).

Sperm banking should be offered to all men likely to suffer gonadal dysfunction. Those accepting the offer should be advised that successful pregnancy depends on the quality and quantity of sperm at the time of storage. If good-quality sperm is stored in sufficient quantities to permit six cycles of artificial insemination, there is a 45% cumulative chance of pregnancy. In contrast, storage of a single ejaculate of poor-quality sperm only offers, at best, a 20% chance (Scammel et al 1985).

Sperm banking has been widely available for some time and many men experiencing gonadal failure as a consequence of treatment will have sperm stored. Nevertheless, studies have shown that there are few requests to use frozen sperm. This may be partly attributable to those men who have already completed their families or those who are not completely recovered and have fears and concerns for the welfare of any subsequent child.

The ability to achieve pregnancy from frozen sperm is also low. This may be because sperm specimens were obtained from unsuitable candidates initially, including those having had previous intensive treatment (Friedman & Broder 1981) (Fig. 18.3).

Strategies for women

Women who develop ovarian failure as a consequence of chemotherapy/radiotherapy have three choices for motherhood. First, if they

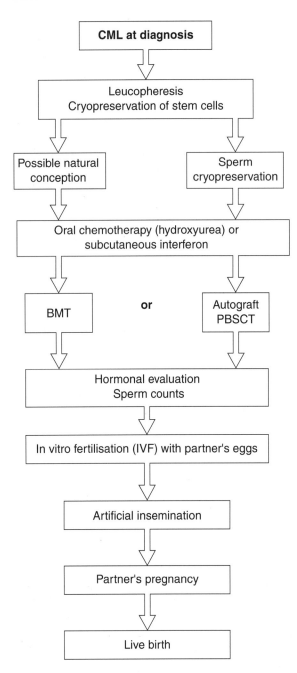

Figure 18.3 Typical pattern of treatment a male patient with CML may follow

have a regular partner and the commencement of treatment can be delayed, ovarian hyper-stimulating oocyte collection, fertilisation and cryopreservation of embryos can be performed. If the start of treatment cannot be delayed, the second option involves fertilisation of donor

eggs by their partners' sperm or donated embryos from an unrelated couple. The third option is the possibility of surrogacy. There are advantages and disadvantages to each approach. However, surrogacy is surrounded by emotional, legal and ethical problems, and is probably the least feasible option (Fig. 18.4).

Embryo cryopreservation

Women wishing to have embryo cryopreservation must undergo superovulation for at least one and possibly more menstrual cycles. This is usually achieved by using one of a variety of protocols to stimulate multiple follicle maturation (e.g. clomiphene alone or in combination with FSH or a GnRH agonist, e.g. buserelin). Eggs are not always retrieved using this procedure and it is not without risk. Women and their partners must therefore be well prepared and counselled before the procedure is undertaken.

If the procedure is successful multiple oocytes can be harvested, enabling several embryos for cryopreservation. The ability to collect and fertilise good-quality oocytes depends on adequate ovarian function at the time of hyperstimulation and a number of other issues, including

- advancing age
- fertility status pre-diagnosis
- underlying disease
- patients' general condition to enable the procedure
- impaired ovarian function due to prior exposure to chemotherapy
- successful superovulation technique
- failure to retrieve eggs
- time available
- more than one stimulation cycle necessary
- quality and quantity collected
- fertilisation and quality of embryos for storage.

Prior exposure to chemotherapy and increasing age will diminish successful collection cycles. A further problem for patients with malignant disease is the time needed for the procedure. Each ovarian hyperstimulation

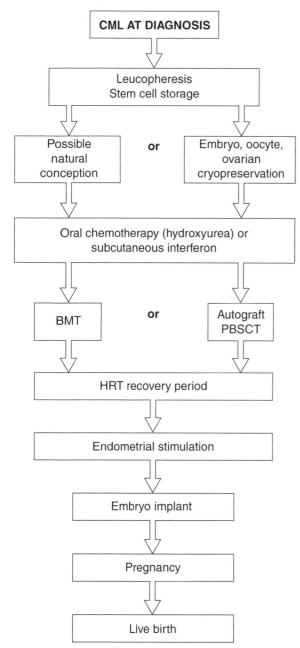

Figure 18.4 Typical pattern of treatment a female patient with CML may follow

cycle requires 4 weeks. For some conditions, such as CML and Hodgkin's disease, this delay in commencing treatment may be reasonable; for others, including the acute leukaemias, it will not be feasible. Treatment may need to be administered before gametes can be harvested and stored, which may affect the quantity and quality of oocyte harvested and, consequentially, the chances of future pregnancies.

Fertilisation of donor eggs

An alternative when time is of the essence is fertilisation of donor eggs with the partner's sperm. Unfortunately, there is a waiting list for donor eggs and a limited supply. Most women undergoing a superovulation programme are understandably often reluctant to donate their eggs for fear of limiting their own chances of future pregnancies. Often family and friends are looked to for help in such situations, but this is not without emotional entanglement and such donors must be fully counselled of the risks involved. Another possible solution is the use of donated embryos from storage after a couple have completed their family. However, it is important to note that any offspring born from donated embryos will not be genetically related to the recipient couple, although they will be considered the parents under UK law (Human Fertilisation and Embryology Act 1990).

Pregnancy after treatment

Spontaneous pregnancies have been reported in patients treated for severe aplastic anaemia by BMT (Schmidt et al 1987), for cancer (Aisner et al 1993) and treated by autologous transplant (Salooja et al 1994). However, for those treated with TBI and BMT such pregnancies are rare (Lipton et al 1993).

The possible use of embryos after transplant is a highly charged ethical and emotional issue. To date there are two known cases of successful pregnancy after BMT utilising embryo implantation, the first with a fresh donor embryo (Rio et al 1994) and the second from a cryopreserved embryo prior to BMT for CML (Atkinson et al 1994).

A review of the published reports of pregnancies after BMT suggests an increased risk of both pregnancy and neonatal complications. In particular the incidence of eclampsia, pre-term labour and low birth-weight infants seems higher than normal (Hinterberger-Fischer et al 1991, Sanders et al 1993, 1996, Atkinson et al

Table 18.4 Complications seen in pregnancy and neonates post-BMT

Pregnancy	Neonates
Multiple pregnancy	Congenital abnormalities
Spontaneous abortion	Pre-term labour
Eclampsia	Low birth weight
Hypertension	Post-natal complications
Placenta praevia	Pulmonary complications
Placental insufficiency	Failure to thrive
Increased Caesarean delivery	Increased susceptibility to malignancies
Disease relapse	

1994, Apperley & Reddy 1995. Complications seen in pregnancy and neonates post-BMT are shown in Table 18.4.

Early clinical relapse, after delivery, has also been reported in some women treated by BMT for CML. These incidences of relapse may have occurred independently; however, it is thought that the immunosuppression associated with pregnancy may reduce the graft versus leukaemia (GVL) effect known to help suppression or eradication of residual disease post-BMT (Sanders 1983, Atkinson et al 1994, Rio et al 1994).

Another problem associated with embryo transfer is the increased risk of multiple pregnancy due to the increased number of embryos transferred at each session. The greater the number of embryos transferred, the higher the incidence of achieving a pregnancy. This is now a great concern of the Human Fertilisation and Embryology Authority (HFEA) who have imposed an upper limit of transferring three embryos at each replacement cycle.

Spontaneous abortion is also common in the first trimester of pregnancy utilising frozen embryos (Van-Steirteghem et al 1987). This risk is thought to increase with advancing age (Austin & Short 1986). Pregnancy and live birth rates have also been reported to be lower with cryopreserved embryos than those following fresh embryo transfer (HFEA 1994). Therefore it

is essential that the maximum number of good-quality embryos are stored to enable multiple attempts at transfer. This may not always be possible in patients awaiting chemotherapy and they must therefore be counselled about the chance of success to avoid disappointment in the future.

Case study 18.1

Gaynor was diagnosed with chronic myeloid leukaemia in 1988 aged 22. She was 8 weeks' pregnant in her second pregnancy, the first having resulted in a spontaneous abortion at 5 weeks' gestation. Gaynor was not given chemotherapy to treat her leukaemia and her white cell count was controlled by leucopheresis. The pregnancy progressed normally and in August 1988 Gaynor delivered a normal healthy female infant weighing 3 kg. She was commenced on hydroxyurea and in 1989 decided she wanted another child. The pregnancy ended in spontaneous abortion at 7 weeks' gestation.

Bone marrow transplantation from her identical HLA sibling was decided upon to treat her leukaemia and embryo storage was chosen by Gaynor and her partner. Superovulation was induced, utilising buserelin and pergonal, and 24 eggs were collected. Normal fertilisation occurred with sperm from her husband, and the resulting 13 embryos were cryopreserved.

In October 1989 Gaynor received her allogeneic BMT. She recovered well with minimal graft versus host disease (GVHD). HRT was commenced 3 months after transplant which controlled her menopausal symptoms but she experienced no menstrual bleeds.

Two and a half years after her transplant Gaynor and her partner decided to attempt a pregnancy. In May 1992 the first embryo transplant was attempted but exogenous endometrial stimulation with routine treatment failed. Gaynor was commenced on prolonged high-dose oestradiol to stimulate endometrial response. A year later in May 1993 a further embryo replacement cycle was attempted. Despite double-dose prolonged treatment the endometrium still failed to respond and at the patient's request embryos were transferred with

Continued

Case study 18.1 *Continued*

progesterone support for endometrial
maintenance.

Twenty eight days following embryo transfer a
twin pregnancy was confirmed. At 10 weeks'
gestation one twin stopped developing. The
remaining fetus continued to develop normally.
Gaynor was closely monitored throughout by
obstetricians and haematologists. The pregnancy
and her haematological status continued
normally until 34 weeks' gestation when during a
routine antenatal visit Gaynor was found to have
pre-eclampsia. She was admitted to hospital and
underwent emergency Caesarean section being
delivered of a live female infant weighing 1.9 kg.

Since delivery, Gaynor's CML has relapsed.
Having received lymphocytes from her sibling
donor she is currently in remission. Her child is
now 4 years old with normal development.

Oocyte and ovarian cryopreservation

Currently, embryo cryopreservation is the only
strategy available to women post-BMT to have
genetic offspring. This option is not offered to
all patients, and it is especially limited for
patients without a regular partner or preme-
narchal girls. For these patients, fertility options
are less straightforward and in the future ovarian cryopreservation may offer further opportunities. Oocyte and ovarian cryopreservation
are the subject of active laboratory research but
are not yet available in clinical practice
(Gosden et al 1994). Additionally, ovarian
cryopreservation involves a minor operative
procedure which may be contraindicated
in the pancytopenic patient and the ability to
fertilise an oocyte appears to be profoundly
affected by freezing.

The collection of oocytes requires at least one
ovarian hyperstimulation cycle and should take
place prior to the start of chemotherapy. This
introduces a delay of approximately 4 weeks
between diagnosis and treatment which may be
neither medically advisable nor acceptable to
the patient and her physician (Apperley &
Reddy 1995).

Ovarian tissue and the ability to collect
oocytes should not be affected by the underlying disease, i.e. the ovaries should not contain
malignant cells and impaired gonadal function
should not be a feature of the disease at
presentation. Again this procedure involves
surgical intervention and may be contraindicated by the patient's general condition.

The advancement of research in this area is
important. To date only two pregnancies from
cryopreservation of oocytes have been
reported (Chen 1986, Van Uem et al 1987). The
complexity of the cryopreservation technique
is thought to be with the oocytes themselves.
Some of the problems are now being
addressed and it is likely that in the near future
the technical difficulties will be overcome and
the procedure will be offered to BMT recipients, with a real likelihood of achieving a successful pregnancy and live birth (Hunter et al
1991, Apperley & Reddy 1995)

NURSING ISSUES

The success of fresh embryo transfer has helped
many infertile couples have children. However,
such procedures raise a number of legal and
ethical issues and procedures are controlled by
legislation. In the UK, HFEA provides guidance
and direction to licensed units providing treatment for infertility, storage of embryos/gametes
and research. Nurses need to be aware of these
legal and ethical issues and be able to address
them with patients and their partners.

Counselling is the key element in the provision of an assisted conception service and is
emphasised in the Warnock report (1985).
Counselling involves helping couples to understand the various options open to them, including medical interventions, as well as coming to
terms with disappointment and failure, possible relapse of their disease and the possibility
of being outlived by their gametes. The availability of effective, informed, independent and
involved counselling is essential, and if done
with warmth and a genuine caring attitude will
help reassure, build trust and confidence, and
help the patient feel cared for whatever the
outcome (Edwards 1996). The nurse's role in
counselling is both supportive and educational,
paving the way for more in-depth and genetic
counselling by trained professionals.

Reflection point

Strategies for maintaining fertility pre-treatment are time-consuming, costly and not easily available or accessible. Consider your unit's current policy relating to this issue. Should the service be offered to all suitable candidates? What are the main constraints in your institution? What is your role in patient education?

The educative role of the specialist nurse is not an easy one. Up-to-date knowledge of current research and developments is necessary to be able to provide realistic, accurate information without giving false hope and to help empower patients to make informed choices. Nurses need to be able to explain the investigations needed before treatment and the process and outcomes of treatment. Handled sensitively this information can help alleviate many fears and worries. Provision of information is an important part of the nurse's role and professional integrity must be maintained. Continuing education is required to keep nurses well informed so that they in turn can inform, counsel, and educate, giving individuals a sense of control over their lives, in spite of the emotional, ethical and legal difficulties associated with assisted reproduction.

CONCLUSION

Gonadal failure and infertility are inevitable consequences of high-dose chemotherapy and TBI. Currently there are a number of strategies for maintaining fertility after treatment. However, these are not without their difficulties, and the issues require to be handled with care and sensitivity.

DISCUSSION QUESTIONS

1. What are the short- and long-term complications of chemotherapy/radiotherapy? Consider this with respect to your unit's policies in the use of both conventional (anti-emetics) and non-conventional (complementary) methods of minimising side-effects.
2. What are the main strategies for maintaining fertility post-treatment and the factors affecting gonadal recovery post-BMT?
3. Which HRT preparations are commonly prescribed in your unit? What are their common side-effects and their short- and long-term benefits and risks?
4. What supporting services are currently available in your unit for patients facing infertility? How accessible are these services?
5. What ethical, legal and emotional issues may be associated with assisted reproduction?
6. Central to the systemic approach to comprehensive and effective follow-up of patients post-transplant is the detection and treatment of potential complications at an early stage. How can nurses in your unit contribute to this in relation to fertility issues?

References

Aisner J, Wienik P H, Pearl P 1993 Pregnancy outcome in patients treated for Hodgkin's disease. Journal of Clinical Oncology 11(3): 507–512

Apperley J, Reddy N 1995 Mechanism and management of treatment related gonadal failure in recipients of high dose chemo-radiotherapy. Blood Reviews 19: 93–116

Atkinson H G, Apperley J F, Dawson K, Goldman J, Winston R 1994 Successful pregnancy following allogeneic bone marrow transplantation for chronic myeloid leukaemia. Lancet i(344): 199

Austin C R, Short R V (eds) 1986 Reproduction in mammals. In: Manipulating reproduction, 2nd edn. Cambridge University Press. London, Ch. 5

Baker J W, Morgan R L, Peckham R J, Smithers D W 1972 Preservation of ovarian function in patients requiring radiotherapy for para aortic and pelvic Hodgkin's disease. Lancet i: 1307–1308

Chapman R M, Sutcliffe B 1981 Protection of ovarian function by oral contraceptives in women receiving chemotherapy for

Hodgkin's disease. Blood 58: 849–851

Chatterjee R, Mills W, Katz M, McGarrigle H H, Goldstone A H 1994 Prospective study of pituitary–gonadal function to evaluate short-term effects of ablative chemotherapy or TBI with autologous marrow transplantation in post menarcheal women. Bone Marrow Transplantation 13: 511–517.

Chen C 1986 Pregnancy after human oocyte cryopreservation. Lancet i: 884–886

Chiodi S, Spinelli S, Cohen A 1991 Cyclic sex hormone replacement therapy in women undergoing allogeneic marrow transplantation: aims and results. Bone Marrow Transplant 8(Suppl 1): 47–49

Choo Y C, Chan S Y, Wong L C, Ma HK 1985 Ovarian dysfunction in patients with gestational trophoblastic neoplasia treated with intensive courses of etoposide (VP16-213). Cancer 55: 2348–2352

Dannie E, Apperley J, Lindsay K 1994 A study of the disease and its treatment on gonadal function in women with chronic myeloid leukaemia. Unpublished dissertation for BSc in Health Studies, University of Surrey

Edwards S D 1996 Nursing ethics. Macmillan Press, London

Fairley F K, Barrie J U, Johnson W 1972 Sterility and testicular atrophy related to cyclophosphamide therapy. Lancet i: 568–569

Friedman S, Broder S 1981 Homologous artificial insemination after long-term semen cryopreservation. Fertility and Sterility 35: 321–324

Giri N, Vowels M R, Barr A L, Mamegham H 1992 Successful pregnancy after total body radiation and bone marrow

transplantation for acute leukaemia. Bone Marrow Transplantation 10: 93–95

Goldman J M 1990 Options for the management of CML. Leukaemia and Lymphoma 3: 159–164

Gonen Y, Casper R F, Jacobson W, Blankier J 1989 Endometrial thickness and growth during ovarian stimulation. A possible predictor of implantation in IVF. Fertility and Sterility 52: 446–450

Gosden R G, Baird D T, Wade J C, Webb R 1994 Restoration of fertility to oophorectomised sheep by ovarian autografts stored at −196° C. Human Reproduction 9: 597–603

Gradishar W J, Schilsky R L 1989 Ovarian function following radiation and chemotherapy for cancer. Seminars in Oncology 16(5): 425–436

Gratwohl A, Hermans J, Neiderwieser D et al 1993 BMT for CML long term effects. Bone Marrow Transplantation 1(2): 509–516

HFEA Human Fertilisation and Embryology Act 1990, Department of Health. HMSO, London

HFEA (Human Fertilisation and Embryology Authority) 1994 Third Annual Report, Department of Health. HMSO, London

Hinterberger-Fischer M, Kier P, Kahls P et al 1991 Fertility, pregnancy and offspring complications after BMT. Bone Marrow Transplantation 199(7): 5–9

Horning S J, Hoppe R T, Kaplan H S, Rosenberg S A 1981 Female reproductive potential after treatment for Hodgkin's disease. New England Journal of Medicine 304: 1377–1382

Hunter J E, Bernard A, Fuller B, Amso N, Shaw R W 1991 Fertilisation and development of

the human oocyte following exposure to cryoprotectants low temperature and cryopreservation: a comparison of two techniques. Human Reproduction 6: 1460–1465

Kolb H J, Bender-Gotze C, Haas R J 1989 Late effects in marrow transplanted patients results of the AG-KMT Munich. Bone Marrow Transplantation (Suppl 3): 31–35

Lipton J H, Derzko C, Fyles G 1993 Pregnancy after bone marrow transplantation. Three case reports. Bone Marrow Transplantation 11: 415–418

Lushbaugh C C, Casarett G W 1976 The effects of gonadal irradiation in clinical irradiation: a review. Cancer 37 (Suppl 2): 1111–1125

Marks D J, Cullis J O, Ward K N 1993 Allogeneic bone marrow transplant for chronic myeloid leukaemia using sibling and unrelated donors. Annals of Internal Medicine 119: 207–214

Morris I D, Shalet S M 1990 Protection of gonadal function from cytotoxic chemotherapy and irradiation. Baillière's Clinical Endocrinology and Metabolism 4(1): 97–118

Quigley M M, Hammond C B 1979 Oestrogen-replacement therapy: help or hazard. New England Journal of Medicine 301: 646–648

Redman J R, Bajorunas D R, Goldstein M C et al 1987 Semen cryopreservation and artificial insemination for Hodgkin's disease. Journal of Clinical Oncology 5: 233–238

Rio B, Letur-Konirsch H, Ajchenbaum-Cymbalista F et al 1994 Full term pregnancy with embryos from donated oocytes in a 36 year old woman autografted for chronic myeloid leukaemia. Bone Marrow Transplantation 13: 487–488

Salooja N, Chatterjee R, Macmillan A K et al 1994 Successful pregnancy in women following simple autotransplant for acute myeloid leukaemia with a chemotherapy ablation protocol. Bone Marrow Transplant 13: 431–435

Sanders J E, Buckner C D, Leonard J M et al 1983 Late effects on gonadal function after cyclophosphamide and total body irradiation and bone marrow transplantation. Transplantation 36: 252–255

Sanders J E, Buckner C D, Amos D et al 1988 Ovarian function following marrow transplantation for aplastic anaemia or leukaemia. Journal of Clinical Oncology 6: 813–818

Sanders J E, Buckner C D, Storb R, Doney K, Sullivan K, Witherspoon R 1993 Pregnancy outcome after bone marrow transplantation for AA or haematology malignancies. Experimental Haematology 21 (Abstr 210): 1067

Sanders J E, Hawley J, Levy W et al 1996 Pregnancy following high-dose cyclophosphamide with or without high-dose busulphan or total body irradiation and bone marrow transplantation. Blood 7: 3045–3052

Scammel G E, White N, Stredronska J, Hendry W F, Edmonds D K 1985 Cryopreservation of semen in men with testicular tumour or Hodgkin's disease. Lancet ii: 31–32

Schmidt H, Ehninger G, Dopfer R, Waller H D 1987 Pregnancy after bone marrow transplantation for severe aplastic anaemia. Bone Marrow Transplantation 2: 329–332

Shalet S M, Hann I M, Lendon M, Morris-Jones P H, Beardwell C J 1981 Testicular function after combination chemotherapy in childhood for acute lymphoblastic leukaemia. Archives of Disease in Childhood 56: 275–278

Sherins R J 1993 Gonadal dysfunction. In: De Vita V T, Hellman S, Rosenberg S A (eds) Cancer: principles and practice of oncology, Vol 2 (4th edn). Lippincott, Philadelphia, pp 2395–2406

Speiser B, Rubin P, Casarett G 1972 Aspermia following lower truncal irradiation in Hodgkin's disease. Cancer 32: 692–698

Studd J W W, Whitehead M I 1988 The menopause. Blackwell Scientific Publications, London

Udall P R, Kerr D N S, Tacchi D 1972 Amenorrhoea and sterility. Lancet i: 693–694

Van-Steirteghem A C, Van der Abeel E, Braeckmans P, Camus M 1987 Pregnancy with a frozen-thawed embryo in a woman with primary ovarian failure. New England Journal of Medicine 317: 113–116

Van Uem J, Siebzehnrubl E, Schuh B, Koch R, Trotnow S, Lang M 1987 Birth after the cryopreservation of unfertilised oocytes. Lancet i: 752–753

Viviani S, Santoro A, Gangi G, Bonfante V, Bestetti O, Bonadonna G 1985 Gonadal toxicity after combination chemotherapy for Hodgkin's disease. Comparative results of MOPP vs ABVD. European Journal of Cancer & Clinical Oncology 21: 601–605

Vose J M, Kennedy B C, Bierman P J 1992 Long term sequalae of autologous bone marrow or peripheral stem cell transplantation for lymphoid malignancies. Cancer 69: 784–789

Wang C, Ng P R, Chan T K 1980 Effect of combination chemotherapy on pituitary–gonadal function in patients with lymphoma and leukaemia. Cancer 45: 2030–2037

Warnock M 1985 A question of life. Basil Blackwell, Oxford

Watson A R, Rance C P, Bain J 1985 Long term effects of cyclophosphamide on testicular function. British Medical Journal 291: 1457–1460

Whedon M B, Wujcik D 1997 Bone and marrow stem cell transplantation: principles, practice and nursing insights, 2nd edn. Jones and Bartlett, Boston

Winston R M L, Handyside A H 1993 New challenges in human in vitro fertilisation. Science 260: 932–936

Further reading

Apperley J, Reddy N (1995) Mechanism and management of treatment-related gonadal failure in recipients of high dose chemo-radiotherapy. Blood Reviews 9: 95–116

This article describes the normal reproductive function relevant to patients at risk of chemotherapy- or radiotherapy-induced infertility. It gives a good overview of the mechanism by which fertility may be affected and preventative measures that may be employed. It also describes methods of IVF from stored gametes, and the legal and ethical aspects of assisted reproduction.

**Barton C, Waxman J 1990
Effects of chemotherapy on
fertility. Blood Reviews
4: 187–195**
This article reviews the effects of
chemotherapy on gonadal
function utilising single and
combination therapy for a variety
of malignant disorders. It also
gives a brief overview of
prevention strategies and
management of gonadal failure.

**Studd W W, Whitehead M I 1988
The menopause. Blackwell
Scientific Publications,
London**
This book gives a good general
overview of the physiological
aspects of the menopause. It is
sensitively written in respect to
distressing menopausal symptoms,
femininity issues and the short- and
long-term side-effects, as well as
the benefits and risks of HRT.

**HFEA Human Fertilisation and
Embryology Act 1990. HMSO,
London**
This Act and its subsequent
frequent reports gives an in-depth
description of the legal and
ethical issues of assisted
conception in respect to the units
that are licensed to provide
infertility treatment, storage of
embryos and gametes and
research involving embryos. It also
states the rights of IVF treatment in
patients with malignancies, and
defines the status of the parties
involved in donation and
reception of embryos or gametes
and outlines the concerns for the
welfare of any children and the
prospective parents.

**Whedon M B, Wujcik D 1997
Fertility and sexuality issues. In:
Blood and marrow stem cell
transplantation, 2nd edn. Jones
and Bartlett, Boston, Ch. 15**
This chapter is written by nurses
working in a BMT unit. It describes
the inevitable consequences of
chemotherapy/radiotherapy on
gonadal function, and the
resulting infertility and
psychosexual issues. It also gives a
good overview of how nurses may
approach this sensitive
subject with patients and their
partners, and interventions that
may be employed to improve
sexual function.

19 *P*sychological issues

JULIA DOWNING

Key points
- The psychological impact of a diagnosis of a haematological malignancy is unique to every individual and their family
- Adapting to a diagnosis of cancer takes time, energy and effort
- Attempts to cope with the diagnosis will echo individuals' previous coping strategies
- Provision of information helps individuals gain control
- Fear of relapse and subsequent death is a major concern for many individuals
- A diagnosis of cancer does not affect the individual alone but their whole family

INTRODUCTION

Cancer strikes with a vengeance, leaving its victims threatened, vulnerable and anxious

Hagopian 1993

The diagnosis of a haematological malignancy is one that will change an individual and their family for life. Cancer is a life-threatening illness: one which emphasises humanity and mortality, and leaves individuals searching for meaning and questioning their attitudes, values and beliefs. Each individual will seek to try and understand their illness and place it in the context of their life and their meaning of life, which has been undermined as their very existence has been threatened (O'Connor et al 1990).

This chapter explores some of the psychological issues for an individual with a haematological malignancy, and their family, from diagnosis, through treatment to remission and the fear of relapse. The psychological impact of the disease and treatment is vast and has an impact on all areas of our care for the individual.

IMPACT OF DIAGNOSIS

Adapting to a diagnosis of cancer takes a lot of time, energy and effort. An individual's entire focus will be on the illness, which demands attention and causes pain, anxiety and uncertainty. Individuals may feel vulnerable, helpless and out of control, and may be facing loss, pain, suffering, anxiety, financial difficulties and a fear of death (Halldorsdottir & Hamrin 1996).

The impact a diagnosis of a haematological malignancy will have on an individual will be unique to them and their family. Factors such as age, diagnosis and prognosis all have an impact; however, there are emotions that will be experienced by many, including:

- grief
- fear
- loneliness
- anger
- powerlessness
- loss of control
- depression
- despair (Kumasaka & Dungan 1993).

Another reaction to a cancer diagnosis is that of denial, a defence that allows an individual to escape unpleasant realities by ignoring their existence. Denial can relieve psychological pain and discomfort, decrease anxiety and protect self-esteem by negating the threat posed by the diagnosis (Hagopian 1993). It is unusual for an individual to deny completely what is happening to them, although some may seek another opinion as they don't want to accept

Reflection point

What impact may an individual's denial of their disease have on your ability to support them through their diagnosis?

that the diagnosis is true. However, some form of denial is common, especially in the early stages of an illness. For example, individuals might accept the diagnosis of a haematological malignancy but deny the seriousness of the illness. Some individuals may try and cope with their diagnosis by comparing themselves with someone else whose condition is more serious.

Attempts to cope with their diagnosis will echo individuals' previous coping strategies; however, these may not be adequate to cope with such a devastating issue. Support will be needed to help individuals build upon and strengthen past coping strategies and enhance their coping skills (Kumasaka & Dungan 1993).

After diagnosis, individuals need to be able to try and understand the disease and its implications. Information needs to be given to individuals at a rate which coincides with their 'need to know', so that they are not overwhelmed. This includes information about the disease, reasons for treatment and procedures, along with expected side-effects. Provision of such information will help individuals gain control in an otherwise 'chaotic' environment (Kumasaka & Dungan 1993). The nurse can act

Case study 19.1

Jane is a 20-year-old university student. She is undertaking a degree in physiotherapy and has always been very fit and active. She and her boyfriend are planning to get married when he finishes his degree in 6 months' time. Since being diagnosed as having Hodgkin's disease 10 days ago she has been very withdrawn and uncommunicative. What are some of the emotions that she might be experiencing and how might you begin to build up a rapport with her?

as a 'coach', providing the individual with information and care and encouraging them to develop inner strengths, by taking what is foreign and fearful to the patient and making it familiar and thus less frightening (Benner 1984). With time, care and concern, individuals can adapt to their diagnosis and move on: for some this may happen quickly; others take longer and are still coming to terms with their diagnosis many months into treatment.

LIVING WITH A HAEMATOLOGICAL MALIGNANCY

Soon after diagnosis, individuals are drawn into the medical world of treatment, investigations, blood counts and central lines. Hardly have they had time to let the word 'cancer' sink in, and they are battling with side-effects of treatment. Their 'normal' environment has been replaced by one of fear, anxiety and helplessness. Not only are they trying to cope with their illness but also with the effects of their illness: for instance, their emotional balance, self-image, uncertainty and changed relationships with friends and family (Hagopian 1993).

Following the discovery of a life-threatening disease an individual will undergo treatment which may be traumatic and cause them considerable physical and psychological distress. These stresses put great demands on the coping capabilities of both the individual and their family. Many will cope by drawing on the support of others, for example family and friends; others may take one day at a time and live in the present, not the future. During treatment some individuals will feel they are on an emotional roller coaster, with moods swinging from optimism, to ambivalence and despair. Suicide may even be thought of as a 'way out', to relieve not only their suffering but that of their families as well, although few will take this option.

Learning to live with cancer is an important part of an individual's search for meaning, and is very personal (O'Connor et al 1990). It may be a time when individuals reappraise their life; they take a second look at their values, attitudes and beliefs. These may be challenged and replaced as a reflection of what is perceived to be important or valuable. The spiritual aspect of an individual's life is important in this search for meaning, whether that be in the form of a religious faith or some other belief (Hagopian 1993). This has been described by some as their strongest support in bringing meaning to their situation (O'Connor et al 1990) (see Ch. 21).

Reflection point

How might you engender hope in what might appear to be a 'hopeless' situation?

Hope, described as the 'expectation of achieving a future goal which seems realistically possible and is personally significant' (Dufault & Martocchio 1985), is very important to the individual suffering from a haematological malignancy. It is vital in their adaptation to their illness and will have an effect on their quality of life, coping skills and adherence to treatment regimes. Despite adverse experiences many individuals are able to maintain hope and regain it if lost, when threatening events, such as the treatment for haematological malignancy, result in feelings of hopelessness (Ersek 1992).

For an individual with a haematological malignancy, treatment may be aggressive; great emphasis is placed on blood results, there is talk of remission, relapse, possible bone marrow or stem cell transplant, possibly even death. All of which are out of the control of individuals thus increasing their sense of helplessness and uncertainty.

Fear of a relapse and therefore death is a major concern for many people with haematological malignancies who are hoping for a transplant while in remission and fear they will relapse before that is possible. An individual's reaction to a relapse will depend on past personal experience and the setting in which the relapse occurs (Mahon & Casperson 1997). Individuals who relapse for the second or third time generally cope better than those who are relapsing for the first time since achieving remission, as they are more hopeful that remission can be achieved again, despite feeling that the threat of death may also be nearer (Dixon et al 1996).

Individuals may go through similar emotions when they relapse as experienced on diagnosis. Along with these emotions, Mahon et al (1990) suggests that at the time of relapse the individual may feel

- the threat of death is more real
- decisions about treatment are harder
- their fear of uncontrollable pain is increased
- greater fatigue
- dissatisfied and angry with the initial treatment choices
- less hopeful than at diagnosis.

Case study 19.2

Peter is a 42-year-old accountant who had a bone marrow transplant for acute myelogenous leukaemia 4 years ago. During this time he was very positive and coped well with the side-effects of the treatment, as the treatment was going to 'cure' him. He has just been admitted to your unit for further chemotherapy having been told that he has relapsed. He is aggressive towards the staff and has said to you that he does not think he can go through 'all that' again. How might you enable him to explore this further and examine his response to being told he has relapsed?

The 'illness career' of an individual with a haematological malignancy, from diagnosis through to death or 'cure', is full of emotional ups and downs related to multiple remission inductions and relapses and is exhausting to both individuals and their families (Scott et al 1983). For many, enhanced coping skills will allow them to move through their experiences with the support of family, friends and healthcare professionals. For others, help from specialist professionals, for example a psychiatrist, may be needed in coming to terms with what is happening to them. Each individual's experience is unique and must be treated as such. Individuals bring with them their own environments, coping skills, attitudes, beliefs and we, as nurses, need to encourage them and support them through their illness in whatever way we can.

PSYCHOLOGICAL ISSUES FOR THE FAMILY

Cancer is an illness that does not affect the individual alone but their whole family and support systems. It halts plans for the future, postpones life events and disrupts the everyday routine of all involved. Family members of patients undergoing a bone marrow or stem cell transplant are particularly anxious, and if their unmet needs are ignored then their ability to support the individual undergoing the transplant can be compromised.

Many of the feelings and emotions experienced by the individual with cancer will also be experienced by the family, for example

- anxiety
- fear
- guilt
- anger
- helplessness
- loneliness
- loss of control.

Hence the families needs may be very similar to that of the individual themselves and the most important of those needs is for information (Wochna 1997).

Some of the psychological issues for the family are due to their altered roles and life styles, how they comfort and support their loved one, or a perceived inadequacy of services. It is impossible to separate the psychological needs and care of the individual suffering from a haematological malignancy from those of their family. Many emotions are similar, although they may be expressed in different ways, and the family are essential in the individual's care (Jassak 1992).

TREATMENT-RELATED ISSUES

Chemotherapy and radiotherapy

Treatment for haematological malignancies is stressful. Regimens are long, aggressive, have many side-effects and may require long terms of hospitalisation (see Chs 8, 9 and 10). Individuals need to be well prepared for such treatment, given the appropriate knowledge and understanding, and be helped to maintain some sense of control over what is happening to them (Manson et al 1993). For some, the existence of, or potential for side-effects of treatment may be more devastating than the disease and treatment itself (Persson et al 1997). The disruption of treatment to daily life is enormous; hence, individuals' distress and anguish may be increased through interference with employment and family life (Andrykowski et al 1990).

Molassiotis (1996) reported that the most distressing symptoms for individuals having treatment are

- alopecia
- sexual difficulties
- tiredness
- lack of stamina
- insomnia
- headaches
- constipation
- irritability
- anxiety
- depressed mood.

Although not life-threatening, many of these can have a significant impact on an individual's quality of life and psychological morbidity (see Ch. 20).

Body image

Both treatment for haematological malignancies and the disease itself can have an impact on an individual's self-esteem and body image. Body image is basic to an individual's self esteem and self-concept and any change in that image implies an individual feels changed physically or psychologically (Burt 1995). Cancer patients may experience an altered body image simply from their diagnosis, without any outward physical changes, as cancer violates part of the body, whether that be a specific organ, or the blood system.

Treatment such as chemotherapy and the resulting changes in appearance such as alopecia can have an enormous affect on an individual's body image. The presence of a Hickman catheter, weight loss, bruising due to thrombocytopenia, a sore mouth or the presence of herpetic lesions can also impact on body image. The self-esteem of some individuals may be based on their physical strength, endurance and productivity, thus causing problems when the side-effects of fatigue and weakness occur. Changes in body image can lead to feelings of worthlessness, unattractiveness and a feeling of being unable to be loved or valued, and this can lead to feelings of anger, depression, pessimism or withdrawal (Dudas 1992).

The impact of the disease and treatment – e.g. chemotherapy, hormone therapy, graft versus host disease – on an individual's body image will be different at different stages of the disease and treatment trajectory as an individual's priorities change. Problems in adjusting to a change in body image may affect an individual's ability to learn, compliance with treatment or role in the family. This adjustment to a changed body image and self-image is important in an individual's recovery and rehabilitation.

Case study 19.3

Betty is a 39-year-old lady with acute myelogenous leukaemia. On initial treatment 3 years ago she was devastated at the prospect of losing her hair, and would never be seen without a wig or a head scarf on. She has recently had a further course of chemotherapy following a second relapse and has once again lost her hair. How might her feelings towards her change in body image have changed since her initial treatment and why?

Bone marrow or stem cell transplantation

Bone marrow or stem cell transplantation has become the treatment of choice for many of the haematological malignancies. The process and experience of transplantation is unique and individuals experience high levels of anxiety related to the unpredictability of progress throughout the transplantation process (Shuster et al 1996). The process is unique in many ways, for instance:

- from a psychological perspective
- length of hospitalisation
- physical side-effects
- risk of infection
- extensive isolation (Gaston-Johansson et al 1992).

It is therefore a hard process psychologically, not only for the individual undergoing the transplant but also their family and friends. Many individuals will feel anxious, depressed, withdrawn, angry, hostile, non-cooperative and suffer from sleep disturbances (Andrykowski 1994). These emotions will vary at different stages of the transplant process, from the decision to undergo a transplant to adaptation to life out of hospital post-transplant. As treatment progresses, individuals and their families are submitted to a consistent sequence of physical and psychological stresses to which they have to find a means of coping.

The decision as to whether an individual should or should not undergo transplant is very stressful. Issues such as the individual's chances of survival, availability of a donor, attaining and maintaining a remission all raise anxiety and may cause mood swings from optimistic to depressed. A great amount of information is given to an individual prior to consent for transplant and, combined with the uncertainty of the transplant process, it is often hard for individuals to take it all in and then respond. The immense side-effects of transplant have an impact on an individual's psychological well-being, triggering distress in the individual and their family and hindering compliance. For the individual's family, watching a loved one go through so much can lead to thoughts of 'should they have gone through with it', 'are they going to die' and feelings of utter helplessness.

Often the transplant centre is far away from an individual's home; thus both the patient and their family may feel isolated, alone and lost without their usual support systems. Long-term relationships often develop between individuals, their families and staff due to the length of hospitalisation and trust and support from staff is therefore very important. Families look to the staff for support but will also vent their anger and frustration towards them, so sensitive handling and emotional support is needed.

Reflection point

How do we as nurses cope with the long-term relationships, and the anger and frustration that can be aimed at ourselves?

Isolation

Prolonged periods of isolation may be experienced by individuals receiving treatment for a haematological malignancy. They are separated from staff, family and friends and may feel physically, socially and emotionally concealed from the external environment (Gaskill et al 1997). Individuals who are isolated during transplantation exhibit distress which can in part be attributed to isolation.

Initially, isolation may not be a problem due to the effects of treatment, but as physical condition improves the impact of isolation has a greater importance (Gaskill et al 1997). Collins et al (1989) identified five areas which were important to individuals in isolation:

1. Previous experience
2. Preparation – knowing and understanding the rationale behind isolation
   – taking their own belongings with them into the room
3. Being inside – the dimensions of the room may be seen as mentally and physically confining
   – the television, video and radio were important along with the view from their window
4. Keeping in touch – was essential
   – not just with family and friends but also the outside world
5. Passing time – to begin with time went quickly but as the physical condition improves, time slows down!

Nurses need to be accessible to individuals, have time to listen and foster hope and above all be honest and open with both them and their families. The experience of isolation can lead to emotional disturbances such as:

- regression
- anxiety
- mild depression
- non-compliance
- sleep disturbances
- demands on staff (Ford 1990).

Small matters assume great importance to the individual in isolation, and their need for privacy is important. Individuals need to be able to pull down the blinds and have some space for themselves without fear of being interrupted by staff or family, however difficult this may seem. The stress of isolation can be reduced by recognising and respecting an individual's unique style of coping and helping them to maintain a sense of control in such an unfamiliar environment.

Case study 19.4

Edward is a 16-year-old boy with acute lymphocytic leukaemia. He is currently undergoing a bone marrow transplant in a cancer centre. His home is 70 miles from the centre and so his mother is staying at the hospital with him; his father travels back and forth as often as he can. He is in contact with some of his school friends by telephone, but conversation is often hard and he gets frustrated as his friends do not know what to say to him. He has been in isolation for 3 weeks and has become very dependent on his mother. What issues do you think his isolation will cause that may affect the way that you care for him and his mother?

CONCLUSION

There are many different factors which influence how an individual will cope psychologically with a haematological malignancy. At all stages of the disease trajectory individuals will cope in different ways and their whole value and belief system will be questioned.

An individual will experience a wide range of emotions and at times these emotions will be in response to several different factors. As nurses we need to recognise and understand these emotions and support the individual and their families, being sensitive to their needs, listening and encouraging good communication between all concerned. Care should be directed towards helping patients to maintain control and make decisions regarding their care. Hence in our psychological care of individuals with haematological malignancies we need to view the individual as a whole person passing through an experience which is unique to them, and experiencing emotions and coping in a way that is unique to them; hence our care must also be unique to the individual.

DISCUSSION QUESTIONS

1. An individual's psychological response may be due to several factors. In our nursing care of that individual is it important that we identify all the factors, or if we support them through one issue will that have an impact on the rest?
2. Does an individual need 'to come to terms' with their illness? and what does this actually mean?
3. Can you remember nursing a patient who was 'in denial' – how did you care for them? How did that feel?
4. Examine your own practice in nursing an individual in isolation – could support for the individual and their family be improved?
5. Is there a role for the psychologist/psychiatrist in the psychological care of individuals with haematological malignancies? If so, when and how would you decide that an individual was 'not coping' and needed support?

References

Andrykowski M A 1994 Psychological factors in bone marrow transplantation: a review and recommendations for research. Bone Marrow Transplantation 13: 357–375

Andrykowski M A, Altmaier E M, Barnett R L, Otis M L, Gingrich R, Henslee-Downey P J 1990 The quality of life in adult survivors of allogenic bone marrow transplantation. Transplantation 50: 399–406

Benner P 1984 From novice to expert: excellence and power in clinical nursing practice. Addison Wesley, Menlo Park, LA

Burt K 1995 The effects of cancer on body image and sexuality. Nursing Times 91(7): 36–37

Collins C, Upright C, Aleksich J 1989 Reverse isolation: what patients perceive. Oncology Nursing Forum 16(5): 675–679

Dixon R, Lee-Jones C, Humphris G 1996 Psychological reactions to cancer recurrence. International Journal of Palliative Nursing 2(1): 19–21

Dudas S 1992 Altered body image and sexuality. In: Groenwald S L, Frogge M H, Goodman M, Yarbro C H Cancer nursing: principles and practice, 2nd edn. Jones and Bartlett, Boston

Dufault K, Martocchio B C 1985 Hope: its spheres and dimensions. Nursing Clinics of North America 20: 379–391

Ersek M 1992 The process of maintaining hope in adults

undergoing bone marrow transplantation for leukemia. Oncology Nursing Forum 19(6): 883–889

Ford R E 1990 Psychosocial and ethical issues. In: Kasprisin C A, Snyder E L (eds) Bone marrow transplantation: a nursing perspective. Karger, Basle

Gaskill D, Henderson A, Fraser M 1997 Exploring the everyday world of the patient in isolation. Oncology Nursing Forum 24(4): 695–700

Gaston-Johansson F, Franco T, Zimmerman L 1992 Pain and psychological distress in patients undergoing autologous bone marrow transplantation. Oncology Nursing Forum 19(1): 41–48

Hagopian G A 1993 Cognitive strategies used in adapting to a cancer diagnosis. Oncology Nursing Forum 20(5): 759–763

Halldorsdottir S, Hamrin E 1996 Experiencing existential changes: the lived experience of having cancer. Cancer Nursing 19(1): 29–36.

Jassak P F 1992 Families: an essential element in the care of the patient with cancer. Oncology Nursing Forum 19(6): 871–876

Kumasaka L M K B, Dungan J M 1993 Nursing strategy for initial emotional response to cancer diagnosis. Cancer Nursing 16(4): 296–303

Mahon S M, Casperson D M 1997 Exploring the psychosocial meaning of recurrent cancer: a descriptive study. Cancer Nursing 20(3): 178–186

Mahon S M, Cella D F, Donovan M I 1990 Psychosocial adjustment to recurrent cancer. Oncology Nursing Forum 17(3) (Suppl): 1201–1208

Manson H, Manderino M, Johnson M H 1993 Chemotherapy: thoughts and images of patients with cancer. Oncology Nursing Forum 20(3): 527–531

Molassiotis A 1996 Late psychosocial effects of conditioning for BMT. British Journal of Nursing 5(21): 1296–1302

O'Connor A P, Wicker C A, Germino B B 1990 Understanding the cancer patient's search for meaning. Cancer Nursing 13(3): 167–175

Persson L, Hallberg I R, Ohlsson O 1997 Survivors of acute leukaemia and

highly malignant lymphoma – retrospective views of daily life problems during treatment and when in remission. Journal of Advanced Nursing 25: 68–78

Scott D W, Goode W L, Arlin Z A 1983 The psychodynamics of multiple remissions in a patient with nonlymphoblastic leukemia. Cancer Nursing 6(3): 201–206

Shuster G F, Steeves R H, Onega L, Richardson B 1996 Coping patterns among bone marrow transplant patients: a hermeneutical inquiry. Cancer Nursing 19(4): 290–297

Wochna V 1997 Anxiety, needs and coping in family members of the bone marrow transplant patient. Cancer Nursing 20(4): 244–250

Further reading

Kumasaka L M K B, Dungan J M 1993 Nursing strategy for initial emotional response to cancer diagnosis. Cancer Nursing 16(4): 296–303
This article examines psychological issues surrounding diagnosis and nursing strategies to help with these.

Dixon R, Lee-Jones C, Humphris G 1996 Psychological reactions to cancer recurrence. International Journal of Palliative Nursing 2(1): 19–21
This article identifies issues around recurrence and the fear of relapse.

Kahn D L. Steeves R H 1995 The significance of suffering in cancer care. Seminars in Oncology Nursing 11(1): 9–16

This article examines issues around 'suffering' and the psychological implications.

Stetz K M, McDonald J M, Compton K 1996 Needs and experiences of family caregivers during marrow transplantation. Oncology Nursing Forum 23(9): 1422–1427 Compton K, McDonald J C, Stetz K M 1996
Understanding the caring relationship during marrow transplantation: family caregivers and healthcare professionals. Oncology Nursing Forum 23(9): 1428–1432

McDonald J C, Stetz K M, Compton K 1996 Educational interventions for family caregivers during marrow

transplantation. Oncology Nursing Forum 23(9): 1432–1439
This is a selection of three articles looking at the involvement of the family and the important part they have to play in psychological care.

Ersek M 1992 The process of maintaining hope in adults undergoing bone marrow transplantation for leukemia. Oncology Nursing Forum 19(6): 883–889
This paper examines the important issue of 'hope' and how we can engender hope. Issues raised can be applied to other situations within haematological oncology.

20 *Social issues*

ALEXANDER MOLASSIOTIS

Key points
- Survivorship is viewed as living with, through and beyond cancer
- Surviving a haematological malignancy may result in an altered perspective on life and change relationships
- Survivorship is related to individual adjustment to life after a cancer diagnosis
- Psychological, physical and social difficulties may affect quality of life after bone marrow transplant
- Nurses have an important role in the social and vocational integration of their patients

INTRODUCTION

Limited literature on social issues dealing exclusively with haemato-oncology patients exists and within this chapter inferences are drawn from other cancer studies which include small numbers of haemato-oncology patients. The more extensive literature on quality of life issues in bone marrow transplant (BMT) survivors is presented in detail. Common patient problems including fatigue, sexual dysfunction and cancer-related employment discrimination are examined and recommendations for nursing practice are outlined.

Research about social issues in cancer is limited, as nursing research has focused mainly on biophysical issues of cancer and its treatments. There are several explanations for this lack of research:

- physical cancer-related problems and treatment complications place social issues in a secondary position

- pessimistic views and misconceptions about long-term survival
- minimal funding of research dealing with social issues in cancer patients
- time constraints and staff shortages
- lack of basic training or language barriers for multicentre studies in Europe (Carter 1989, Molassiotis 1997).

However, nursing interest in quality of life, long-term adjustment and psychosocial issues is high. These issues are identified as priorities for future research in both stem cell and bone marrow transplant (Haberman 1997), and also rank among the top ten oncology nurses' research priorities in the USA and in Europe (Oberst 1978, Degner 1987, Molassiotis 1997). These research priorities may reflect professional nursing attitudes that involve a multidimensional model of physical, psychological, social and spiritual care.

SURVIVORSHIP ISSUES

The concept of survivorship is relatively new in cancer nursing practice. Crude markers of survival, such as surviving for 5 years after an initial diagnosis of cancer, being in remission, needing no treatment or being cured from cancer, dominated the survival literature several decades ago but are now insufficient to describe survivorship. Nowadays, survivorship is viewed as a dynamic process, involving not only a disease-free life, but living with, through and beyond cancer (Herbst 1995). Certainly such a point of view is extremely important for nursing practice, as it can be used as a reflective model of care that could improve the humane and holistic way we treat and care for our patients.

Shanfield (1980), Mullan (1985) and Dow (1990) described the process of surviving cancer and they named the different stages 'seasons of survival'. Four main seasons are identified:

1. *Surviving the diagnosis and treatment* predominantly refers to the initial cancer treatment. Most of the cancer nursing research deals with this season, as great attention is focused on physical complications of the disease and treatment and their nursing management.

2. *Extended survival* refers to the time after treatment, where patients go through a 'wait-and-see' period. During this season, fear of relapse is the main feature (Carpenter et al 1989, Welch-McCaffrey et al 1989, Dow 1990).

3. *Surviving with uncertainty* – that is, dealing with the unknown. Avoidance of long-term plans and taking life as it comes dominate this season.

4. *Permanent survival*, where the likelihood of recurrence or relapse is so small that the disease is considered permanently arrested, and patients try to re-start their lives.

Bushkin (1993) stated that to survive is to learn to live, because the skills and attributes of survivorship are learned rather than innate. Haemato-oncology nurse specialists are in a unique position to enhance such skills in individuals and improve their psychosocial adjustment, either by promoting new health behaviours that can prevent additional risks (Rose 1989) or by teaching new coping skills and introducing social rehabilitation in long-term survivors.

Many individuals perceive post-treatment wellness as being 'normal' (healthy) or being the way they were before the cancer diagnosis. Dow (1990) disagrees, and states that getting well does not mean getting back to normal, because lives can be drastically changed by cancer. This is another important consideration in planning care. Many individuals have high expectations from their lives after treatment that, in some cases, will lead to frustration.

The nursing role is to help prevent such unnecessary frustration by providing accurate information and discussing with patients their outlook on life, future plans, perspectives and expectations.

Surviving a haematological malignancy may produce a sense of vulnerability, change in life priorities, heightened appreciation of life and fear of relapse and death. It may also involve changes in social relationships, relationships with health-care professionals, adjustment to physical complications, alterations in social support systems, isolation, and sexual and psychosexual problems. Finally, it may cause employment discrimination, insurance problems, uncertainty and emotional stress (Shanfield 1980, Welch-McCaffrey et al 1989, Haberman et al 1993, Ferrell et al 1995, Molassiotis et al 1995a).

Survivorship is closely related to how patients adjust to everyday life after a diagnosis of cancer – physically, psychologically and socially. The degree of and perception of adjustment is described by another multidimensional concept, quality of life (QoL).

 Reflection point

What assessment data do you think you need to collect in order to meet patients' survivorship needs? What might these needs be?

QUALITY OF LIFE

There is no universal definition of QoL. It has been described as

- satisfaction with physical, psychological, social, functional, material and structural aspects of life (Hörnquist 1982)
- a global evaluation of an individual's satisfaction with life (Szalai 1980)
- shaped by physical symptoms, treatment toxicity, body image, mobility, mental state, interpersonal relationships, spiritual, financial, cultural, political and philosophical issues (Caplan 1987).

Few studies examine QoL exclusively in patients with haematological malignancies: most only

Reflection point

What do you think are the factors that contribute to the quality of life of your patients?

include some patients with leukaemia or lymphomas in their samples (Greaves-Otte et al 1991, Ferrell et al 1995). Despite achievements in the treatment of Hodgkin's disease (HD) and leukaemias in adults and children, psychosocial aspects of the illness seen as significant issues affecting QoL have been neglected (Yellen et al 1993).

QoL has been associated with a positive attitude to life, which is dependent on interpersonal relationships and autonomy by individuals with leukaemia (Bertero & Ek 1993). Security, support, respect, information and conversation were related to interpersonal relationships and autonomy. Additionally, eight core concepts have been reported as defining QoL by long-term BMT survivors (Ferrell et al 1992a):

- having family and relationships
- being independent
- being able to work/financial success
- having a heightened appreciation for life
- being normal
- being healthy
- being alive
- being satisfied and fulfilled with life.

These themes were also confirmed in a later qualitative study of chronic myeloid leukaemia BMT survivors (Molassiotis & Morris 1998).

QoL in bone marrow transplant survivors

Several studies, using a wide range of outcome variables, address psychosocial issues related to QoL in BMT survivors. However, earlier studies, especially those before 1991, suffered from methodological difficulties with small sample sizes, limited quantification of outcome variables, failure to conceptualise QoL, retrospective study designs and unsuitable control groups. These weaknesses have been addressed

in more recent studies. However, these methodological limitations should be considered when reviewing studies.

Both physical and psychological problems have been reported as affecting QoL post-BMT. Hengeveld et al (1988) found that many patients felt unprepared for the emotional and sexual problems they faced immediately after discharge. Their daily lives were hampered by illness-related physical complications, sexual problems, infertility and/or failure to return to employment. However, despite these problems, the majority of participants reported positive changes in their personality, outlook on life and social relationships. These results should be viewed with caution as the reliability of the study is not reported, although other studies also report positive changes on life following BMT, including greater spiritual well-being and appreciation for life (Ferrell et al 1992b, Haberman et al 1993, Molassiotis & Morris 1998).

Other studies examining QoL in BMT survivors have found physical status and employment issues to be the main concerns (Belec 1992). Experiencing physical difficulties, losing relationships, having unfulfilled goals and being financially distressed worsened QoL (Ferrell et al 1992a). Additionally, subjects had considerable difficulty in re-establishing their lives, dealing with the physical complications of BMT, adjusting to their social environment and returning to work. Dealing with physical symptoms, family and friends and work/education issues, together with altered body image, were the most distressing aspects of their adjustment (Haberman et al 1993). Finally, problems with health and functioning had the most negative impact on QoL (Ferrell et al 1992b, Gaston-Johansson & Foxall 1996).

Younger age, a higher level of physical functioning, greater social support and self-esteem have been found to be predictors of better QoL (Baker et al 1994). Furthermore, more physical symptom distress has been reported following allogeneic BMT than after autologous BMT (Molassiotis et al 1995b, 1996).

Length of time post-transplant also has an impact on QoL. In one study 67 allogeneic BMT patients demonstrated maximum physical dysfunction 90 days post-BMT, but their functioning returned to pre-transplant levels 1 year later. After 2 years 68% had returned to full-time work/education, increasing to 91% after 4 years (Syrjala et al 1993). In a further study, most of the 162 adults (mean time post-BMT 5 years) and 50 children (mean time post-BMT 6 years) were doing well in the domains of QoL examined, with younger age being associated with better adjustment (Schmidt et al 1993). Approximately three-quarters of the study subjects had returned to employment, although a minority of respondents reported difficulties with sleeping or sexual activity.

Conversely a prospective study of allogeneic BMT patients showed that many experienced long-term problems of physical, emotional, occupational and cognitive functioning with little change over time (Andrykowski et al 1989). It is interesting that comparison of BMT and renal transplant patients revealed few differences between the two groups in post-transplant QoL, with both groups reporting impaired QoL following transplant (Andrykowski et al 1990).

Marital problems

Marital problems have been reported in several studies. Wasserman et al (1987) found that lymphoma patients had higher divorce rates when compared with healthy others of a similar age and race in the USA. Furthermore, survivors of childhood cancer have been found to be more reluctant than sibling controls to marry, and have fewer children, irrespective of reproductive difficulties (Tooter et al 1987). Yellen et al (1993) found that HD survivors avoid intimate relationships for fear of an uncertain future and those already in a relationship often have difficulty communicating their disease-related concerns. Several studies have shown that patients' spouses often experience depression, distress and sexual difficulties when dealing with their partners' illness (Schmale et al 1983, Kissane et al 1994). However, other studies have shown that marital relationships strengthened after the diagnosis of HD (Hannah et al 1992).

Sexual functioning

BMT survivors often become infertile due to aggressive chemotherapy and total body irradiation. Males more often experience impotence and females somatic symptoms (i.e. dyspareunia). Both may experience altered body image, decreased sexual satisfaction and low sexual desire (Auchincloss 1991, Mumma et al 1992, Molassiotis et al 1995a, 1996). Cancer patients, in general, have worse sexual functioning (in terms of desire, satisfaction with sexual life, somatic symptoms or body image) compared to sexually active young adults from the general population (Molassiotis 1998). These experiences limit their QoL. Thus, nursing interventions should be directed toward sexual/psychosexual rehabilitation. Sperm/ova banking before chemotherapy and/or radiotherapy may help BMT recipients (see Ch. 18).

If psychosexual problems exist, psychosocial/psychiatric support may improve the patient's QoL. In the UK psychosocial support is patchy and further resources are required. Patients at greater risk of psychosexual dysfunction (i.e. unmarried or younger patients) should receive therapy at an early, or preventative stage (Molassiotis et al 1995a, 1996).

Case study 20.1

Eight months after treatment for acute myeloid leukaemia with a BMT, a 28-year-old man wrote a letter to the unit's sister asking for her advice about the impotence he was experiencing. He stated that, although his wife was very understanding and was not putting any pressure on him, he felt 'embarrassed and incomplete'. He asked what was wrong with him. He also wrote that he did not mention this problem to his consultant, as he was 'too shy'. He visited the unit at his follow-up clinic appointment 2 weeks later and some issues were discussed with him. Further to this, an investigation of his sexual hormonal levels was ordered, revealing that the hormonal levels (serum FSH, LH, testosterone) were within the normal range. Physiological dysfunction was therefore unlikely. An alternative explanation was impotence as a result of extreme stress and difficulties related to his post-treatment period. Together with his wife, he agreed to see a sex therapist. Two months later he called in the unit to thank the Sister and tell her that his problem no longer existed.

Effects on activities of daily living

Individuals treated with maintenance chemotherapy have reported a poorer QoL than those treated with BMT (Molassiotis et al 1996): however, 64.8% reported their QoL as good to excellent. Activities like shopping or climbing stairs were impaired among some patients in both groups, with social and domestic adjustment being most compromised when compared with healthy adults. In their study of lymphoma survivors, Wallwork and Richardson (1994) noted that patients' social activities decreased. Despite the small sample size the authors reported that although many patients' lives had changed they adjusted their lives to accommodate these changes. Wallwork and Richardson called this 'subtle survivorship'.

Fatigue

Fatigue seems to be the main problem in long-term survivors of haematological malignancies. Some studies estimate that 25–35% of patients with leukaemia and lymphomas report moderate to severe fatigue (Molassiotis et al 1996, Molassiotis & Morris 1998). Additionally, in a group of patients with haematological cancers, lack of energy and tiredness (used as descriptors of fatigue) could be predicted by the combined effects of psychosocial and physical symptoms (i.e. shortness of breath, headaches, difficulty concentrating or social maladjustment), suggesting that the concept of fatigue is multidimensional (Molassiotis 1999).

However, fatigue research is relatively recent and many questions remain. Its prevalence and impact on patients' lives requires that nurses be aware of it, assess it regularly and test different interventions to combat it. Such interventions include periods of inactivity, sleep, exercise and stress management programmes, rearranging activities to conserve energy or manipulating the environment to allow undisturbed time for rest and sleep (Irvine et al 1991). Anecdotal data and clinical observations also link fatigue to periods of febrile illness, and alleviating fever may be helpful in decreasing fatigue.

Attentional fatigue manifesting as difficulties with concentration, memory and insomnia are frequently reported in QoL studies (Wallwork &

Richardson 1994, Molassiotis et al 1996, Molassiotis 1999). Unless treated this can lead to social withdrawal, inability to work, maladjustment and even suicide. Nurses should assess such problems regularly and accurately. Training in the recognition and assessment of such symptoms may be necessary. Planned interventions should be flexible to meet each patient's needs.

 Case study 20.2

A 33-year-old nursing sister received a BMT after failing to respond to conventional treatment for paroxysmal nocturnal haemoglobinuria. Approximately 1 month after BMT she developed symptoms thought to be indicative of graft versus host disease (GVHD). She was also complaining of short-term memory problems, episodes of crying and insomnia. She did not have a sustained depressive affect and refused antidepressants which were also contraindicated because of her liver dysfunction. She was referred to the Psychological Medicine Department. However, she did not keep her appointment.

Later she was admitted to hospital with an acute psychotic episode. Her mental state had severely deteriorated since her last clinic visit. She had also attempted suicide. Her liver dysfunction made it difficult to prescribe medication and she was provided with 24-hour psychiatric nursing. Symptoms eventually subsided and prior to discharge her mental state showed an improvement. A week later she was admitted to hospital with further physical problems but mentioned that she still had short-term memory problems. A few months later she started work as a part-time nurse teacher and eventually a full-time one. However, she had problems coping with work, possibly due to her short-term memory loss. Her family were also concerned about her and she was referred to the hospital psychiatrist. Before the appointment she committed suicide.

Although extreme, this scenario (Molassiotis & Morris 1997) highlights the need for regular assessment and appropriate support. Nurses should provide patients and their families with realistic expectations for the chronic phase after treatment and assist them with realistic goal-setting. Teaching and reinforcement of patients' health-promoting activities may lessen their health concerns. Supporting families could help keep them together during the stressful and difficult times occurring throughout the disease trajectory. Encouraging patients to use their own coping mechanisms or teaching them to use effective coping skills may improve their adjustment. Counselling is important for patients and their families as it enhances social support and allows them to ventilate their feelings. Cognitive-behavioural interventions can improve long-term QoL, although different patients may need different types of interventions (i.e. progressive muscle relaxation, meditation or psycho-educational techniques).

Discrimination in employment and financial issues

A major component of QoL is the vocational adjustment of cancer survivors. Although many studies have reported work-related problems in survivors of haematological cancers (Fobair et al 1986, Carpenter et al 1989, Greaves-Otte et al 1991, Wingard et al 1991, Molassiotis et al 1995b, 1996), many methodological inconsistencies exist, complicating the interpretation of results.

Despite methodological limitations, employment discrimination is a major problem for cancer survivors, compromising further their QoL and social adjustment. Fobair et al (1986) reported that, among 403 survivors from HD, up to 42% had problems in their workplace. Job problems included denial of insurance (11%), denial of other benefits (6%), denial of a job offer (12%), termination of employment following treatment (6%), conflict with supervisors and co-workers (12%) and rejection by the military (8%). A recent study with chronic myeloid leukaemia survivors also reported that over 10% of the sample had increased problems with co-workers as a result of their illness (Molassiotis & Morris 1999). HD survivors in another study perceived their careers had been compromised as a result of their illness (Cella & Tross 1986). Survivors interviewed by Koocher & O'Malley (1982) reported job refusals, being denied benefits and conflict with supervisors. Furthermore, 76% of 422 cancer patients

surveyed indicated that they were working at the time of diagnosis; this number decreased to 56% after diagnosis (Rothstein et al 1995).

Reflection point

Why might employers be reluctant to employ cancer survivors?

Individuals with leukaemia and lymphoma along with those with lung and head and neck cancers and those aged over 45 years have been shown to have lower return-to-work rates than other cancer survivors (van der Wouden et al 1992, Berry 1993). In a recent study, 26% of patients with haematological cancers receiving maintenance chemotherapy ($n=73$) and 19.3% of BMT patients ($n=91$) had not returned to work an average of 40 months post-initial treatment or BMT, respectively (Molassiotis et al 1996). Although a major limitation in such a finding is that employment type and status before treatment was unknown, data shows that unemployment after cancer diagnosis requires further attention, possibly through vocational rehabilitation services.

Reports of unemployment in other studies of BMT survivors ranges from 15% (Wolcott et al 1986) to 50% (Hengeveld et al 1988). Job discrimination in long-term BMT survivors has been shown to be independently associated with lack of and loss of employment (Wingard et al 1991). In the latter study, job discrimination was reported even among those who had been working, as 57% of subjects reporting substantial discrimination were employed full-time. Furthermore, a large study of 566 survivors in two rehabilitation centres showed that, in general, most patients seem either to resort to early retirement or are able to resume their occupational activity without special occupational training (Weis et al 1994). This same study demonstrated that medical rehabilitation had a negligible influence on vocational integration of cancer patients. In agreement with other reports, blue-collar workers returned less frequently to their former places of work, being more likely to take early retirement. Type of occupation has been found to be the main determinant of whether patients were employed after diagnosis (Rothstein et al 1995).

It is surprising that survivors of haematological or other types of cancers are discriminated against in their employment, as most of them are able to resume their previous work and are very willing to return to work, except those who experience physical complications from their disease or treatment. Cancer survivors appear to have similar productivity rates to other workers (Wheatley et al 1974). Several myths contribute to employment discrimination, including cancer is a death sentence (i.e. banks deny loans, assumption of short-term life), cancer is contagious and cancer survivors are an unproductive drain on the economy, as employers are afraid that insurance premiums will increase (Hoffman 1989).

Unemployment and employment discrimination, together with expenses associated with travelling to oncology centres for treatment, may have a negative impact on patients' financial status. Studies indicate that HD survivors may experience negative socioeconomic effects. Factors enhancing this negative effect include being male, earning less than US$15 000 (£9375) per year, being unemployed or unmarried, having had serious illnesses since treatment completion and being less educated (Kornblith et al 1992). Unfortunately such studies have yet to be conducted in the UK.

Reflection point

What measures would you take to enable one of your patients to obtain and/or continue work?

CONCLUSION

BMT survivors often experience problems with physical health, sexual functioning, unemployment and dysfunction in social adjustment. Positive changes with social relationships also occur. However, more rigorous research with patients with haematological malignancies is needed.

Nurses working in haematological oncology can play an important role in the social and vocational integration of their patients. Nurses can serve as their patients' advocates by making realistic assessments of patients' capacities and guiding them towards appropriate resources, such as employment counsellors, social workers, support groups and governmental agencies (Hoffman 1989). The existence of legislation for equal opportunities for all individuals with a cancer history is an important step in decreasing employment discrimination, and professional nursing bodies could advocate for this (i.e. the Royal College of Nursing in the UK or the Oncology Nursing Society in the USA). Further, nurses can assist their patients to plan a return-to-work schedule, as they can understand and assess the nature of the relationship between the patient's work responsibilities and the effects of treatment (Berry 1993). Being supportive, listening, assessing patients' needs and abilities, planning long-term care services and referring patients to other appropriate agencies can enhance patients' QoL and contribute to an easier patient transition from the sick role to post-cancer social integration and psychosocial adjustment.

DISCUSSION QUESTIONS

1. What assessment data would you need to collect from a long-term survivor of leukaemia or lymphoma? What would be the priorities in your care planning?
2. How could the specialist haemato-oncology nurse enhance the adjustment of his/her patients and support their families? Discuss individual interventions based on evidence.
3. What measures are you taking in your practice to assess and treat fatigue and sexual dysfunction in your patients?
4. Is there a role for a mental health nurse in the care of haemato-oncology patients?
5. How can the family be involved in the care of their relative? What are the objectives of such an involvement?
6. How could you increase awareness about social care among your colleagues?

References

Andrykowski M A, Henslee P J, Barnett R L 1989 Longitudinal assessment of psychosocial functioning of adult survivors of allogeneic bone marrow transplantation. Bone Marrow Transplantation 4: 505–509

Andrykowski M A, Altmaier E M, Barnett R L, Otis M L, Gingrich R, Henslee-Downey PJ 1990 The quality of life in adult survivors of allogeneic bone marrow transplantation. Transplantation 50: 399–406

Auchincloss S S 1991 Sexual dysfunction after cancer treatment. Journal of Psychosocial Oncology 9: 23–42

Baker F, Wingard J R, Curbow B et al 1994 Quality of life of bone marrow transplant long-term survivors. Bone Marrow Transplantation 13: 589–596

Belec R H 1992 Quality of life perceptions of long-term survivors of bone marrow transplantation. Oncology Nursing Forum 19: 31–37

Berry D L 1993 Return-to-work experience of people with cancer. Oncology Nursing Forum 20: 905–911

Bertero C, Ek A C 1993 Quality of life of adults with acute leukaemia. Journal of Advanced Nursing 18: 1346–1353

Bushkin E 1993 Signposts of survivorship. Oncology Nursing Forum 20: 869–875

Caplan K C 1987 Definitions and dimensions of quality of life. In: Aaronson N K, Beckmann J (eds) The quality of life of cancer patients. Raven Press, New York; pp 1–9

Carpenter P, Morrow G, Schmale A 1989 The psychosocial status of cancer patients after cessation of treatment. Journal of Psychosocial Oncology 7: 95–103

Carter B J 1989 Cancer survivorship: a topic for nursing research. Oncology Nursing Forum 16: 435–437

Cella D F, Tross S 1986 Psychological adjustment to survival from Hodgkin's disease. Journal of Consulting and Clinical Psychology 54: 616–622

Degner L 1987 Priorities for cancer nursing research: a Canadian replication. Cancer Nursing 10: 319–326

Dow K H 1990 The enduring seasons in survival. Oncology Nursing Forum 17: 511–516

Ferrell B, Grant M, Schmidt G M et al 1992a The meaning of quality of life for bone marrow transplant survivors. Part 1: The impact of bone marrow transplant on quality of life. Cancer Nursing 15: 153–160

Ferrell B, Grant M, Schmidt G M et al 1992b The meaning of quality of life for bone marrow transplant survivors. Part 2: Improving quality of life for bone marrow transplant survivors. Cancer Nursing 15: 247–253

Ferrell B R, Dow K H, Leigh S, Ly J, Gulasekaram P 1995 Quality of life in long-term cancer survivors. Oncology Nursing Forum 22: 915–922

Fobair R, Hoppe R T, Bloom J, Cox R, Varghese A, Spiegel D 1986 Psychosocial problems among survivors of Hodgkin's disease. Journal of Clinical Oncology 4: 805–814

Gaston-Johansson F, Foxall M 1996 Psychological correlates of quality of life across the autologous bone marrow transplant experience. Cancer Nursing 19: 170–176

Greaves-Otte J G W, Greaves J, Kruyt P M, van Leeuwen O, van der Wouden J C, van der Does E 1991 Problems at social re-integration of long-term cancer survivors. European Journal of Cancer 27: 178–181

Haberman M R 1997 Nursing research in blood cell and marrow transplantation. In: Whedon M B, Wujcik D (eds) Blood and marrow stem cell transplantation, principles, practice and nursing insights, 2nd edn. Jones and Bartlett, Boston, pp 497–505

Haberman M, Bush N, Young K, Sullivan K M 1993 Quality of life of adult long-term survivors of bone marrow transplantation: a qualitative analysis of narrative data. Oncology Nursing Forum 20: 1545–1553

Hannah M T, Gritz B R, Wellisch D K 1992 Changes in marital and sexual functioning in long-term survivors and their spouses: testicular cancer versus Hodgkin's disease. Psycho-Oncology 1: 89–103

Hengeveld M W, Houtman R B, Zwaan F E 1988 Psychological aspects of bone marrow transplantation: a retrospective study of 17 long term-survivors. Bone Marrow Transplantation 3: 69–75

Herbst S 1995 Survivorship: redefining the cancer experience. Oncology Nursing Forum 22: 527–532

Höffman B 1989 Cancer survivors at work: job problems and illegal discrimination. Oncology Nursing Forum 16: 39–43

Hörnquist J O 1982 The concept of quality of life. Scandinavian Journal of Social Medicine 10: 57–61

Irvine D M, Vincent L, Bubela N, Thompson L, Graydon J 1991 A critical appraisal of the research literature investigating fatigue in the individual with cancer. Cancer Nursing 14: 188–199

Kissane D W, Block S, Burns W I, McKenzie D, Posterino M 1994 Psychological morbidity in the families of patients with cancer. Psycho-Oncology 3: 47–56

Koocher G P, O'Malley J E 1982 The Damocles syndrome: psychosocial consequences of surviving childhood cancer. McGraw-Hill, New York

Kornblith A B, Anderson J, Cella D F 1992 Hodgkin's disease survivors are at increased risk for problems in psychosocial adaptation. Cancer 70: 2214–2224

Molassiotis A 1997 Nursing research within bone marrow transplantation in Europe: an evaluation. European Journal of Cancer Care 6: 257–261

Molassiotis A 1998 Measuring psychosexual functioning in cancer patients: psychometric properties and normative data of a new questionnaire. European Journal of Oncology Nursing 2: 194–205

Molassiotis A 1999 A correlational evaluation of tiredness and lack of energy in survivors of haematological malignancies. European Journal of Cancer Care 8: 19–25

Molassiotis A, Morris P J 1997 Suicide and suicidal ideation after marrow transplantation. Bone Marrow Transplantation 19: 87–90

Molassiotis A, Morris P J 1998 The meaning of quality of life and the effects of unrelated donor bone marrow transplants for chronic myeloid leukemia in adult long-term survivors. Cancer Nursing 21(3): 205–211

Molassiotis A, Morris P J 1999 Quality of life in patients with chronic myeloid leukemia after unrelated donor bone marrow transplantation. Cancer Nursing 22(5): 340–349

Molassiotis A, van den Akker O B A, Milligan D W,

Boughton B J 1995a Gonadal function and psychosexual adjustment in male long-term survivors of bone marrow transplantation. Bone Marrow Transplantation 16: 253–256

Molassiotis A, Boughton B J, Burgoyne T, van den Akker O B A 1995b Comparison of the overall quality of life in 50 long-term survivors of autologous and allogeneic bone marrow transplantation. Journal of Advanced Nursing 22: 509–516

Molassiotis A, van den Akker O B A, Milligan D W et al 1996 Quality of life in long term survivors of marrow transplantation: comparison with a matched group receiving maintenance chemotherapy. Bone Marrow Transplantation 17: 249–258

Mullan F 1985 Seasons of survival: reflections of a physician with cancer. New England Journal of Medicine 313: 270–273

Mumma G H, Mashberg D, Lesko L M 1992 Long-term psychosexual adjustment of adult leukemia survivors: impact of marrow transplantation versus conventional chemotherapy. General Hospital Psychiatry 14: 43–55

Oberst M T 1978 Priorities in cancer nursing research. Cancer Nursing 1: 281–290

Rose M 1989 Health promotion and risk prevention: application for cancer survivors. Oncology Nursing Forum 16: 335–340

Rothstein M A, Kennedy K, Ritchie K J, Pyle K 1995 Are cancer patients subject to employment discrimination? Oncology 9: 1303–1306; discussion 1311–1312, 1315

Schmale A M, Morrow G R, Schmitt M H et al 1983 Well-being of cancer survivors. Psychosomatic Medicine 45: 163–169

Schmidt G M, Niland J C, Forman S J et al 1993 Extended follow-up in 212 long-term allogeneic bone marrow transplant survivors. Transplantation 55: 551–557

Shanfield S 1980 On surviving cancer: psychological considerations. Comparative Psychiatry 21: 128–134

Syrjala K L, Chapko M K, Vitaliano P P, Cummings C, Sullivan K M 1993 Recovery after allogeneic marrow transplantation: Prospective study of predictors of long-term physical and psychosocial functioning. Bone Marrow Transplantation 11: 319–327

Szalai A 1980 The meaning of comparative research on the quality of life. In: Szalai A, Andrews F M (eds) The quality of life, comparative studies. Sage, Beverly Hills, CA, pp 7–21

Tooter M A, Homes G E, Homes F F 1987 Decisions about marriage and family among survivors of childhood cancer. Journal of Psychosocial Oncology 5: 59–68

van der Wouden J C, Greaves-Otte J G, Greaves J, Kruyt P M, van Leeuwen O, van der Does E 1992 Occupational reintegration of long-term cancer survivors. Journal of Occupational Medicine 34: 1084–1089

Wallwork L, Richardson A 1994 Beyond cancer: changes, problems and needs expressed by adult lymphoma survivors attending an out-patients clinic. European Journal of Cancer Care 3: 122–132

Wasserman A L, Thompson E I, Williams J A, Fairclough D L 1987 The psychological status of childhood/adolescent Hodgkin's disease. American Journal of Diseases in Childhood 141: 626–631

Weis J, Koch U, Kruck P, Beck A 1994 Problems of vocational

integration after cancer. Clinical Rehabilitation 8: 219–225

Welch-McCaffrey D, Hoffman B, Leigh S, Loescher L, Meyskens F 1989 Surviving adult cancers. Part 2: Psychosocial implications. Annals of Internal Medicine 111: 517–523

Wheatley G M, Cunnick W R, Wright B P, van Keuren D 1974

The employment of persons with a history of treatment for cancer. Cancer 33: 441–445

Wingard J R, Curbow B, Baker F, Piantadosi L 1991 Health, functional status and employment of adult survivors of bone marrow transplantation. Annals of Internal Medicine 114: 113–118

Wolcott D L, Wellisch D K, Fawzy I F, Landsverk J 1986 Adaptation of adult bone marrow transplant recipient long-term survivors. Transplantation 41: 478–484

Yellen S B, Cella D F, Bonomi A 1993 Quality of life in people with Hodgkin's disease. Oncology, 7: 41–45

Further reading

Andrykowski M A 1994 Psychosocial factors in bone marrow transplantation: a review and recommendations for research. Bone Marrow Transplantation 13: 357–375
This article presents a critical analysis of all the existing literature at the time on the psychosocial issues of bone marrow transplantation. It highlights the important findings as well as the limitations of some studies. It also gives valuable directions for future research.

Auchincloss S S 1989 Sexual dysfunction in cancer patients: issues in evaluation and treatment. In: Holland J C, Rowland J H (eds), Handbook of psycho oncology. Oxford University Press, Oxford
This chapter provides detailed information on research into sexuality and cancer patients and highlights important considerations in the assessment and measurement of sexual dysfunction and different treatment options, based on individual requirements.

de Haes J C J M, van Knippenberg F C E 1985 The quality of life of cancer patients: a review of the
literature. Social Science and Medicine 20: 809–817
Although not a recent article, it is very well written and provides a good background on definitions about quality of life, its assessment and methodological issues.

Greenberg D B, Kornblith A B, Herndon J E 1997 Quality of life for adult leukemia survivors treated on clinical trials of cancer and leukemia group B during the period 1971–1988. Cancer 80: 1936–1944
This is a large study of QoL in leukaemia survivors an average of 5 years post-treatment. It identified predictors of greater psychological distress, including less education, younger age, poor family function, medical problems post-treatment and anticipatory distress during chemotherapy treatment. It also provides a post-traumatic stress disorder model for leukaemia survivors.

Molassiotis A 1997 A conceptual model of adaptation to illness and quality of life for cancer patients treated with bone marrow transplants. Journal of Advanced Nursing 26: 572–579
This article investigates the theory behind stress and adaptation,
and proposes a new theoretical framework for assessment and interventions for patients with haematological malignancies in relation to their quality of life.

Molassiotis A, van den Akker O B A, Boughton B J 1997 Perceived social support, family environment and psychosocial recovery in bone marrow transplant long-term survivors. Social Science and Medicine 44: 317–325
This multicentre comparative study presents data from both patients with haematological malignancies treated with maintenance chemotherapy and bone marrow transplant survivors. It assesses the effects of social support and family environment on the psychosocial adjustment of long-term survivors.

Nail L M, Winningham M L 1995 Fatigue and weakness in cancer patients: the symptoms experience. Seminars in Oncology Nursing 11: 272–278
This article distinguishes fatigue and weakness and reviews symptom management for both. The limited research on fatigue and the development of interventions are discussed, as well as the implications for nursing practice.

21 Death, bereavement and spiritual issues

ROBERT LLOYD-RICHARDS

Key points

- For those facing impending death the nurse–patient relationship must be one of trustworthy friend
- Being alongside individuals who face a bleak future requires a genuineness of presence and an informed skill
- Spirituality is not always associated with religious observance
- Key ingredients of spiritual distress are meaninglessness coupled with a sense of isolation
- There may be special demands on oncology nurses in terms of their own spirituality
- Nurses need to be clear about their own spirituality before they can be effective in supporting others

INTRODUCTION

Nursing in oncology appears to demand more of carers at a personal level than in some other nursing contexts. This chapter considers some of those special demands, and highlights the need to understand bereavement processes in the context of patient spirituality and religion, and proposes that the nurse–patient relationship must be one of trustworthy friend – an amicus mortis – a friend unto death.

THE *AMICUS MORTIS*

Ivan Illich, writing in the *British Medical Journal* in late 1995, wrote

> The old Mediterranean norm – that a wise person needs to acquire and treasure an *amicus mortis*, one who tells you the bitter truth and stays with you to the inexorable end – calls for revival.
>
> *Illich 1995*

Illich reminds us that what in 1974 he first called the 'medicalization of death' has profoundly changed our awareness of the relationship between living and dying. 'Medicalization led people to see themselves as two legged bundles of diagnosis' claims Illich, and he goes on to suggest that the growing trend towards seeing our lives as not only part of a 'system' but also an actual system itself has blunted self-perception. Oncology nursing is about patient-centredness, which addresses all the needs of the whole person. There is something profoundly humbling in being with someone who suddenly realises that their life-threatening illness is not just the running down of a biological system but is also the opportunity to make sense of what being a person has been all about. It is at this point that holistic care becomes less the management of the system (although that is not to deny the importance of such things as pain management) but is more, in Illich's words, 'the staying with to the inexorable end'.

Being alongside individuals who are facing bleak futures requires two things of the *amicus mortis*: a genuineness of presence and an informed skill. Genuineness of presence means a quality of trust and empathy within a therapeutic relationship with the patient, so that the patient knows that here is a nurse, or a team of nurses, who will reliably stay to the inexorable end. To inform nursing skill there has to be a knowledge of the processes that are underway and an understanding of how those processes may be expressed by the patient. These processes range from how the patient is reacting to the real possibility of loss, to the coping strategies that are being employed by the patient and family, to the nature and range of emotions that are being felt by both the carers and the cared for. Hagopian (1993) reminds us that adapting to a diagnosis of cancer 'requires much time, energy and effort'. She highlights for us the cognitive adaptations that patients make, one of which is in the context of the patient's spirituality, which she calls the 'vital force'. The use of such a phrase suggests how difficult it is to pin down the whole idea of spirituality, as it is equally difficult to comprehend the power of ultimate questions about living and dying: not just what has life been about, but what has *my life* been about, and what lies in the future.

'TYPES' OF SPIRITUALITY

Religion and prayer sometimes play important roles during cancer diagnosis and treatment and can facilitate emotion focused and problem focused coping. To some, religion and prayer offer an explanation for what has happened and provide solace.

Hagopian 1993

Here we find a common confusion between religion and spirituality, and it would be wrong to assume that only those with a formal religious allegiance use prayer in this way. It is possible to identify three 'types' of patient spirituality:

1. Those for whom personal spirituality is seen as *unconnected* with religious observance.
2. Those whose personal spirituality is seen as connected to formal religious observance, but where spirituality uses religion as only *one* means of expression.
3. Those where spirituality is rarely expressed *other than* through religious practice; individual spirituality is seen as part of a greater corporate religious faith, usually expressed in acts of worship.

In other words, some patients express their spirituality without formal religious language and without any link with a religious group while others dip in and out of religious structures and sometimes use religious language if it seems appropriate or meaningful. The third 'type' see no distinction between their spirituality and their religion and religious activities. The practice of prayer is common to all three groups. However unorthodox a patient's belief system (unorthodox in the sense of not neatly fitting into the belief system of a formal religion), the use of prayer can be part of a patient's process of making sense of their situation and finding some meaning in it.

It is difficult for those who are caught up in tragic circumstances to believe that their life was not worth it, or even that it had no worth in it, because that implies that there is no meaning to be found in its dying. meaninglessness coupled with a sense of isolation are the key ingredients of spiritual distress as patients try to reflect on their history, as well as on their present predicament. In order to support such patients it is useful to have some idea of what 'type' the patient is, although no one will fit neatly into only one. Isolation and meaninglessness can be as much the result of feeling one's religion has let one down as it can be the result of regretting not having a firm faith. Entering into the world of the patient must mean understanding the patient's perception of their own spirituality. Tables 21.1, 21.2 and 21.3 illustrate some of the issues of spiritual distress that feature in each *type* which we have just discussed.

For those who already have a habit of prayer, the ability to reflect and make sense of their history is already, at least partly, in place. Lichter (1993) shows that the skilled helper can help the patient to compile a biography, through which a new perspective emerges on personal history, and to banish any sense of meaninglessness. The constructive use of memory, especially if this is coupled to a sensitive use of sacred objects – such as a photograph, a book of verse, a cross, or a sacred text – also adds to self-esteem and value. Some have suggested that

Table 21.1   Type one: personal spirituality seen as *unconnected* with religious observance

The spiritual life	The religious life	Kinds of religious or spiritual distress	The management of spiritual distress
Striving for inspirations, reverence, awe, meaning and purpose, even for those who do not believe in any God. The spiritual dimension tries to be in harmony with the universe, strives for answers about the infinite and comes into focus when the person faces emotional stress, physical illness or death (Murray & Zentner 1989, p 259)	Little or no formal religious practice, no shared formal belief system, doctrinal agreement with others or common belief in God	1. The experience of illness challenges the individual's understanding of the meanings of themselves as persons 2. A sense of disjointedness with the world around them, heightened if in hospital (away from home context, support) 3. A sense of anger at a world/society that has let them down 4. Loss of confidence (many aspects) because the sense of spiritual well-being is linked to a sense of physical well-being 5. Facing serious illness or death without ever having considered it as a serious reality	1. Work to minimise the sense of isolation 2. Deal directly with the *whole* person, especially feelings and fears. Valuing the patient 3. Reliability, trustworthiness and honesty in dealing with patients. Unqualified regard, non-judgemental 4. Show the patient that care is as much about the art of healing (i.e. the whole person) as it is about physical curing (e.g. pain/symptom control). Be clear yourself that healing is not always the same as curing 5. Offer help (and know who to involve) in this process. See it as another part of the spiritual journey

the use of dreams might also have an important role (Dombeck 1995).

Reflection point

Think about individuals you have cared for recently or are currently caring for. Identify how knowledge of the 'types' of spirituality could help you understand individuals' perceptions of their own spirituality.

NURSES AND SPIRITUALITY

Patients suffering from haematological malignancies are frequently treated over long periods of time. A therapeutic relationship is often built up between patient and carers which makes hope realistic in optimistic moments, and which prevents sadness turning to despair when the future looks bleak. Unlike in many other branches of nursing there seem to be special demands on oncology nurses in terms of their own spirituality.

Before nurses or any health carers can hope to be effective in supporting others in their spirituality they must be clear about their own. This is especially difficult when the carer is distanced from the patient either in terms of age or through lack of personal traumatic experience. Nevertheless, much of the literature on counselling implies that, at least in the majority of counselling situations, the ability to create a relationship which is therapeutic is crucial to a successful outcome. Relationships are of course

Table 21.2 Type two: personal spirituality seen as connected to religious observance but spirituality uses religion as *one* means of expression

The spiritual life	The religious life	Kinds of religious or spiritual distress	The management of spiritual distress
Share many of the aspirations of group 1 (Table 21.1) but often focus it in religious action or allegiance. This group might be equally comfortable expressing their spirituality inside or outside the structures of institutional religion	Religious practice used to express an aspect of spiritual awareness; e.g. religious ritual used as a 'rite de passage', such as baptism, funerals, marriage, 'last rites'	1. In this group many of the feelings of spiritual distress are similar to those in group 1 2. Even though a sense of spiritual well-being remains essentially individualistic, some link is seen *in crisis* with formal religious practice. Distress is caused if requests for anointing by a dying patient (even when previous offers to be visited by a chaplain have been dismissed) are not respected 3. Distress can result (paradoxically) from a return to religious practice, prompted by illness; e.g. prayer that doesn't result in miracles	1. All of the strategies for group 1 are also appropriate to this group 2. Listen to the spiritual language of the patient, often coded. Always take their requests for something 'religious' seriously, while at the same time understanding the process that is underway. Avoid cynicism of seemingly arbitrary religious requests. Take prayers seriously, even if they seem like expletives! 'O God help me!' 3. In confusion reassure patients that you have access to people who have skills to support people in spiritual distress

two-way things and nurses who enter into a therapeutic relationship with the dying have to have sufficiently robust emotional lives as well as an understanding that however difficult it is to pin down the idea of spirituality it is none the less a powerful force. This is no less true when nurses are faced with the actual death of a patient. The nurses who are able to stay to the inexorable end, the patients' death, are those who have attended to the skills of understanding the transcendent needs of patients. These range from making sense of, and finding meaning in, the past life, to the final letting go. Anecdotal evidence suggests that such nurses not only cope more easily with the grief

of the family but also with their own grief. Inevitably, carers are more effective when they have genuinely entered into their patients' frames of reference, remaining alongside patients who are self-grieving, that is bereaved of themselves. Evans (1994) may want to call such premature grieving 'terminal response'; however, in self-grief a process that is certainly an expression of bereavement is often seen in the time before dying.

It is relatively easy to categorise such reactions in the light of loss models. Worden (1982) emphasises the phases of bereavement, accepting the reality of the loss, experiencing the pain of the loss, adjusting to the loss, and finally

Table 21.3 Type three: spirituality is rarely expressed *other than* through religious practice

The spiritual life	The religious life	Kinds of religious or spiritual distress	The management of spiritual distress
Clearly focus their understanding of the spiritual life in the teaching of a worshipping community. Often strive to remain 'orthodox' in belief. Sometimes see their allegiance primarily to a subgroup (e.g. Christian denomination, reformed or orthodox Judaism, Sunni or Shia Moslems, etc.)	Commonly shared religious actions such as prayer, worship, hymn singing, communion, etc., gives a strong bond with other members, believers. Personal spirituality worked out in the context of shared belief and practice. Spiritual life becomes the personal understanding of a corporate activity. Religion	1. A sense of isolation from a home worshipping community 2. When religious discipline has to be modified because of illness (e.g. when regular prayers become physically difficult, reading the Bible lapses or when confined to bed/house getting to church is impossible) 3. The realisation that the spiritual life is also a personal journey and that the isolation of illness, at home or in hospital focuses on the realisation that not much work has been done on personal faith over the years as opposed to the joining in of the corporate life of the worshipping community 4. Facing serious illness or death highlights the fact that many things have been taken for granted. A painful reassessment of faith in terms of personal meaning	1. Encourage the things that link the patient with their community. House communion (if at home) or bedside communion (if in hospital). Involve chaplains, clergy, family visitors in the explicitly spiritual care of the patient. Show that *you* think that it is important 2. Encourage the patient to use the time forced upon them by illness constructively. Be alert to the patient's 'sacred objects', from the obvious (e.g. a rosary or a Sikh ceremonial sword) to the less obvious (e.g. a favourite photograph) 3. Reassure patients that even if the personal aspect of their spiritual journey has been neglected, it is never too late to start again. Illness may be seen as a constructive challenge 4. Be alert to the need to involve chaplains, clergy or others in spiritual counselling

reinvesting the energy of loss in the future. In Worden's second edition (1991) he changes this final task to *emotionally relocating the deceased and moving on with life*. Bowlby (1986), on the other hand, sees the same process in terms of feelings. Numbness gives way to yearning, searching, disorientation and despair, which finally resolves into reorganisation. Loss mod-els are best used as tools to understanding the 'story' that is being told, perhaps being modi-fied and of course still being lived. This is true for the family as it is for the dying patient. In those whose grief is for themselves there is the awesome knowledge that the story is coming to an end. Some of the earlier story may be being re-evaluated or re-expressed. Self-grief is part of anticipating the writing of the final chapter.

The final chapter of life's story has a range of new characters, and not least among them are the nurses who nurse the dying to their end. Some of the family members also take on a new role in the story because they emerge as carers, copers or non-copers, more practical or more tearful than the patient imagined. Suddenly the dying patient's own story has to be modified in the light of these discoveries and the potential for distress and confusion increases because making sense of the new story is being attempted with less and less time remaining.

So-called loss models (for example, Worden 1982, 1991, Schneider 1984, Bowlby 1986, Lindemann 1986, Corr & Doka 1994) are tools to understand the perplexity of the grieving process; they are not rigid frameworks to be imposed on someone else's experience. Most if not all loss models mirror the transition experience that is common to us all. The one that is remembered most acutely is the transition from childhood to adulthood. Confusion and lack of control feature strongly in the teenager, and once reintegrated as an adult there is no going back, for, as St Paul reminds us, we put away 'childish things'! Among many minor transitions in life we are likely to find a few major and more difficult ones: moving from being single to a couple relationship; changing jobs, especially through unexpected redundancy; moving from childlessness to parenthood are just a few examples. The experience of confusion in the transition period is often typified by lack of control: Are we an 'item' yet? Will I ever work again? Am I a parent yet? Our greater understanding of transition is easily illustrated in the last case. If a couple have a baby and the child later dies or is stillborn no one who understands the nature of the transition experience would want to call the couple 'childless' but 'parents whose child has died' because a key feature of transition is that there can never ever be any going back.

The realisation that an illness is life threatening puts a patient into transition. Between relative good health and death there is the period of confusion and lack of control, and this of course is not helped by the uncertainty of remission and the sense of disintegration and sadness that may follow a relapse, nor by the further lack of control that results from simply becoming an inpatient. The patient, uncertain about their patient 'role', may be confused as to whether he or she is a dying person, or someone living as fully as possible until death. Distress and suffering are heightened when any transition is 'out of time', such as when a young person receives a catastrophic prognosis. Unwritten rules of life are challenged when imminent death is out of time; our sense of fairness is offended.

Nursing individuals with underlying malignancy as I observe it, with the relative detachment of a hospital chaplain, is at its most effective when the good management of physical symptoms is married to a genuine understanding of suffering. Here there are tensions between banishing and controlling physical pain, and living with, and in, the patient's suffering. The natural response to physical pain is to relieve it, but the paradox of spiritual pain is that it can only be relieved by experiencing it and living in it. Significant bereavement, probably the greatest insult to our spirituality, may sometimes be postponed but can never be avoided, and, some would say, never ever quite finally be resolved. Alison Grey (1994) sums up the challenge in quoting Frankl (1987): 'Man [sic] is not destroyed by suffering, he is destroyed by suffering without meaning'. Grey (1994) goes on to remind us that dying patients may *for the first time* be in touch with their own spirituality. This is also true for some nurses in haemato-oncology, especially those first entering this special field of care, in that they may find it not only professionally challenging but also an opportunity for personal growth and spiritual maturing.

Entering into the suffering of a patient – into the hope and into the confusion which is part of the growing awareness of imminent loss – as well as sharing in the bereavement that follows with the family, makes special demands on the oncology nurse in terms of boundary making. Peteet et al (1992) asks the deceptively simple question: 'Can a clinician be a friend?'. In this study 70% of staff (the majority being nurses) stated that relationships with patients in the oncology setting were different from those in previous working environments in health care Among the many rewards in working in oncology 27% specifically cited an insight and a positive perspective that directly informed their own personal lives. Personal growth through nursing in oncology leads to greater empathy, better skills and more sensitive patient care, but there is some potential danger that some may enter this field of nursing to fulfil their own personal needs.

Spiritual distress can be a reality in both the patient's hope and in the patient's confusion, as accepted meanings in life's story appear to be challenged, and the story comes to its end. The oncology nurse has two tasks: first, to help patients 'make sense' of their feelings and emotions, their hopes and their fears; and, secondly, to give back to the patient as much control of the situation as is practicable. Families also move into transition on hearing 'bad news', and parallel skills are needed to help the family make sense of a changed life story (their own and the patient's) and to facilitate control by the patient of the situation (Fryback & Reinert 1993). The most difficult part of this task can be in preventing the family, or specific family member, from taking control from the patient, even trying to limit information to the patient. This can happen at the very time when the patient needs to feel the confidence that flows from exercising personal control, not least over one's own life, and especially over a dying life. In this task the nurse can not act alone but should be able to draw on the skill of other health-care professionals, not least, in spiritual support, those of a chaplain.

CONCLUSION

For patients with haemato-oncological disorders perhaps Illich is right to encourage us to rediscover the role of the *amicus mortis*. For some, a key family member or a few close relatives together take on the role. This in no way detracts from the nurse's professional role as *amicus mortis*, as someone who tells the truth with compassion and can be relied on, with colleagues, to stay to the inexorable end. What Illich is also saying to us is that dying itself and the grief that follows are not diseases but are natural processes, however sad they are when cruelly early or when unexpected. When caring for the dying is not primarily about curing, it has to be about healing the battered spirit. Strong faith makes sense of such healing with clearly expressed religious hope. It can be a comfort. Having no formal faith does not mean that there can be no hope, because hope also springs from knowing someone cares and cares enough to stay to the inexorable end.

DISCUSSION QUESTIONS

Issues of spirituality have a special focus in death and bereavement.

Consider the following questions and identify what special demands are made in haemato-oncology nursing:

1. In dealing with the potential death of a patient how would you address their anticipatory grief?
2. How could you use the loss models to help to identify how different family members may be differently bereaved?
3. Is it important that nurses are aware of their own spirituality? What are the reasons for your answer?
4. Do serial deaths lead to accumulative bereavement in carers? Is it always recognised?
5. How can nurses be supported in their role as an *amicus mortis*?

Reflection point

Consider your role as an *amicus mortis*.
Identify areas for future personal growth and development.

References

Bowlby J 1986 Attachment and loss: sadness and depression. Springer, New York

Corr C A, Doka K J 1994 Current models of death, dying and bereavement. Critical Care Nursing Clinics of North America 6(3): 545–557

Dombeck M T B 1995 Dream telling: a means of spiritual awareness. Holistic Nursing Practice 9(2): 37–47

Evans A J 1994 Anticipatory grief: a theoretical challenge. Palliative Medicine 8: 159–165

Frankl V E 1987 Man's search for meaning, 5th edn. Hodder and Stoughton, London

Fryback P B, Reinert B R 1993 Facilitating health in people with terminal diagnosis by encouraging a sense of control. Med Surg Nursing 2(3): 197–201

Grey A 1994 The spiritual component of palliative care. Palliative Medicine 8: 215–221

Hagopian G A 1993 Cognitive strategies used in adapting to a cancer diagnosis. Oncology Nursing Forum 20(5): 759–763

Illich I 1995 Death undefeated. British Medical Journal 311(7021): 1652–1653

Lichter I 1993 Biography as therapy. Palliative Medicine 7: 133–137

Lindemann E 1986 Symptomatology and management of acute grief. American Journal of Psychiatry 101: 141

Murray R B, Zentner J B 1989 Nursing concepts for health promotion. Prentice Hall, London

Peteet J R, Ross D M, Medeiros C, Walsh-Burke K, Rieker P 1992 Relationships with patients in oncology: can a clinician be a friend? Psychiatry 55: 223–229

Schneider J 1984 Stress loss and grief. United Press, Baltimore

Worden J 1982 Grief counselling and grief therapy. Springer, New York

Worden J 1991 Grief counselling and grief therapy, 2nd edn. Springer, New York

Further reading

Adam J 1995 Caring for the 'new' family in palliative care. British Journal of Nursing 4(21): 1253–1254 and 1271–1272
This article shows that a knowledge of societal changes within the family and bereavement theories increases the nurses' understanding of the loved ones' needs in palliative care. The encouragement of self-awareness and reflective practice facilitates staff to support the new family or patient's partner effectively.

Atkinson J M 1993 The patient as sufferer. British Journal of Medical Psychology 66(2): 113–120
The use of the term 'sufferer' to replace 'patient' has become increasingly common. This paper examines the varied meanings implicit in the word sufferer from the Judaeo-Christian perspective.

This includes the biblical themes of suffering as human nature, as punishment, as a test, as atonement and as liberation and deliverance. The consequences of these themes for the sufferer's role are examined, particularly the sufferer as accepting and the sufferer as victim. It is argued that replacing the medical model, implied by 'patient' with a theological model, implied 'sufferer' does not free the person from the constraints of a damaging label.

Dukes R L, Denny H C 1995 Prejudice toward patients living with a fatal illness. Psychological Reports 76, 3(2): 1107–1114
A challenge to our understanding of 'normal' and 'health'.

Hamel R P, Lysaught M T 1994 Choosing palliative care: do religious beliefs make a difference? Journal of Palliative Care 10(3): 61–66
An exploration into religious beliefs in the context of palliative care. Compare with the typology of spiritual care.

Kaye J, Robinson K M 1994 Spirituality among care givers. Image 26(3): 218–221
Can carers deal with spiritual distress without understanding their own spirituality?

Kelly J D 1992 Grief: re-forming life's story. Journal of Palliative Care 8(2): 33–35
An article that challenges us to think of our lives as a narrative – a story to be told. Where in a crisis one can adapt and review the story rather more objectively than when we feel overcome by ongoing events.

Nyatanga B 1993 Emotional pain in terminal illness: A dilemma for nurses. Senior Nurse 13(3): 46–48
Attachment and distancing in caring.

Ross L A 1994 Spiritual aspects of nursing. Journal of Advanced Nursing 19(3): 439–447
Is spiritual care-giving a nursing role?

Roy D J 1993 Biology and meaning in suffering. Journal of Palliative Care 9(2): 5–13
The importance of making sense of pain

Smith-Regogo P 1995 'Being with' a patient who is dying. Holistic Nursing Practice 9(3): 1–3
The challenge of sharing in the patient's journey to the end of life.

Wallace B 1995 Suffering, meaning, and the goals of hospice care. American Journal of Hospice and Palliative Care 12(3): 6–9
This article highlights, from an American perspective, the nature of the hospice and explores its future.

22 Ethical issues

GOSIA BRYKCZYNSKA

> **Key points**
> - Conflicting opinions regarding the nature of treatment may result in ethical problems
> - Ethical problems may result from some nursing acts which, although beneficial in the long term, inflict pain in the short term
> - Knowledge of moral reasoning can help us reach decisions based on calm, rational thought
> - Ethical issues must be considered if an individual is participating in research or innovative treatments
> - 'Informed consent' is one of the most frequent ethical issues arising in nursing

INTRODUCTION

All aspects of nursing have ethical implications and present ethical issues for consideration. Some areas of nursing, such as haematological oncology, by its very nature, present to the professional and the patient serious and thought-provoking issues for consideration.

Morality and ethics concern themselves with various aspects of being human, human conduct and concerns, and these need to be discussed calmly. As Beverley Taylor (1994) comments. '...Essentially, being human is about living in the world of other people and things...' It is when these other people and things start to impinge on *our* thoughts and conduct and affect *our* reasoning and behaviour that we enter the domain of ethics and professional moral discourse.

THE NATURE OF ETHICAL ISSUES

Ethical problems in health-care work fall into several fairly distinct categories: human interaction/conflict of interests, the morality of the act itself and metaphysical considerations.

Human interaction/conflict of interests

Various problems arise from interaction with other people: some of these problems are probably unavoidable given that we function in society as social beings and have differing needs, desires and aspirations. In the context of haematological nursing a conflict of opinion concerning the nature of treatment may pose an ethical problem, and nurses can feel obliged to act as advocates for the patient or the family or even the interests of the oncology team (Gates 1994). For some individuals, blood products from *another* individual are not an acceptable treatment option, due to religious convictions, even if accepting this treatment may mean a greater likelihood of survival, or faster recovery rate. For the haematology nurse such a treatment preference by the patient may pose considerable moral problems. This may be because the nurse would wish the best medical treatment option for the patient and does not share the patient's religious values. Here the moral problem is accentuated by a conflict of values and interests with the nurse assuming a paternalistic view that she knows what is in the patient's best interest. Yet, if the nurse is to accept the patient's right to autonomy then the patient must be provided with sufficient information to be allowed to make an informed decision about treatment (Faden & Beauchamp 1986, Dworkin 1988). Once a decision is made it should be respected

Case study 22.1

Child B and the limitations of the courts
After extensive treatment for AML, a 9-year-old
school girl from Cambridgeshire relapsed yet
again. Cambridgeshire Health Authority, after
seeking expert opinion from paediatric oncology
centres, decided that it was not in the child's best
interest to undergo yet another round of stressful,
painful and for the Trust, expensive treatment
(around £75 000). The physicians treating the girl
felt that no further treatment could benefit the
child. They suggested changing the treatment
plan from aggressive curative mode to a more
gentle palliative care approach. The child's
father disagreed and challenged
Cambridgeshire Health Authority in court. The
case, highlighted by the media, drew attention
to the lack of resources in oncological services
and went to the Court of Appeal, where the
decision was that, however complicated and
sad the particulars of the case, 'it was
nevertheless misguided to involve the court in a
field of activity where it is not fitted to make a
decision favourable to the patient'. The Court of
Appeal felt that medical decisions (even health-
care resource allocations) were a matter for
health-care professionals to decide. In the event
the child's father found a sponsor who was willing
to privately fund experimental treatment for the
girl. Sadly, in spite of initial promise of remission,
the girl died in May 1996. This case illustrates
much of the angst and real life complexities of
cancer nursing in the context of financial
restraints and limited professional capabilities.

Reflection point

As members of the oncology health-care team,
how can haematology nurses contribute to
minimising the pain and stress involved in treatment modalities and how can they facilitate
better patient/family/staff communication?

unavoidable infliction of pain on a patient
when administering a powerful cytotoxic drug.
The nursing act is intended to bring long-term
benefit to the patient, but in the short term the
nurse may inflict pain in terms of the side-
effects of treatment. This example illustrates
the theory of double effect, where good is
intended but adverse effects also occur.
Inflicting pain on a person is a form of harm
and in some instances a host of potential long-
term counterproductive side-effects, such as
infertility, may also be inflicted. It is difficult
sometimes to justify such moral behaviour
especially if one is striving *not* to inflict harm
and to promote maximum good (Reiser 1992,
Corner 1997).

Even though moral philosophers, especially
moral theologians, talk about the theory of
double effect and try to assuage the guilt feelings of well-intended nurses, this does not
diminish the immediate stress caused to the
nurse or the actual physical and psychological
pain caused to the patient (Blustein 1991,
Smith 1992). Mostly the theory of double effect
is brought forward to justify a subsequent negative outcome, e.g. death, but where the actual
primary moral act was good, e.g. administration of potent analgesics (Beauchamp &
Childress 1994). Such nursing acts bring into
question the primary admonition to all health-
care workers that whatever else you do you
should not cause the patient harm.... That is,
a basic exhortation to uphold the principle of
non-maleficence, probably the oldest and most
persuasive bioethical principle that is used by
health-care workers.

In the last few years a new type of ethical
problem has arisen concerning the unavoidable infliction of harm, and that is the problem

by all health-care professionals, even if it con-
flicts with their own beliefs and values (Smith
1992). Sometimes the conflict of interests is quite
obvious, as in the much publicised Child B case.

Highly publicised cases such as this tend to
arouse strong emotions which affect our reasoning. Knowledge of moral reasoning can
help us reach decisions based on calm, rational
thought rather than emotion.

The morality of the act itself

These problems may be due to the intrinsic nature of the moral act itself, e.g. the

Case study 22.2

An obligation to do good
Robert McFall was diagnosed with aplastic anaemia. After initially testing members of his family for HLA compatibility, his cousin Mr Shimp was found to be a close tissue match. However, Mr Shimp, although aware of the consequences of his action, decided he was not prepared to be a bone marrow donor for his cousin. Mr McFall tried to cajole his relative into cooperation, but to no avail and eventually took his cousin to court, to persuade the courts to make a judgement enforcing his cousin (even against his will) to potentially contribute to saving his life, by being a bone marrow donor. The court, however, could not do this. The judge in the concluding statement said that the 'law did not allow him to force Shimp to engage in such acts of positive beneficence ...' but that the action of Mr Shimp was 'morally indefensible'. Although we have a moral obligation not to do harm – that is, to refrain from actively inflicting harm on others – a principle upheld in law, we do not have an equally strong imperative to actively intervene to promote 'good'. Good acts and certainly supererogatory acts (i.e. those deemed above and beyond the normal call of duty and interpersonal relationships and, therefore, heroic), are commendable but can never be obligated or morally demanded and/or enforced. Altruism must come from the moral stance of the individual; it cannot be legislated or forced on someone (Beauchamp & Childress 1994 (Ch. 4, pp 189–258), Culliton 1978).

Reflection point

In the course of preparing patients and potential donors for bone marrow/peripheral stem cell transplants, how can the haematology nurse working in the multidisciplinary oncology team assure the well-being and respect of all parties involved?

of the increased possibilities of the existence of secondary cancers (particularly haematological cancers) several years following the successful treatment of the first cancer. Likewise there are problems with long-term negative side-effects due to the treatment regimen for the cancer. With increased survival chances for the patients, minimising side-effects has become an increasingly more important moral aspect of both oncologists' and nurses' work. As moral agents we attempt to do good, and to promote happiness, but we are positively *obligated* by

our profession and common understanding of morality to strive to avoid inflicting harm on others (Amnesty International 1993, Beauchamp & Childress 1994, Edwards 1996).

Metaphysical considerations

A third group of ethical problems stem not from the social nature of nursing and our very existence, nor as a result of the consequences of our direct actions, but from a deeper consideration of ethical issues (Gaylin 1976, Dworkin 1988, Blustein 1991, Brallier 1992, Brykczynska 1997, Smith 1997). This is a moral anxiety which stems from the considered reflection of metaphysical questions (Teichman & Evans 1995). Pivotal questions related to life and death are often posed, such as what is the nature of *truth*, or should we treat *all malignant diseases*, or what are the *limits* of confidentiality or our obligation to help others. These essentially moral intellectual activities can often highlight further hitherto unconsidered potential moral problems and present a form of moral debate and examination (Gaylin 1976, Bok 1978, Edwards 1996). Some of this intellectual moral activity is present during the deliberations of ethics committees, at presentations of scientific papers at conferences, in the writings of bioethicists, in the case study analysis of nurses in professional journals, in academic programmes of study and finally by the age-old method of purposeful and deliberate discussion and debate among concerned individuals. This latter method can take place anywhere and at any time but certainly structure and leadership during the discussion helps for clarity of outcome (Teichman & Evans 1995).

HAEMATOLOGICAL ISSUES

Some moral issues are specific to haematological nursing precisely because they relate to specific haematological cancers, and very specific treatment options such as bone marrow transplant (BMT) or peripheral blood stem cell transplant (PBSCT). Examples of such issues include:

- dissemination of information on histocompatibility of family members may contravene aspects of medical confidentiality
- treatment decisions or priorities among already vulnerable groups, such as patients with Down's Syndrome suffering from acute lymphocytic leukaemia (ALL) and the elderly with haematological malignancies.

Bone marrow/peripheral blood stem cell transplantation

Some proposed treatment hits at the core of human individuality and psyche and often, additionally, undermines accepted social and cultural understandings of the human body, its workings and indeed limitations. Such an ethical minefield is still posed by various aspects of BMT. In these cases, the often quite moral act, from the health-care practitioner's perspective, of trying to save a life, becomes highly immoral from the public's or even the patient's point of view. One of the aspects of BMT that is a constant problem is the difficulty of finding a good haematological match for the ill patient and the resultant reliance on *known donors* with all the ensuing unavoidable problems, especially of a psychological nature, that this can entail (Wochna 1997).

Recently, there has been an increase of cases in the press where parents of a child with haematological cancer have contemplated conceiving another child in order to be able to obtain stem cells from this planned baby. The hope is that the unborn child's tissue type would be more compatible with the ill child's than that of either parent. The multitude of problematic issues in these situations make it extremely difficult to see how this can ever be ethically condoned, except by virtue of the parents' enormous anxiety levels and wish to do anything that might help the existing child with cancer. Nonetheless, from an ethical perspective, human beings must always be treated as meaningful ends in themselves, not as means to an end, as the latter approach can demean the integrity of the individual and treats them simply as vehicles to some other projected goal.

Obviously, it would be very rare that parents planned to treat a new baby solely as a means to cure an already existing child, but the arguments of some desperate parents come pretty close to this position. It should also be said that nowhere in the parents' arguments, as presented to the public, is there evidence of clear thinking as to the physiological and subsequent psychological effect on the child-donor, at what one must presume to be quite an early age, and without their consent. There certainly have been cases of minors being coerced to be donors, especially vulnerable minors – e.g. those with learning disabilities. This is an area where nurses' advocacy skills may be put to the test (Gates 1994).

Research trials and innovative treatments

Due to the inordinate stress levels that those with haematological cancers may experience they often agree to participate in research trials (Solzhenitsyn 1968, Faden & Beauchamp 1986). Research trials and the ethics of research modalities in the context of cancer treatment are a very complex matter. Often the only treatment offered is within the context of a research trial and the patient feels they have no option but to agree to the treatment/research. In instances like this, the entire health-care approach rests on the ethical integrity of the health-care team (Marks-Maran 1994). Louise de Raeve (1996), a palliative care nurse and ethicist, brings out some of these issues very nicely in a most thought-provoking recent publication on this very topic, relating to ethical issues in nursing research.

It is clear that treatment must be evidence-based but the evidence must be obtained ethically and legally and there are fortunately many documents and guidelines addressing just these issues, so that ignorance of the accepted required norms on how to assure the ethical conduct of research is no defence (Amnesty International 1993, Marks-Maran 1994, de Raeve 1996).

Informed consent

One of the most frequent ethical problems arising in nursing is the problem of informed consent. The problem most often facing the haematology nurse, however, is not a lack of understanding as to what constitutes 'informed consent', or even how informed a patient needs to be for 'informed consent' to exist, but the vexed issue of conflict of interests. It is part of the nature of cancer that it invokes strong feelings and passions, and it is not that infrequent to find a conflict of interests between members of a family, members of the health-care team, even members of the public as to whether to proceed with treatment or not and how to phrase the proposition for treatment so that the 'patient' consents to therapy (Faden & Beauchamp 1986, Dworkin 1988, Beauchamp & Childress 1994). It is not just a coincidence that all three case studies that are included in this chapter, although addressing different issues in haematological oncology nursing, all involve in their resolutions the fundamental issue of freely given and uncoerced informed consent to treatment.

The nurse's role, especially that of the clinical nurse specialist, in discussing treatment options and obtaining informed consent from the patient is to get to know the patient sufficiently to be able to say conscientiously that the consent given was valid and ethically sound. This is not that easy in practice as few

> **Case study 22.3**
>
> Jolene Tuma was a registered nurse and clinical tutor at a school of nursing. In 1979 working with an elderly lady suffering from chronic granulocytic leukaemia and about to administer to the lady her prescribed dose of chemotherapy, she became aware of the woman's concerns about the efficacy of the proposed treatment. At the request of the woman, Jolene explained the treatment options, probabilities of success, and discussed alternative treatments. The woman declined to have the chemotherapy and requested that the nurse talk with her family and discuss matters as she had with herself. Subsequently, at the complaint of a family member, the treating physician requested that the Idaho Board of Nursing revoke the nurse's licence to practice for intervening in the physician–patient relationship. She was dismissed from work and the Idaho Nursing Board found her to have 'engaged in unprofessional conduct'. After much legal activity, the nurse was eventually reinstated. This case is illustrative of several moral and legal issues. It is sobering to think about the arbitrariness of the Board's decisions, the power of the family in such complaint procedures, the authority of the physicians, the vulnerability of evidence/scholarship and the need for more open and constructive communication among professionals and patients and their families.

patients, however intelligent, really thoroughly understand the available options. The real world of disease and infirmity is messy and relentless (Reiser 1992, Smith 1992). Thus, most patients want to proceed with treatment, but few wish to be treated *at any cost*. (For a beautiful description of this issue read Ch. 6 of Solzhenitsyn's *Cancer Ward*.) Psychological well-being and spiritual health are equally important for many patients (Brallier 1992, Taylor 1994, Corner 1997, Brykczynska 1997, Smith 1997). In reality the health-care team must be convinced, in spite of the awkwardness of the real-life situation, that the patient is intellectually capable of giving consent for treatment, is capable of rational thought, understands the likely consequences of their decisions, and indeed wishes to undertake a decision (Faden & Beauchamp 1986, Dworkin 1988, Marks-Maran 1994, Edwards 1996, de Raeve 1996). Most patients over the age of 5 are capable of *some degree of participation* in the process of obtaining informed consent, with the exception of the unconscious patient.

It is inordinately hard psychologically for the health-care team to know that a therapeutic action could have been taken, but this was rejected by the patient (Smith 1992). However, if someone is of sound mind, or even of sufficiently sound mind to understand the notion of 'discontinued treatment', as the patient in Case study 22.3, this needs to be respected.

Reflection point

Case study 22.3 occurred almost 20 years ago; consider the extent to which things have changed. How could the call for evidence-based practice help prevent such an occurrence happening again and to what degree are academic and clinical studies in oncology nursing helping to redress the climate in which such cases can take place?

Traditionally, informed consent has been regarded as freely given consent for a particular treatment management strategy necessary because of the disease process or the current treatment protocol. Thus, a patient must be 'rescued' with a BMT after irradiation and chemotherapy, for the treatment of AML, otherwise to start the treatment without a prospect of transplant would be akin to manslaughter (see Ch. 10). However, a new problem is arising with informed consent, where patients may be asked to consent to prophylactic treatments, often of an experimental nature, for potential and future problems, that of themselves are not life threatening, and may not in fact be necessary, although the proposed treatment is irreversible. This is the case with the proposal to remove germ cells from patients undergoing aggressive courses of chemotherapy and 'or BMTs' for the purpose of re-implanting them into the patient at a later date, or holding them

in storage until they might be needed (see Ch. 18). For the sentient recovered patient, removal of sperm or ova by themselves may not be a major ethical problem, as the ova themselves do not even represent potential life and are therefore morally insignificant. The moral issue is that more often than not it is not single ovum, or even ova, that are stored but embryos, as these tend to keep longer and in a better condition. Here the problem is of what to do with the stored embryos that might not be needed for many years, if ever, and to what extent should next of kin and relatives have a say about the future of these embryos.

These are new problems that are urgently awaiting answers. The treatments are already being proposed to patients and already several cases have been presented to the High Court, to contest decisions about implantation and disposal of embryos and use of sperm after the death of the patient. Additionally, the experimental nature of the procedure cannot be underestimated, since the effects of long-term freezing on an embryo are largely unknown as are the effects of the parent's medical condition.

CONCLUSION

The purpose of this chapter has been to demonstrate that we already tend to approach moral issues in a far more structured way than may appear at first and that we already have much understanding of ethical reasoning and a more than adequate moral aptitude to tackle most ethical problems. What is often lacking, however, especially among nurses, is the courage and confidence to go through with a moral decision, which is basically an issue of personal moral development and personal integrity (Brykczynska 1997).

It is the personal integrity of a particular nurse that will effect a change for the better or worse for an individual patient (Corner 1997). Thus, our aim must always be to have both a healing and restorative effect on our patients. The caring haemato-oncology nurse will be both competent in her craft *and* ethically aware. This will not only promote her own moral development but will also contribute to the re-integration and healing process of the 'fragmented' patient (Gaylin 1976, Blustein 1991, Taylor 1994, Corner 1997, Smith 1997). Holistic nursing of the haematology cancer patient needs to begin with the increased moral sensitivities of the nurse.

DISCUSSION QUESTIONS

1. What is the nurses role as patient advocate in the process of informed consent and decision making in relation to treatment options?
2. What nursing acts undertaken in your area of practice involve the theory of double effect?
3. What are the ethical considerations for blood and marrow donors?
4. What are the ethical problems which arise most commonly in your area of practice?

References

Amnesty International 1993 Ethical codes and declarations relevant to health professions, 3rd edn. Amnesty International, London

Beauchamp T L & Childress J F 1994 Principles of biomedical ethics, 4th edn. Oxford University Press, New York

Blustein J 1991 Caring and commitment. Oxford University Press, Oxford

Bok S 1978 Lying: moral choice in public and private life. Vintage Books, New York

Brallier L W 1992 The suffering of terminal illness: cancer. In: Starck P L, McGovern J P (eds) The hidden dimension of illness: human suffering. National League for Nursing Press, New York, NY, pp 203–226

Brent N J 1997 Nurses and the law: a guide to principles and applications. Tuma V. Board of Nursing 1979. W B Saunders, Philadelphia, p 354

Brykczynska G (ed) 1997 Caring: the compassion and wisdom of nursing. Edward Arnold, London

Corner J 1997 Beyond survival rates and side-effects: cancer nursing as therapy. The Robert Tiffany Lecture. Cancer Nursing 20(1): 3–11

Culliton B J 1978 Court upholds refusal to be medical Good Samaritan Science 201, 18th August: 596–597

de Raeve L (ed) 1996 Nursing Research: an ethical and legal appraisal. Baillière Tindall, London

Dimond B (ed.) 1996 Child health care provision and service oraganisation. In: The legal aspects of child health care. Mosby, London, pp 40–42

Dworkin G 1988 The theory and practice of autonomy. Cambridge University Press, Cambridge

Edwards St D 1996 Nursing ethics: a principle-based approach. Macmillan Press, Basingstoke

Faden R, Beauchamp T L 1986 A history and theory of informed consent. Oxford University Press, New York

Gates B 1994 Advocacy: a nurses' guide. Scutari Press, London

Gaylin W 1976 Caring. Knopf, New York

Marks-Maran D 1994 Nursing research. In: Tschudin V (ed) Ethics: education and research. Scutari Press, London, pp 40–71

Re B (a minor) [wardship, medical treatment] 1981, 1 WLR 1421

Re B v. Cambridge and Huntingdon Health Authority, Times, Law Report 15/3 1995

Reiser St J 1992 Technological environments as causes of suffering: the ethical context. In: Starck P L, McGovern J P (eds) The hidden dimension of illness: human suffering. National League for Nursing Press, New York, pp 43–52

Smith J W 1997 Cultural and spiritual issues in palliative care. Journal of Cancer Care 5(4): 175–178

Smith P 1992 The emotional labour of nursing. Macmillan Press, Basingstoke

Solzhenitsyn A 1968 Cancer ward. Penguin Books, Harmondsworth

Taylor B J 1994 Being human: ordinariness in nursing. Churchill Livingstone, Melbourne

Teichman J, Evans K C 1995 Philosophy: a beginner's guide, 2nd edn. Basil Blackwell, Oxford

Wochna V 1997 Anxiety, needs, and coping in family members of the bone-marrow transplant patient. Cancer Nursing 20(4): 244–250

Further reading

Brykczynska G 1995 Reflective practice : an analysis of nursing wisdom. In: Jolley M, Brykczynska G (eds) Nursing: beyond tradition and conflict. Mosby, London, pp 9–28
This chapter looks at the necessary moral disposition of the nurse and analyses the qualities necessary to facilitate practice.

Brykczynska G (ed) 1997 Caring: the wisdom and compassion of nursing. Edward Arnold, London

This is a recently published nursing book – consisting of a series of essays, written from several perspectives – on the nature of caring modes in nursing practice. It is an excellent, reflective text that re-affirms and extends the ideas raised in the present chapter.

Craven M 1967 I heard the owl call my name. Picador, London
Margaret Craven's free biography of her brother is a beautifully lyrical account of the last 2 years in the life of a curate who is diagnosed with a haematological cancer and sent by his bishop to work among the Native Americans in the Canadian Pacific Northwest. It is through reading such literature that nursing sensitivities and ethical awareness can be raised and much processing of emotions take place.

23 *Staff support and retention*

TIMOTHY JACKSON

Key points
- Investment in staff begins in the recruitment phase
- Positive working initiatives are a means of recruiting and retaining staff
- Information portraying a positive image of the area should be developed as a marketing tool
- Well-supported staff are more likely to be retained
- A well-planned orientation programme is essential for all new staff
- Preceptorship and clinical supervision are important means of supporting staff
- Investing in education and training is important in supporting nurses

INTRODUCTION

The following chapter outlines strategies for good practice in promoting a positive working environment in which staff perceive they are achieving personal and professional growth and feel 'invested in'. Staff who feel they are developing personally and professionally are likely to remain in the workplace; this provides the benefits of an experienced nurse, which ultimately enhances the overall experience and outcome of patient care and the working dynamics of the multidisciplinary team. The following strategies have been successfully used within the author's unit.

RECRUITMENT

Staff investment begins in the recruitment phase and emphasis on personal and professional growth when marketing the workplace is paramount. Marketing the image of the nursing service, and the delivery, development and management of nursing are vital in attracting high-quality dynamic nurses, as nurse recruitment, especially of some specialist nurses, is a major problem.

The recruitment crisis is not universal; shortages vary between regions and nurse specialities (Daly 1998). However, many managers are currently having difficulty filling vacancies, which increases workloads for existing staff, escalates stress levels and predisposes to higher levels of job dissatisfaction, sickness and potential burnout. This places a responsibility on managers to maintain a full complement of staff, which may prove difficult given the current shortage of nurses.

In January 1997 former Conservative Health Minister Stephen Dorrell launched a £32 million action agenda for nursing, aimed at recruitment, retention and attracting nurses to return to practice following career breaks. The campaign focused on 'hard to recruit' specialities such as mental health, learning disabilities, paediatrics, cancer and palliative care nursing. At the launch of this campaign Mr Dorrell stated:

> In order to attract some of the best and brightest young people into an NHS Nursing Career, the health service must compete with a wide variety of alternative career opportunities. Once attracted, it must work hard to keep them. These

national initiatives will help the NHS to do so.

Department of Health 1997

Mr Dorrell also stated:

I am absolutely committed to reinforcing and expanding the role of the nursing profession within the NHS.

Department of Health 1997

He believed that this new initiative would provide an important boost to the recruitment and retainment of nurses. However, nurse recruitment and retention continues to be problematic and in the early months of 1999 the Labour government launched a further £5 million recruitment campaign. Early response to the campaign has been encouraging although local initiatives based on the national agenda are needed to continue the recruitment drive.

Positive working initiatives

One method of recruiting and retaining staff is the development of positive, flexible, working practice initiatives such as part-time work or job shares and carers, paternity and domestic leave policies; this promotes evidence of supportive management to nurses with child care and other responsibilities (Department of Health 1996).

The haematology unit itself also has a responsibility in providing flexible working patterns according to individual needs and circumstances. Once recruited, *self-rostering* is a democratic way for all staff to have a say in which shifts they want to work. Additionally, involvement in decision making in the work environment enhances job involvement and an understanding of team work. Ground rules may need to be established by the team – for example, skill mix per shift, number of staff on annual leave/study leave – to provide the right number and quality of nurses to look after patients. In some units this is further developed where individual nurses decide whether they prefer to work conventional early, late, night duty shifts or double shifts.

Reflection point

How could flexible working patterns be developed within your unit to attract nurses with child care or other domestic commitments?

Marketing

First impressions count! Information produced by the haematology unit should be sent out with application forms. Suggestions for the contents may include:

- the unit's nursing philosophy
- numbers of patients treated annually
- treatment modalities used
- number of procedures/transplants performed per annum
- nursing skill mix
- flexibility of working patterns
- names and role of key nurses, consultant medical staff and other professionals working within the unit.

This information can help create a positive image of how the unit operates and is managed. A brief description of professional development opportunities available to registered nurses within the unit/hospital should also be included. Compilation of the above information may initially take some time and effort but once designed it can easily be stored on a computer database and is an essential marketing tool to attract potential nurses, reflecting the positive, professional image of the nursing team.

Individual units need to compete with other units to recruit and retain staff or they will fail to deliver a quality service and meet service

Reflection point

Consider what resources you would require to produce an information booklet promoting your unit. What local strategies could be introduced to help attract those nurses not currently working to return to practice?

level agreements. Advertising in the local and national press in addition to professional journals can be an effective way of recruiting specialist nurses, especially those contemplating a return to work following a career break.

RETENTION AND SUPPORT

Orientation

The process of advertising, interviewing and staff selection is time consuming and expensive, so once registered nurses have been successfully recruited, a well-planned orientation programme is essential to prepare them for their new role. A 2–3 week orientation programme may be considered expensive in the short term but is a good investment in the long term. Matthews & Nunley (1992) demonstrated that a well-structured orientation reduced turnover rate by 17% over a 6-month period.

University College London NHS Trust operate a 2-week orientation programme that allows the registered nurse to become acquainted with policies and procedures and undergo statutory and Trust training; for example, lifting and handling, fire training, and health and safety. Integral to this is time spent undergoing orientation to the haematology unit, essential for meeting key people and for the new nurse to be assigned their preceptor – or for the more experienced nurse – a facilitator. This programme has been successfully evaluated by the personnel department.

A well-planned orientation programme allows nurses to be well informed and prepared, enabling them to function more effectively in their new role. According to Cherniss (1980), research has also shown the orientation process to be a successful method of preventing burnout among human service professionals.

STAFF SUPPORT

Preceptorship

The United Kingdom Central Council for Nursing, Midwifery and Health Visiting (UKCC) (1995) recommend that all staff in a new role

whether they are a newly registered nurse or a senior nurse manager *must* be assigned a preceptor during their first 4–6 months in post. The preceptor works closely with the preceptee on a regular basis to discuss performance issues as well as any other concerns. As nurses begin to feel more confident and competent in their new role, preceptorship can be reduced and replaced with individual performance review, learning contracts and clinical supervision. Ashton and Richardson (1992) conclude

> Overall the introduction of preceptorship should be seen to offer the potential for a smoother and more supportive introduction to the process of continuous professional development.

 Reflection point

As a preceptor, what would you include in a new RN's orientation programme?
What do you think are the qualities of a good preceptor?
What are the responsibilities of a preceptee?

Clinical supervision

Clinical supervision is a further means of supporting staff:

> Clinical supervision brings practitioners and skilled supervisors together to reflect on practice. Supervision aims to identify solutions to problems, improve practice and increase understanding of professional issues.
>
> *UKCC 1996*

Supervision is an integral part of practice for midwives, counsellors and social workers but it has only recently been introduced into nursing, enabling staff to learn through their own practice and develop as practitioners. Clinical supervision supports nurses and helps them survive the tremendous pressures of a demanding profession and encourages a high standard of care to patients (Wilkin et al 1997). Examples of good practice exist where supervisors meet regularly with the nurse to reflect on practice, discuss critical incidents, practice-based issues, problem solving and resolution of practice and professional and personal issues. Supervision can be undertaken on an individual or a group/team basis. The potential positive impact of clinical supervision on the nursing profession is far reaching as the UKCC 1996 outline:

> Indicators of benefit could include safer practice; reduced untoward incidents and complaints; better targeting of educational and professional development; better assessment of patient/client opinion; increased compliance with post-registration education requirements; increased innovation/practice development; reduced stress among staff; improved levels of sickness or absenteeism; improved confidence and professional development; greater awareness of accountability; better input into management appraisal systems; better managed risk and better awareness of effective evidence-based practice.

Evaluation of the impact of clinical supervision nationally will be of interest in the future.

Reflection point

How do you feel clinical supervision does or could support nurses in your area?

Clinical competence

Developing clinical competence in haematology, where clinical practice is significantly expanded from generic nurse training, can be overwhelming and stressful for the nurse new to the speciality. The nursing team needs to match the skills and knowledge of nurses to meet the care requirements of individual patients.

Benner's (1984) concept of novice through to expert haematology nurse can be used as a model for professional development if supported with appropriate education and used in combination with preceptorship. The five phases of Patricia Benner's (1984) skill acquisition framework link favourably to the British clinical grading structure:

1. 'Novice' D grade
2. 'Advanced beginner' E grade
3. 'Competent' F grade
4. 'Proficient' G grade
5. 'Expert' H grade.

Clinical competence, skills and knowledge can easily be matched to the above phases of development and incorporated into the unit's nursing development strategy. This could be interpreted as being too simplistic, as the clinical grading system may not be adhered to in all units and, currently, grading does not necessarily correlate with a defined level of competence. However, given the current situation, Benner's framework may be a useful professional tool for determining clinical competence. It also has the potential to be used as a framework for developing a much needed clinical career structure for nurses, which might also positively influence nurse retention within the speciality.

Clinical competence can be further developed through an educational strategy, such as the advanced practitioner role outlined by the English National Board's (ENB's) 10 key characteristics of expert practice.

The 10 key characteristics of expert practice (ENB 1991) are

- accountability
- clinical skills
- use of research
- team work
- innovation
- health promotion
- staff development
- resource management
- quality of care
- management.

Although this framework is generic, with the help of educationalists and the provision of appropriate courses it can be adapted for the preparation of expert haematology nurses. This would allow both clinical and personal development, encouraging nurses to meet ongoing learning objectives and remain within the speciality.

Education and training

Investing in staff through education and training is vitally important in supporting nurses and helping them to feel valued. Managers and practitioners need to be creative with education and training budgets in both purchasing and developing specialist clinical modules. Sheperd (1994) states:

> Training needs analysis has been identified as an essential part in the development of continuing education programmes and their implementation into practice.

The unit manager and nursing team should perform an annual training needs analysis which allows the team to determine what skills and knowledge individual nurses need to function within their unit. This aids in meeting the needs of both the service and the wider professional, educational and health agendas.

The RCN Cancer Nursing Society (1996a,b) offer positive guidance on 'A structure for cancer nursing services' and 'Guidelines for good practice in cancer nursing education'. Both these documents consider professional and political agendas as outlined in the Policy Framework for Commissioning Cancer Services Report (Calman Hine Report) (Department of Health 1995). This guidance has been enhanced by the positive merger and movement of post-registration nurse education into universities and centres of higher education, enabling haematology units to access a wider portfolio of specialist modules than previously available, with courses being offered from certificate level through to masters degree level.

Despite the increased range of courses offered, they may not be viable options for everyone. Individual haematology units need to recognise and value their own contribution to nurse education and training. With innovation and careful planning, units can organise their own study days and may find support and sponsorship from external agencies.

Networking

Encouraging networking with others working in the same speciality can be a further source of support for nurses. The NHS Executive (NHSE) document 'Networking, a guide for nurses, midwives and health visitors and the professionals allied to medicine' (NHSE 1994) has enormous value. Networking may be undertaken for a particular purpose or as an ongoing process. It is suggested that networking is used for exchanging information and ideas, understanding the organisation for which you work, making work more productive, developing your skills and your career.

> Each of these activities are invaluable, increasing your power and influencing changes to the service that your patients receive
>
> *NHSE 1994*

Tremendous opportunities exist, given all the current professional, specialist and political agendas (Department of Health 1995).

At a grass roots level, it can mean organising multidisciplinary, ward/unit/directorate-based seminars; on a wider level, it means establishing and developing links with other nurses and professionals within similar units, either locally, nationally or internationally. Membership of organisations such as the European Bone Marrow Transplantation Group can be a useful way of developing links.

Links can also be developed through professional organisations such as the Royal College of Nursing, who have practice-based societies/forums such as the Cancer Nursing Society, Palliative Care and Haematology and Bone Marrow Transplant. These groups consist of dynamic specialist nurses who hold local and national meetings, as a focus for sharing ideas, establishing protocols and standardising practice: for example, guidelines for skin tunnelled catheters (RCN 1995).

Newsletters and conferences are also organised by these forums and are a positive way of networking and preventing professional isolation. The European Bone Marrow Transplant (UK) Nurses and Allied Professional Group was established in June 1997 as a forum to establish working parties who explore national issues and recommend solutions in relation to blood and marrow transplant nursing. One group is currently focusing on the subject of recruitment and retention of nurses in this speciality.

Encouraging and facilitating nurses to network and attend professional interest group meetings may help them feel valued and increase job satisfaction.

Further means of staff support

Haematology is an intensive, rapidly moving speciality; patient throughput is high, length of hospital stay is longer than the average general patient and associated with repeated admissions. This places unique and often impossible demands on the haematology nurse, physically, emotionally and professionally. Nurses frequently develop strong relationships with patients and their carers, and invest a lot of themselves which can be exhausting emotionally and physically. The patient population tends to be younger and there is a high mortality rate due to the nature of the disease and treatments.

It is therefore important to provide regular time out for the nurse; obvious solutions are regular planned annual leave and study leave. Time out of direct patient care for reflection both as an individual or as a team is important. Various options are available, i.e. individual clinical supervision, staff support groups, or access to bereavement counsellors and complementary therapists. However, support groups require a good facilitator and staff need to make their own decisions either as individuals or as a team as to how their needs will be met. Imposing staff support groups is not the answer and within the author's unit support group meetings are often poorly attended.

Molassiotis & Haberman (1996) claim that a:

staff support programme, acknowledges nursing stress and offers a variety of services which nurses individually or as a team, can utilise to manage possible sources of working stress.

In attempting to support staff, the ward manager needs to provide clear leadership, where staff feel valued and treated fairly. In inpatient areas nurses tend to remember patients who relapse or who are repeatedly readmitted with problems and often forget the patients who have done well as these patients are more likely to be seen in an outpatient setting. This can result in huge emotional stress, causing nurses to leave and eventually leading to burnout. To prevent this, staff may benefit from a change of working practice – a move to an area such as outpatients, where patient care is similar but the focus different, may be useful. This allows the nurse to develop a holistic and balanced focus to care, which may be forgotten when nursing inpatients only.

Conflict between medical and nursing teams can arise in any working environment and regular informal meetings where teams discuss day-to-day organisational issues is a productive way of problem solving and reducing conflict. Weekly or monthly meetings are a means by which the team can take ownership of unit problems. Once problems are identified, a problem-solving approach is adopted so that immediate action is taken. This approach has been adopted by University College London Hospitals NHS Trust team and, although formal evaluation is required, anecdotal evidence suggests that this has led to both improved working relations and communication within the multidisciplinary team.

CONCLUSION

Supporting and retaining staff is dependent on creating a work force which values all members of the team at every level. There needs to be flexibility, creativity and fairness not only in meeting the needs of the service but also in attempting to meet the holistic needs of the nurse and their family. By achieving a balance a unit could be transformed into a people-centred workplace, where nurses will want to continue to work and develop both professionally and personally.

DISCUSSION QUESTIONS

1. Given current resources, what measures could be taken to make your clinical area a place where nurses are eager to work?
2. How could nurses in your clinical area be further supported both personally and professionally?

3. What opportunities are available for education and training within your workplace? How can the education and training available be accessed?
4. What are the local and national opportunities for networking?

References

Ashton P, Richardson G 1992 Preceptorship and Prepp. British Journal of Nursing 1(3): 145

Benner P 1984 Excellence and power in clinical nursing practice: from novice to expert. Addison Wesley, Menlo Park, CA

Cherniss G 1980 Professional burnout in human services organisation. Praeger, New York

Daly N 1998 A tonic for the nurses. Personnel Today Journal, 12 February, p 13

Department of Health 1995 A Policy Framework for Commissioning Cancer Services. A report by the Expert Advisory Group on Cancer to the Chief Medical Officer of England & Wales. Department of Health, London

Department of Health 1996 Women in the NHS Opportunity 2000. Implementation guidance for second phase to 30 September 1998. Department of Health, London

Department of Health 1997 Dorrell launches £32 million agenda for nursing. Press release. Department of Health, London

English National Board for Nursing, Midwifery and Health Visiting 1991 Framework for continuing professional education for nurses, midwives and health visitors. A guide to implementation. ENB, London

Matthews J J Nunley C 1992 Rejuvenating orientation to increase nurse satisfaction and retention. Journal of Nursing Staff & Development 8(4): 159–164

Molassiotis A, Haberman M 1996 Evaluation of burnout and job satisfaction in marrow transplantation nurses. Cancer Nursing 19(5): 360–367

National Health Service Executive 1994 Networking: a guide for nurses, midwives, health visitors and the professionals allied to medicine. Opportunities Towards a Balanced Workforce 2000. NHS Executive, London

Royal College of Nursing Haematology and Bone Marrow Transplant Forum 1995 Skin tunnelled catheters, guidelines for care, 2nd edn. RCN, London

Royal College of Nursing Cancer Nursing Society 1996a A structure for cancer nursing services. RCN, London

Royal College of Nursing Cancer Nursing Society 1996b Guidelines for good practice in cancer nursing education. RCN, London

Sheperd J C 1994 Training needs analysis necessity or luxury. Journal of Nursing Management 3(6): 319–322

United Kingdom Central Council for Nursing, Midwifery and Health Visiting 1995 The UKCC's position concerning a period of support and preceptorship. Registrar's letter 3. UKCC, London

United Kingdom Central Council for Nursing, Midwifery and Health Visiting 1996 The UKCC position statement on clinical supervision for nursing and health visiting. UKCC, London

Wilkin P, Bowers L, Monk J 1997 Clinical supervision, managing the resistance. Nursing Times 93(8): 48–49

Further reading

The following selected reading has been recommended by the author, as it gives guidance to nurses at all levels on the issues *that are paramount as we move into the millennium. The focus of the documents is in the area of recruitment and retention, in that* *they attempt to encourage and motivate nurses to be innovative in their approach to practice and flexible working. Embracing these issues should encourage local initiatives that may result in the retention of a dynamic group of health-care professionals who will benefit both patient care and the wider health-care team.*

Department of Health (1999) Making a difference: strengthening the nursing, midwifery & health visiting contribution to health and health care. Department of Health, London
  Ch. 1: Making a difference
  Ch. 3: Recruiting more nurses
  Ch. 4: Strengthening education

and training
  Ch. 6: Improving working lives

Laurie J, Mullins L J 1995 Management and organisational behaviour, 3rd edn. Pitman Publishing, London
  Ch. 6: The nature of groups
  Ch. 8: The nature of leadership
  Ch. 14: The nature of work motivation
  Ch. 15: Job satisfaction and work performance

NHS Executive 1994 Networking: a guide for nurses, midwives, health visitors and

the professionals allied to medicine. BAPS Health Publications Unit, Heywood, Lancs

United Kingdom Central Council for Nursing, Midwifery and Health Visiting 1996 Position statement on clinical supervision for nursing and health visiting. UKCC, London

United Kingdom Central Council for Nursing, Midwifery and Health Visiting 1997 PREP and you. UKCC, London

24 *Future developments*

DAMIAN HERON

Key points
- Haemato-oncology is a speciality of rapid scientific development
- Advances in medical research will have a major influence on future developments
- Health policy and economics are likely to produce a greater shift towards day care and care in the community
- In the future there is likely to be significant role enhancement for nurses within the speciality of haemato-oncology

INTRODUCTION

This chapter attempts to discuss some technological advances and their likely impact on nursing. In addition to the influence of technology there are a variety of more general issues which it is believed will effect the future of nursing within the speciality of haematological oncology, namely the Expert Advisory Committee on Cancer: Policy Framework for Commissioning Cancer Services Report (Calman Hine Report, Department of Health, 1995) economics and the development of specialist nursing posts.

TECHNOLOGICAL ADVANCES

The speciality of haematological oncology is undoubtedly one of rapid scientific development, a fact that gives the speciality a particularly strong 'medical' influence over the treatment and care protocols utilised. It may be fair to say that much future development both

in the speciality and the nursing therein will, inevitably, be dictated to a large degree by medical research and medicine in general.

Another factor by no means unique to haematological oncology, but of particular relevance to the speciality within the United Kingdom, is cost. Health care worldwide is proving prohibitively expensive and oncology is notorious for its extremes. The drive behind the use of growth factors and high-dose therapy in the late 1980s and early 1990s found increased momentum based on the potential for reduced costs (Pettengell et al 1993).

The use of growth factors and high-dose therapy with stem cell rescue has been revolutionary, with the use of such treatments both together and separately seeing an expansion of diseases being treated, a reduction in morbidity and a reduction in hospitalisation (Sheridan et al 1992, Pettengell et al 1993). The fallout from these developments is probably not yet complete in the United Kingdom, but the effect on both patients and organisations is being recognised and addressed through the redeployment and reconfiguration of resources. Perhaps one of the most graphic examples of this is the widespread re-evaluation of isolation facilities and the nursing processes that have accompanied them.

The above developments (particularly the use of growth factors and stem cell rescue) have been significant for some disease groups; but in general, they have failed to induce long-term remission in those patients suffering from haematological malignancy such as acute leukaemia. The challenge in providing these patients with a long-term remission through whatever means must remain one of the key areas for development in the speciality for years to come.

It would seem that the options for cure for the two-thirds of leukaemia patients without a matched sibling donor remain essentially the same as they were 5, even 10 years ago. Therefore areas for development must include increased precision of tissue typing, expansion of the donor registries, particularly among the ethnic minorities, and control of graft versus host disease (GVHD).

Returning to the role of biotherapy, there may be an increased curative and supportive role through utilisation of umbilical cord stem cells (Gale et al 1994) and stem cell factor, the latter having possible use in the recovery of gastrointestinal tissue post-induction chemotherapy. Like the work in biotherapy a decade ago, gene therapy, though in its early developmental stages, looks as if it may offer less toxic alternatives to certain regimens currently utilised in the treatment of a range of diseases (Cline 1994, Gale et al 1994).

Many of these developments will have a major effect on the role nurses play and continue to play in the haematological/oncology speciality: from supporting the patient through clinical trials to supporting the patient through transplant, their contribution will be vital to a successful outcome.

What is already clear from clinical experience is a new balance in workload needs to be achieved. Workload needs to be planned so that staff resources can cope with both the rapid throughput of large numbers of patients receiving autologous stem cell transplants and those patients undergoing comparatively difficult and lengthier allogeneic procedures.

Previously, units were able to plan for a limited number of patients treated over a long period of time. Now they must address the issue of large numbers of patients having treatments of shorter duration, an equation more familiar to other specialities within the health service. However, it is not just an issue of increased numbers and turnover. For some units there will remain the clinically difficult and labour-intensive allogeneic transplants who may draw upon much of their resources already committed to the opposite experience of the number/time equation attributed to autologous stem cell transplants.

For some units this transition has not been an easy one as few have been prepared for the rise in day-case and outpatient attendances resulting from early discharge. Add to this scenario of rapid patient turnover a complex procedure such as an unrelated allogeneic bone marrow transplant and staff and resources may soon become unreasonably stretched.

HEALTH POLICY AND ECONOMICS

A policy framework for commissioning cancer services (the Calman Hine Report 1995)

At the time of writing the Calman Hine Report is 4 years old and as such one may question its validity as a future development. It is true to say that so far most of the newly opened or newly designated cancer units have concentrated upon solid tumour management such as carcinoma of the breast, lung and colon. However, it is also true that some units are expanding into haematological malignancy or high-dose treatment of solid tumours.

It is the key aim of the Calman Hine Report to provide access to cancer services that has begun to drive purchasers to ask if the more specialised treatments or diseases cannot be 'retrieved' from the centres and treated locally.

It is not a question of if this geographical shift happens, but when. The cancer centres with their high-cost transplant units may face loss of revenue and loss of patients and as such could face shrinkage or a need to broaden their service into more research-based, experimental activity. The effect on nurses in the centres could be one of insecurity through bed closures or an increasingly experimental workload.

However, the greatest effect of this development will be on the nurses within the cancer units who will be required to care for diseases they, at least initially, will be unfamiliar with. The ability of the units to deliver services previously provided by specialist centres will depend heavily on the ability of nurses to learn, adapt and deliver and the education, training and support provided for them.

Economics

There has been in recent years a move towards ambulatory and outpatient care in a setting that previously dictated lengthy admission, often utilising expensive and, for the patient, restrictive isolation procedures. The greatest development has been seen in North America, where for several years ambulatory care has existed and is now being extended to outpatient high-dose therapy.

Ambulatory care has not, as yet, been adopted to the same extent in the United Kingdom, a fact that probably reflects the particular reasons behind the development in American institutes. In the United States it has virtually been a necessity to have ambulatory facilities available at or near treatment centres due to the extreme distances involved between the transplant centres and the patient's local hospital or home (Jones 1992, Wujcik 1994, Dunleavey 1996).

However, the United Kingdom may wish to move more emphatically towards such developments on the grounds of economics. This move would in part develop from the current usage of growth factors and high-dose stem cell rescue, which having reduced the need for expensive supportive costs might become more attractive to those authorities purchasing such services (Pettengell et al 1993).

It is possible that the practical evolution of the 1995 Calman Hine Report and the drive for a primary-led health-care system will lead purchasers and commissioners to seek methods of reducing costs on what must be considered an exceptionally expensive service. It is this difficulty with costs that is more likely to drive care back to the day care and community setting.

Nursing has already recognised the need and benefit of seeing patients, in the past hospitalised, in their own community or home (Jones 1992). Several Trusts and commercial organisations have commenced home-based chemotherapy delivery schemes. For example, Dougherty (1998) outlines the use of highly trained nurses among specific patient groups.

These projects show promise but highlight a significant problem regarding primary care in that community-based nursing services are simply not yet equipped with nurses skilled for the tasks traditionally associated with haematological oncology. As such, any community-based projects are generally small in number and more expensive than necessary.

The lack of finance available to the NHS has always been thought to be insufficient and unless there is radical redevelopment of NHS funding the perceived shortage of finance will continue. It may therefore be safe to say that the aforementioned relocation of patients and reduction of costs, coupled with the development of the service to meet this change, are likely to be the major development for the future (Baggott 1994).

NURSE SPECIALISTS

Perhaps the clearest development for nursing in the future is the continued development of the specialist nurse. The United Kingdom Central Council (UKCC) through 'The Scope of Professional Practice' (1992) and the Department of Health through the 1991 'New Deal' mechanism have encouraged the development of nursing down the route of autonomous, advanced practice. Both the UKCC and the government have demonstrated further commitment to the development of nursing through the proposals for a 'Higher level of practice' (UKCC 1998) and the introduction of consultant nurse posts (Department of Health 1999).

Within the technically difficult and complex environment of haematological oncology nurses gain advanced skills as a matter of necessity. With this facet and the likely future developments already discussed there is likely to be a significant role enhancement for nurses within the speciality. Evidence of a significant benefit to patients and the service as a whole is already available from the few posts developed in the United Kingdom to date, with nurses developing their role to insert Hickman lines, perform bone marrow harvests and coordinate bone marrow transplant programmes

(Fitzsimmons 1995). This is likely to be further enhanced by the consultant nurse who will integrate education and research with clinical practice.

Such an expansion of specialist nurses would seem to have many positives, although continued expansion may require a cultural change. Some commentators express concern at the fragmentation of care and the increased liking among nurses for technology, often evoking criticism from their medical counterparts. As a manager, the author too has concerns that the growth of nurse specialists cannot be sustained both financially and in relation to recruitment.

CONCLUSION

Any discussion of future developments, especially in the field of haematological oncology depends largely on the time frame involved, the speciality being one of constant research and rapid change.

This said, foreseeable development in relation to nursing is likely to reflect three particular themes: the development of cancer services across the country; the continued financial difficulty faced by the NHS; and the advancing development of the autonomous, specialist nurse. All three of these factors provide huge scope for development and change and as such make the next 5 to 10 years a time of intense challenge and interest.

DISCUSSION QUESTIONS

1. What technological advances in medicine are likely to occur and how will they impact upon nursing and the organisation?
2. How much will the redeployment of cancer services take place and how will it effect the balance of services?
3. With the redeployment of services, what will be the impact on nurses in both cancer centres and cancer units?
4. As money becomes more pressurised, what will the effect be upon the speciality?
5. What effect will the drive to ambulatory and community-based care have upon both hospital-based and community-based services?
6. Is the rise of the clinical nurse specialist an advance, and is it one that can be sustained? Is there enough money to pay this ever-expanding group and is the expansion too great for available manpower?

References

Baggott R 1994 Health and healthcare in Britain. St Martins Press, London

Cline M 1994 Bone marrow transplantation in the 21st century. In: Forman J et al (eds) Bone marrow transplantation. Blackwell Scientific Publications, Boston

Department of Health 1991 NHS (ME) The New Deal. Department of Health, London

Department of Health 1995 Expert Advisory Committee on Cancer Report to the Chief Medical Officer for England and Wales: A Policy Framework for Commissioning Cancer Services. Department of Health, London

Department of Health 1999 Making a difference, strengthening the nursing, midwifery and health visiting contribution to health and healthcare. Department of Health, London

Dougherty L 1998 Establishing ambulatory chemotherapy at home. Professional Nurse 13(6): 356–358

Dunleavey R 1996 Isolation in BMT: a protection or a privation. British Journal of Nursing 5(11): 663–668

Fitzsimmons L 1995 Percutaneous insertion of tunnelled intra clavicular central venous catheters by a clinical nurse specialist. Unpublished paper

Gale P, Juttner C, Henon P 1994 Blood stem cell transplantation. Cambridge University Press, Cambridge

Jones S 1992 Establishing a new role to meet the need of adult leukaemia patients and their families. Journal of Cancer Care 1(1): 41–45

Pettengell R, Morgenstern G R, Wohl P J et al 1993 Peripheral blood progenitor cell transplants in lymphoma and leukaemia using a single apheresis. Blood 82(12): 3770–3777

Sheridan W P, Begley C G, Juttner C A et al 1992 Effect of peripheral blood progenitor cells mobilised by filigrastim (G-CSF) on platelet recovery after high dose chemotherapy. Lancet 339: 640–644

United Kingdom Central Council for Nursing, Midwifery and Health Visiting 1992 The scope of professional practice. UKCC, London

United Kingdom Central Council for Nursing, Midwifery and Health Visiting 1998 A higher level of practice: consultation document. UKCC, London

Wujcik D 1994 Advances in bone marrow transplantation. Seminars in Oncology Nursing 10(1): 1–71

Further reading

The author does not wish to highlight any specific text but recommends further reading on the financial constraints within the NHS, NHS policy-making regarding health commissioning, the latest discussion on nurse specialists and any documentation regarding medical developments within haematological oncology.

Appendix: useful resources

Anthony Nolan Research Centre
PO Box 1767
The Royal Free Hospital
London
NW3 4YR
Tel: 020 7284 1234
Fax: 020 7284 8226
Website: www.anthonynolan.org.uk

BACUP
3 Bath Place
Rivington Street
London
EC2A 3JR
Tel: 020 7696 9003
Fax: 020 7696 9002
Website: www.cancerbacup.org.uk

British Bone Marrow Donor Appeal
18 Warwick Street
Rugby
Warwickshire
CV21 3DD

CancerHelp UK
Living with Cancer CRC Institute for Cancer Studies
University of Birmingham
Birmingham
Website:http://medweb.bham.ac.uk/cancerhelp

CancerLink
17 Britannia Street
London
WC1X 9JN
Tel: 020 7833 2451
Fax: 020 7833 4963

Compassionate Friends
National Secretary
6 Denmark Street
Bristol
BS1 5DR
Tel: 0117 953 9639
Fax: 0117 966 5202

European Bone Marrow Transplant Group (UK)
Nurses & Allied Professions Group
c/o PPW6 University College London Hospital
Grafton Way
London
WC1E 6AU

International Myeloma Foundation, UK Office
9 Gayfield Square
Edinburgh
EH1 3NT
Tel: 0800 980 3332
Website: www.myeloma.org.uk
Email: TheIMF@myeloma.org.uk

Leukaemia Care Society
14 Kingfisher Court
Venny Bridge
Pinhoe
Exeter, Devon
EX4 8JN
Tel: 0345 673203 or 01392 464848
Fax: 01392 460331
Email: leukaemia.care@ukonline.co.uk

Leukaemia Research Fund
43 Great Ormond Street
London
WC1N 3JJ
Tel: 020 7405 0101
Email: lrf@leukaemia.demon.co.uk

Lymphoma Association
PO Box 386
Aylesbury
Bucks
HP20 2GA
Helpline: Freephone 0808 808 5555
Office: 01296 619400
Website: www.lymphoma.org.uk

OncoLink
University of Pennsylvania Cancer Center
3451 Walnut
Philadelphia
PA19104
USA
Tel: 215 898 5000
Website: http://cancer.med.upenn.edu

Paediatric Oncology Nurses Forum
Royal College of Nursing
20 Cavendish Square
London
W1M 0AB
Tel: 020 2647 3610
Fax: 020 2647 3420
Website: www.rcn.org.uk

Index

Numbers in **bold** refer to tables or illustrations